BLOOD BROTHERS

1

BLOOD BROTHERS

Siblings As Writers

WITHDRAWN

Edited by

Norman Kiell

International Universities Press, Inc.
New York   New York

Library of Congress Cataloging in Publication Data
Main entry under title:

Blood brothers.

    Bibliography: p.
    Includes index.
    1. Authors, English—Psychology—Addresses, essays,
lectures. 2. Authors—Family relationships—
Addresses, essays, lectures. 3. Brothers—Addresses,
essays, lectures. 4. Sibling relations—Addresses,
essays, lectures. 5. Sibling rivalry—Addresses,
essays, lectures. 6. Creation (Literary, artistic,
etc.)—Addresses, essays, lectures. 7. Psychoanalysis
and literature—Addresses, essays, lectures. I. Kiell,
Norman.
PR106.B56 1983   820'.9'353   83-12677
ISBN 0-8236-0545-0

Manufactured in the United States of America.

In fond memory of my brother Aaron
and
for my two terrific sons, Jonathan and Matthew

Contents

Chronology

1828	Dante Gabriel Rossetti	1882
1829	William M. Rossetti	1919
1842	William James	1910
1843	Henry James	1916
1852	Willie Wilde	1899
1854	Oscar Wilde	1900
1853	Herbert Beerbohm Tree	1917
1872	Max Beerbohm	1956
1871	Heinrich Mann	1950
1875	Thomas Mann	1955
1880	Lytton Strachey	1932
1887	James Strachey	1967
1882	James Joyce	1941
1884	Stanislaus Joyce	1955
1887	Julian Huxley	1975
1894	Aldous Huxley	1963
1893	Israel Joshua Singer	1944
1904	Isaac Bashevis Singer	
1898	Alec Waugh	1981
1903	Evelyn Waugh	1966
1912	Lawrence Durrell	
1925	Gerald Durrell	
1926	Anthony Shaffer	
1926	Peter Shaffer	

Contributors

KARL BECKSON (Ph.D., Columbia University) is Professor of English at Brooklyn College of the City University of New York and editor or coeditor of *Aesthetes and Decadents of the 1890s; Oscar Wilde: The Critical Heritage; Max and Will: Max Beerbohm and William Rothenstein, Their Friendship and Letters, 1893–1945; The Memoirs of Arthur Symons: Life and Art in the 1890s;* and *Henry Harland: His Life and Work; Letters of Arthur Symons.* As Lecturer of English in Psychiatry, Cornell University Medical College, he codirects (with Simon Grolnick, M.D.) a seminar on psychoanalysis and literature in the Department of Psychiatry, North Shore University Hospital, Manhasset, Long Island, a teaching unit of Cornell Medical College.

HOWARD M. FEINSTEIN is a psychiatrist and historian who holds both an M.D. (1955) and a Ph.D. in American Intellectual History (1977) from Cornell University. He has published widely on psychobiographical issues and is at present completing a full-length interpretive biography, *Becoming William James.* A Fellow of the American Psychiatric Association and Adjunct Professor of Psychology at Cornell, his research has been supported in part by the Josiah Macy Jr. Foundation, the National Institute of Health, and the National Endowment for the Humanities.

JULES GLENN, M.D., acquired his interest in twins when a number of them became his analytic patients. His expertise alerted him to the twinlike traits of the protagonists in the Shaffer plays. An analyst of children and adults, Dr. Glenn is a graduate of the New York Psychoanalytic Institute. He is a training and supervising analyst at The Psychoanalytic Institute, New York University Medical Center, and Clinical Professor of Psychiatry at N.Y.U. He is editor of *Child Analysis and Therapy* and coeditor (with Dr. Mark Kanzer) of *Freud and His Self-Analysis* and *Freud and His Patients.* Dr. Glenn is also Assistant Editor of the *Journal of the American Psychoanalytic Association* and former President of the Long Island Psychoanalytic Society.

NIGEL HAMILTON was educated at Westminster School and Trinity College, Cambridge, where he took an Honors Degree in History. His biography of Heinrich and Thomas Mann, *The Brothers Mann,* was published in this country in 1979 by Yale University Press. In 1977 he began work on the authorized biography of Field Marshal Lord Montgomery of Alamein, the first volume of which (*Monty: The Making of a General 1887–1942*) won the Whitbread Literary Award. The second volume is currently in preparation.

NORMAN KIELL has for twenty-five years treated college-age students in individual and group therapy, and has lately specialized in the treatment of the obese. He is Professor Emeritus, Psychological Services, Brooklyn College of the City University of New York, and is currently affiliated with the Peninsula Counseling Center in Woodmere, Long Island. He is author of *The Adolescent Through Fiction; The Universal Experience of Adolescence; Varieties of Sexual Experience*; and the two-volume bibliography, *Psychoanalysis, Psychology and Literature.* He has also published the articles, "The Very Private Eye of Ross Macdonald" and "The Characterological Effects of Asthma on Theodore Roosevelt."

JEAN KIMBALL is in the Department of English Language and Literature in the College of Humanities and Fine Arts of the University of Northern Iowa. She has published articles on both Henry James and James Joyce, several of which have appeared in the *James Joyce Quarterly.*

ROBERT J. KLOSS holds a doctorate in clinical psychology from Columbia University and spent five years in postdoctoral study at Columbia's Psychoanalytic Clinic for Training and Research. Currently he teaches psychoanalytic literary criticism at The William Paterson College, Wayne, New Jersey. Coauthor of *The Unspoken Motive,* he has published in *Psychoanalytic Review, American Imago, Literature and Psychology,* and *South Carolina Review.*

JOSEPH C. LANDIS is Professor of English at Queens College of the City University of New York. Founder of the Queens College Yiddish Program and also of the Queens College Jewish Studies Program, he chaired both from 1970 to 1980. From 1966 to 1969, he was Jacob D. Berg Visiting Professor of Yiddish Literature at Brandeis University. His numerous articles in Yiddish as well as in English on both English and Yiddish literature have appeared in various scholarly and critical journals. He has also published numerous translations of Yiddish prose and poetry, including *The Great Jewish Plays*. Editor of *Yiddish*, a quarterly journal devoted to Yiddish language and literature, and coeditor of the *Modern Jewish Studies Annual*, he is currently Secretary of the American Association of Professors of Yiddish.

JANE LAGOUDIS PINCHIN is Associate Professor of English at Colgate University, where she teaches women's studies and modern fiction and poetry. She is the author of *Alexandria Still: Forster, Durrell, and Cavafy*, published by Princeton University Press in 1977. Another piece on Lawrence Durrell, "Durrell's Fatal Cleopatras," has appeared in *Modern Fiction Studies*.

MURRAY H. SHERMAN was formerly Managing Editor of the *Psychoanalytic Review* and now sits on its editorial board. He has edited *Psychoanalysis and Old Vienna: Freud, Reik, Schnitzler, Kraus; Psychoanalysis in America: Historical Perspectives*; and *A Rorschach Reader*. With Marie C. Nelson, he is coauthor of *Roles and Paradigms in Psychotherapy*.

ROBERT VISCUSI is currently Assistant Professor of English and Faculty Associate of the Humanities Institute at Brooklyn College of the City University of New York. At New York University he wrote a doctoral dissertation on Max Beerbohm, and he has recently completed a book-length manuscript on the same subject.

STANLEY WEINTRAUB is Director and Research Professor of the Institute for the Arts and Humanistic Studies at Pennsylvania State University. He is editor of *Shaw: The Annual of Bernard Shaw Studies*, and author or editor of more than thirty books, many of them biographical. These include *Private Shaw and Public Shaw*, *Beardsley* (a 1967 National Book Award nominee), *The Last Great Cause, Journey to Heartbreak, Whistler, Four Rossettis: A Victorian Biography*, and *The London Yankees*. He is an American Council of Learned Societies grantee, a Guggenheim Fellow, and a visiting professor at U.C.L.A. and the Universities of Hawaii, Malaya, and Singapore.

PHILIP WEST, Associate Professor of English at Skidmore College, has published articles in *College English, Monastic Studies*, and *Salmagundi*. Trained at Rutgers University as a specialist in Old English and Anglo-Latin literatures, West teaches classics, linguistics, and medieval studies. He has also taken postdoctoral work at Albany Medical College in Gestalt and transactional therapies.

Then the Lord said to Cain, "Where is Abel your brother?" He said, "I do not know; am I my brother's keeper?" And the Lord said, "What have you done? The voice of your brother's blood is crying to me from the ground. . . ."

Genesis 4:9–10.

Introduction

NORMAN KIELL

The twelve biographical essays in this collection—on brothers who are writers—attempt to show how kinship affects creativity. Knowledge of the sibling rivalry of these men may not be essential to an understanding of their individual works (to extrapolate from Nigel Hamilton's comments on the Manns), but it is essential to an understanding of their achievement. Still, *The Importance of Being Earnest*, as Karl Beckson shows, is based on the dark ravelings of the rivalry braiding Oscar Wilde's life with that of his brother Willie. Many other works reveal similar motivation. Evelyn Waugh's bitterness and anguish over being a second son, for instance, probably contributed to the biting satire found in some of his novels and most certainly gave rise to his lifelong resentment of his older brother Alec.

The extent of the succorance needs of one sibling for the other varies with each pair of brothers. The Huxleys' dependence on one another—almost entirely structured on intellectual stimulation—is greatly at variance with that of the Rossettis'; William relied on Dante Gabriel for literary and artistic stimulation, while the latter was almost entirely dependent on William for his bread and butter and a roof over his head. Although William James's comments on Henry's fiction were gratuitous and pejorative, the brothers had unbounded empathy for one another's physical

3

and emotional woes, which were legion. Stanislaus Joyce bankrolled his profligate brother but salvaged his own identity in so doing. By contrast, Thomas and Heinrich Mann just barely resolved their bitter fraternal rivalry, reflected in their lives, works, and politics. And it was only after I.J. Singer died that Isaac Bashevis Singer was able to express, at least publicly, his debt to his older brother, and his love for him.

Bonds between twins, to which Howard Feinstein compares the Jameses' relationship, epitomize the prodigious difficulties experienced with individuation. Twinship affects nearly all the efforts of the Shaffers, Anthony and Peter, who are fraternal twins. Fraternal complementarianism also affected the Strachey brothers, Lytton and James, and the Durrells, Lawrence and Gerald.

Robert Viscusi, in his chapter on the Beerbohms, tells us of an interview Max Beerbohm gave which appeared in the London *Sketch* (Leverson, 1895). In it Max says that he is "writing a treatise upon the 'Brothers of Great Men,' including a series of psychological sketches of Mr Willie Wilde, Mr Austen Chamberlain, and others." "You are," the interviewer asks, "a brother of Mr. Beerbohm Tree, I believe?" "Yes; he is coming into the series."[1]

With what prescience did Max's facetious remark anticipate the present volume, though it has taken nearly a century for the idea to bear fruit! "As the study of life history emerges from that of case histories," Erikson has somewhere written, "it will throw new light on biography and thus on history itself." Freud, in his speech accepting the Goethe Prize for Literature in 1930, said:

> It is unavoidable that if we learn more about a great man's life we shall also hear of occasions on which he has in fact done better than we, has in fact come near to us as a human being. Nevertheless, I think we may declare the efforts of biography to be legitimate. Our attitude to father and teachers is, after all, an ambivalent one since our reverence for them regularly conceals a component of hostile rebellion. That is a psychological fatality; it cannot be altered without forcible suppression of truth and is bound to extend to our relations with the great men whose life histories we wish to investigate. [p. 210]

The behavioral repertoire of the blood brothers discussed in this book

---

[1] What Max was doing here was displacing hostility which should have been directed against his brother Herbert onto wampus Willie Wilde, for whom he had much contempt. Although Max said that "Herbert was (then and always) a hero to me" (Pearson, 1950, p. 3), Max felt a lifelong rivalry.

is as diverse, and as universal, as the behavior of siblings anywhere. The points of contact through which the brothers matured and developed their genius seem to suggest certain general patterns of interaction, which will be outlined in the sections to follow.

Psychoanalysis and Biography

Although psychoanalytic psychology is approaching its centennial, it was only twenty-five years ago that Edel (1957) pointed out the confusions and misunderstandings which still existed between literature and psychology. Academics resented the atmosphere of the clinic in the library, and critics and biographers were "no less inexpert than the psychoanalysts on *our* ground" (p. 93).

More recently, Edel asked, "What . . . qualifies a student of literature to practice literary psychology? The answer is: when he trains himself thoroughly in both literature and psychology. . . . He must learn to understand his own dreams, his instincts, his anxieties" (1981, pp. 464–465). Although there is still resistance to the analytic interpretation of literature or biography, there is growing acceptance of the relatedness of the disciplines. This may be because more psychoanalysts are becoming students of literature and more critics and biographers are studying psychoanalytic psychology in postdoctoral seminars as well as experiencing psychoanalytic treatment themselves. In the novel with the punning title *Shrinking*, Lelchuk (1978) plaintively asks, "Why don't psychiatrists read more serious literature?" (p. 28). But Coles (1980) does not think it "melodramatic to suggest that literary talent, in its inspired forms, has obsessed if not haunted psychoanalytic psychology" (p. 207).

The discovery of the relationship between literature and his own psychological work was an important element in Coles's growth during his years in the South. He found that the medical and psychiatric modalities he had relied on were insufficient to the task before him. "I have learned to draw upon a book like Ellison's *Invisible Man* instead of a book called *The Mark of Oppression*, which offers 'in depth'—of course!—psychiatric case studies of the Negro. I have learned that one does not have to be a political or social or philosophical 'romantic' to comprehend and appreciate the truth that binds a Faulkner to a Tolstoy, an Agee to a Bernanos, a Simone Weil to an Orwell" (1972, pp. 21–22).

Skura (1981) reinforces Edel's dictum but with a caveat, for she insists there is a true dichotomy between psychoanalytic and literary criticism, though of course many parallels obtain. She recognizes the inevitability of psychoanalysis in biography: both are interpretive arts, both developed in the same century, and they adopted one another's techniques and terminology.

> Nonetheless, no matter how close their parallel paths, critic and analyst have seldom met with much satisfaction. Although the real similarities between the two have made them especially promising resources for one another, the superficial familiarity is misleading and has served more to keep them apart than to bring them together. Familiarity . . . has dampened curiosity and encouraged complacency. . . . [But] the analyst's work can indeed be both different and relevant, provided that it is not taken as a substitute for the critic's investigations but rather as a separate investigation that can supplement the critic's work in various ways. . . . The analyst reminds us that there is always more in a text than we normally see, and much more that would surprise us. . . . The analytic stance gives the critic more to work with . . . so long as he does not use it reductively. . . . Ultimately . . . psychoanalysis provides not only a tool for practical criticism but also for understanding how literature works. The strategies employed in the psychoanalytic process . . . provide the techniques, the categories, and the vocabulary for examining the conditions of meaning and for studying the way we make sense of things—or fail to do so. . . . We can come closer [to finding new meanings in old texts] and to individual insights psychoanalysis can afford—only if critic and analyst each understand—really understand—what the other is doing. [pp. 272–275]

Psychoanalysis and literature have been closely linked ever since Freud borrowed from Sophocles a name for the most famous of his discoveries: the Oedipus complex. In the early days of psychoanalysis, when Freud was attempting to formulate and corroborate his far-reaching concepts about the nature of man, the clinical material at his disposal was severely limited, and he turned respectfully to the analysis of masterworks of art and literature and to the lives of exceptionally creative people. He believed that great works of art and literature contained universal psychological truths. In his interpretation of Wilhelm Jensen's novel *Gradiva*, Freud (1907) wrote of the creative writer, "The description of the human mind is indeed the domain which is most his own; he has from time immemorial been the precursor of science, and so too of scientific psychology. . . . The creative writer cannot evade the psychiatrist nor the psychiatrist the creative writer" (pp. 43–44). D.H. Thomas's novel *The White Hotel* (1981), contains a long chapter, "Frau Anna G," a mimetic case history in which the author has Freud say, "Long may poetry and psychoanalysis continue to highlight, from their different perspectives, the human face in all its nobility and sorrow" (p. 143).

The essays in this volume may cover familiar psychiatric turf, but the observations are refreshingly atypical of psychoanalytic prose. Clinical experience and literary perception lend vitality to each other when used constructively. Clarity and grace of style reflect the twin disciplines which nurture most of the contributors. Their origins were either English literature or psychology; subsequent experience taught them to incorporate the two into an organic whole. An exciting illustration of this is to be found in Karl Beckson's chapter on Oscar and Willie Wilde. In establishing persuasive connections between Oscar's *The Importance of Being Earnest* and his relations with his brother Willie, Beckson has merged classical psychoanalytic theory with his own important contribution: Beckson, I believe, has uncovered a basis for the very writing of the comedy.

Untangling the labyrinthine relations between some of the other sibling pairs is at this time nearly impossible. In many cases there is so little personal data—letters, diaries, journals, or autobiographies—that some men must be studied for the most part on the basis of their published work and secondary sources. All of Aldous Huxley's papers, for example, went up in fire. But the contributors are wary of the not uncommon occupational risk for psychological biographers: hindsight fitted to a know-it-all theory. These writers are free of meretricious psychobiography and are well qualified, indeed, for their task. A broad spectrum of psychological orientations is represented here, ranging from psycholinguistic and cognitive approaches to Jungian and Freudian psychoanalysis.

Sibling Bonds

Sibling bonds in adult life are in many ways the most unusual of family relationships. Often the foci of ego development, they are the longest lasting and the least studied (Adams, 1981). Researchers have explored a broad spectrum of childhood sibling relations for more than a century, starting with Sir Francis Galton's *Hereditary Genius*, published in 1869, and continuing with Ellis's 1904 study of English genius and Cattell's 1917 data on 855 American scientists.

Ever since, psychological studies of childhood sibling variables have been made to a fare-thee-well, as a cursory survey of the *Psychological Abstracts* shows. The studies include birth order, spacing, sex distribution, sex role preference, sibling status, sibling role concept, sibling constellation, interaction, intelligence, maturity, rivalry, academic achievement, physical development, succorance needs, symbiotic dependence, fraternal complementarianism, children's perception of their siblings, fantasy family relationships, psychological distance between family members, parental referee roles, and on and on. But all of these studies deal with children or adolescents. It is as if sibling relations came to an end with the onset of maturity.

Perhaps more research has been done on the effect of birth order than on any other area of sibling relationships. Fifty years ago, Jones (1933) listed about one hundred research articles in which birth order was treated as a primary independent variable. Three decades later, in the year 1964–65, more than seventy-five such articles appeared in American journals alone (Bayer and Folger, 1967). As recently as 1977–1980, two hundred fifty studies were published, the majority suggesting that birth order is a significant factor in many kinds of behavior (Markus, 1981).

Harris (1964) demonstrated the predominance of first sons among eminent poets. His list includes Browning, Byron, Cowper, Donne, Dryden, Gray, Housman, Keats, Kipling, Marlowe, Milton, Pope, Shakespeare, Shelley, Spenser, and Yeats among the English. Other first sons are Baudelaire, Dante, Claudel, Goethe, Heine, Lorca, Pasternak, Pushkin, Rilke, Schiller, Aiken, Hart Crane, Frost, Pound, and William Carlos Williams. There are, naturally, noted second and even later sons, among whom are T.S. Eliot, Poe, Whitman, and Tagore, but the list is not nearly as extensive.

The small population of siblings in *Blood Brothers* proves little about the preeminence of first-born sons. Of the twenty-four brothers treated here, four—Lawrence Durrell, James Joyce, Lytton Strachey, and Dante Gabriel Rossetti—are undeniably more famous than their younger siblings. Whether William—the elder—or Henry James is the more famous perhaps depends on the discipline one favors. And then Anthony Shaffer is five minutes older than his twin Peter.

Whether preeminence is characteristic of the first-born or not, order of birth is undeniably of great importance. As an illustration, Alec Waugh (1967) reveals the resentment his precocious brother Evelyn felt as a second child. At the age of six, for example, Evelyn questioned their mother as to which child was more loved (Robert Kloss reports this conversation in detail). Alec writes of another incident, showing that Evelyn's feeling of being second-best was persistent: when Alec's own return from school was celebrated with a sign, " 'Welcome home to the heir of Underhill,' the six-year-old Evelyn remarked, 'When Alec has Underhill and all this in it, what will be left for me?' My father never put up the notice again" (p. 164). The influence of the chance of birth order on Evelyn Waugh's work is apparent in *Winner Take All*, his black comedy of primogeniture, and in all of the works where children occur in excess of statistical probability (Hinchcliffe, 1966). Birth order, among other factors, played havoc with Evelyn.

It is only with the 1980s that serious studies dealing with adult sibling relations have been published (Lamb and Sutton-Smith, 1982; Milgram and Ross, 1982; Bank and Kahn, 1982). Bank and Kahn categorize three types of adult sibling relations: (1) sibling solidarity, a kind of cohesiveness in which the siblings offer each other a modest degree of support in time of trouble; (2) fervent sibling loyalty, involving an irrational process of putting one's siblings first and foremost, prompted by parents who are physically or psychologically unavailable while the children are growing up; and (3) the persistence of rivalry, almost inevitable in children, into adulthood.

Milgram and Ross (1982) found that a pattern of rivalry sometimes took shape when a young sibling accepted an older one as mentor and then discovered that the mentor was not too disposed to praise the younger sibling's accomplishments. This is seen plainly in the William and Henry James relationship (Edel, 1969). "Harry is a queer boy," William once wrote to his wife, "so good and yet so limited, as if he had taken an oath not to let himself out to more than half his humanhood in order to keep the other half from suffering, and had capped it with a determination not to give anyone else credit for the half he resolved not to use himself.[2] Really, it is not an oath or a resolve, but helplessness" (p. 322). As Edel notes, Henry was "helpless" only in William's presence.

Sutton-Smith and Rosenberg (1970) found personality differences based on birth position: second-born children acquire characteristics of depending conformity and affiliation like their older siblings, while first-born children are less affected by their siblings. James and Stanislaus Joyce exemplify this.

The sibling relationship is a lifelong process, highly influential throughout the life cycle, in one form or another. The support offered Gabriel Rossetti by his brother William approaches symbiosis; at the outset William was netted in Gabriel's trap, however unconsciously, by the glamour of the literati attracted to Gabriel and then, subsequently, out of brotherly loyalty and solidarity. "Siblings are likely to serve each other as models, spurs to achievement, and yardsticks by which to measure accomplishments. . . . The sibling relationship remains alive in some sense" (Adams, 1981, p. 47). The positive aspect of sibling relations, according to Kernberg and Richards (1982), is that they provide a

> source of enjoyment, stimulation in play, mutual learning, teaching relationships, natural partners for the displacement and discharge of oedipal strivings, [and] play and fantasy as an experience in paving

---

[2] See the section on Twins for further clarification of William's perception of "half."

the way for actual function of future roles. . . . Negative affects are safer when not experienced as directed toward the parents, on whom the child must depend, but displaced on to siblings. Siblings provide opportunity for exercising actual and fantasied expression of aggression. Through sibling interaction, mastery systems, cooperation and competitiveness are facilitated. [p. 5]

How do siblings generally feel about each other when they are adults? Do childhood rivalries stop? Is there more or less love than when they were children? Do old competitions, jealousies, and feelings of superiority or inferiority continue into adulthood? According to Cicerelli (1981), there is some evidence that "siblings actually feel closer in adulthood than they did when growing up, when they were faced with petty irritations and conflicts of daily living. Obviously, not all siblings feel equally close. . . . Feelings of sibling rivalry appear to mellow as people mature. . . . Feelings of competition are strongest between brothers" (p. 23). Regardless of whether sibling relationships can be labeled "love," with all its affectionate connotations, bonds between siblings tend to be deep and abiding (Harrison and Harrison, 1981).

The mellowing process of sibling rivalry in adulthood did not seem to hold for Max Beerbohm and his half-brother, Herbert Beerbohm Tree, probably because Max was nineteen years junior to Herbert. Robert Viscusi, in his chapter on the Beerbohms, tells us that Herbert was already a very successful actor when Max reached adolescence, and that he had climbed to the heights of actor-managership by the time Max was at Oxford. Much of Max's imagination reflects Herbert's nature and career; their relationship was a clear oedipal triangle, which Viscusi illustrates with numerous citations from Beerbohm's published work and from private sources.

The form the relationship took has absorbing twists. The most intriguing is a competition that developed as Max began to have his own success. He hammered home in many essays the point that while the actor's success dies with his body, the writer's fame lives forever. Herbert began to attempt writing and might have achieved a fair measure of success had he not died early. He published in fact three "very forgettable books," according to Viscusi. One shows particularly deep parallels between his aesthetic and Max's. Another contains tales that reveal to the attentive reader how profoundly Max had managed to shake the complacency of his very triumphant half-brother. Without rehearsing the whole argument here, it may suffice to say that Herbert inspired Max to treat writing as a form of acting; and Max inspired Herbert, in his turn, to treat acting as a form of writing. As far as the competition was concerned, there was no contest: Herbert's tales make clear that the victor was Max.

To be sure, the relationship between James and Stanislaus Joyce did not mellow as they grew older. Rather, they grew further apart. In *Finnegans Wake*, Mercius boasts to his brother Justius of being a "pariah, cannibal Cain" (p. 193). This is what James Joyce himself had been, according to Cixous (1972):

> [He] fully and selfishly, his whole life, [used] others to feed his work. The victim who suffered most from the cannibal was certainly Stanislaus, from whom Jim took or borrowed everything, from his clothes to his smallest ideas, for nearly twenty years, without thinking of showing any gratitude. Stanislaus, his life, personality and desires, were all taken over by Joyce, until about 1915, with the full consent of the victim. . . . Stannie by his involuntary absence (being interned from 1915 to 1919) became useless and therefore temporarily non-existent; when he was released by the Austrian authorities in 1918, there was no place left for him in his brother's life or works. They met again, briefly and coldly, in 1919, then James left for Paris and the publication of *Ulysses*. The brothers only saw each other three times after that [a record only slightly bettered by the Waugh brothers and the Wildes]. Stannie, guardian, servant and accomplice as long as they were together, became the accuser, traitor and false brother in Joyce's secret and personal mythology; he was the necessary prey that never escapes. [pp. 119–121]

In the preface to Stanislaus's autobiography, *My Brother's Keeper*, T.S. Eliot (1958) expresses our good fortune in having James's boyhood and youth in Dublin observed and studied by a brother so "sedulously, admiringly, and jealously, as no one else ever observed or studied him . . ." (p. ix).

Jean Kimball, in her chapter on the Joyces, sees the brothers' relationship in the frame of Jung's typology, both as to attitude and function. James's basic attitude is that of the introvert, one in whom the ego is "the continuous and dominant note of consciousness" and who is correspondingly removed from "relatedness or proneness to affect." This attitude informs James's life and works to an extraordinary degree. Stanislaus, on the other hand, is almost as clearly an example of the extravert, for whom the accent lies more on "the continuity of his relation to the object and less on the idea of the ego." The complementarity in the dominant and inferior functions is less clear-cut, according to Kimball, but still demonstrable, with James's dominant function falling into the area of thinking and intuition, Stanislaus's into that of feeling and sensation.

The fact, then, she concludes, that the brothers lived so closely with one another for so many years turns this natural psychic complementarity into a compensatory relationship, important for both of them and for the character of James's work. Italo Svevo and other Triestine friends inevitably referred to Stanislaus as playing Sancho Panza to his brother's Don Quixote (Ellmann, 1958, p. xvii). Stanislaus sensed the absurdity of his thralldom, and their paths separated after 1920. What Aldous Huxley called a "hostile symbiosis" existed between the two brothers; yet, after James's death, Stanislaus became his most ardent defender.

Isaac Bashevis Singer's relationship with his older brother Israel Joshua was a singular one. In all of his anecdotal autobiographies (1966, 1969, 1976, 1978, 1981a), there seems to be a curious dichotomy between what he says he feels about Joshua and how he behaves. There is no question but that Joshua indelibly affected his life, influencing him at almost every turn: yanking him out of the desolate Polish *shtetl* of his father into the literary and intellectual stream of Warsaw, securing him writing jobs that kept him from starvation, plotting with him means to escape the dreaded military conscription, and guaranteeing his survival in alien America. These were the material necessities with which Joshua succored Isaac. Perhaps the intellectual underpinnings he provided were more important: leading the way for a break with the traditional, stultifying orthodoxy of their father's pious home, opening up the flood gates of Western enlightenment by bringing books on science and technology and works by non-Jewish authors to Isaac, introducing him to the Warsaw public libraries, and holding lengthy discussions of a philosophical nature in which everything was questioned and nothing held sacred.

Isaac stood in awe of Joshua, afraid to displease him; if he felt his behavior or ideology might, he wrote, "I actually avoided him" (Singer, 1978, p. 32). The avoidance response seems to be the benchmark of Isaac's relations with Joshua. Of Isaac's five available autobiographies, all mention Joshua but briefly. In *In My Father's Court* (1966, p. 51), for example, Isaac writes, "My mother's brothers, as well as her mother, urged her to divorce this dreamer [Bashevis's father], but my mother already had children, my sister Hinde Esther and my brother Israel Joshua." There is a chapter entitled "A Boy Philosopher" (pp. 207–212) which begins by relating Joshua's youthful maunderings, and which leads the reader to believe it will tell more about Joshua, but instead it simply provides a springboard for Isaac's own intellectual forays. Some forty years later, when Isaac was sixty-two, he had not changed: in his introduction (1965) to a posthumous reissue of Joshua's short novel *Yoshe Kalb*, he writes with brotherly respect but keeps running off on tangents. In yet another volume, early resentments are recalled: "My brother had mentioned the philosophers, and although he said that I could learn nothing from them, they had to know something, after all. Otherwise, why were they called philosophers? But where did one get such a book? I could have asked my brother, but first of all, he seldom came home now, and secondly, he often forgot what I asked for and it took him weeks to remember . . ." (Singer, 1976, p. 75).

Still later, Isaac was to write that he forbade his mistress, Gina, "this woman [who] might easily have been my mother" (Singer, 1978, p. 3), to search him out at the Writers Club in Warsaw. "I was too shy to be seen with her by the older writers. I felt that everyone would be able to tell from my face that we were having an affair. Most of all, I was ashamed before my older brother with his knowledge of life and sense of irony. My shyness at that time assumed the character of a neurosis" (p. 15). Some time later, after Joshua had married and achieved a base of familial and financial stability, Isaac wrote that "from earliest childhood I had felt a powerful desire to be with my brother. Now that I had begun to write I was anxious to show him my work and consult with him. My brother was more than willing to help me but I was ashamed to face him both on account of my dealing with women and because of my writing" (pp. 131–132).

Kresh (1979), a biographer of Singer, comments on this ambivalence toward Joshua:

> In his memoirs Isaac talks gratefully of the financial help and moral support his brother offered him. He writes of him always with admiration, even with reverence. Yet he also avoided seeing much of him. . . . There also seems to have been a measure of envy in Isaac's attitude toward Joshua that he has never openly admitted in talking about him; envy not only of the stability of Joshua's life but of his literary achievement. When he was writing *Steel and Iron*, Joshua had shared the manuscript with Isaac, but Isaac had not shown Joshua beforehand either of the stories he published the same year in *Literary Pages*. When Joshua was working on his next book, *Yoshe Kalb*, in the early thirties, he again shared the experience with Isaac. . . . "Once in a while," Isaac says, "he asked me for advice." Isaac would comb the libraries for texts of old incantations his brother wanted for the book while Joshua threw himself into the task of gathering and assembling background information of nineteenth-century life in Galicia. "In this," Isaac observes, "he resembled all the great realist writers who never feel that they can know enough." Even then, however, Isaac did not return the compliment by showing his own work to Joshua. He feared that his brother would only laugh at what he was doing. [pp. 108–110]

The emotional distance that Isaac maintained with Joshua is reversed in the relationship between Lytton and James Strachey. Seven years James's senior, Lytton was adored and idealized by his younger brother, who confided in him his homosexual affairs. Often the two informed one another of likely partners. And where Lytton had been, James was sure to follow: they attended the same university (at different times), lived in the same dormitory room, belonged to the same secret fraternal order, began their careers working for the *Spectator*, were conscientious objectors in World War I, and belonged to the Bloomsbury group.[3] Physically, emotionally, and sexually, there are fraternal similarities: both men were over six feet tall, slender, with delicate constitutions; both were remarkably intelligent and literary; and both were homosexuals, Lytton all his life, James until marriage.

The Siblings' Reactions to One Another's Work

The way the various pairs of brothers reacted to one another's work may often be a clue to how they felt toward each other. Although Isaac Bashevis Singer was overwhelmed by his brother's writing ability and felt his own was trivial and inconsequential by comparison, he had "already proved in *Satan in Goray* that he could match that power while leavening the cruelty with humor, irony, and fantasy. Even so, he emulated the structure and realism of his brother's family novels in his next three novels, *The Family Moskat, The Estate*, and *The Manor*" (Kresh, 1979, p. 175). In 1944, in New York, Israel Joshua Singer died of a heart attack, as had his father before him. To Isaac, Joshua's death was "the greatest misfortune of my entire life. He was my father, my teacher. I never really recovered from this blow. There was only one consolation—whatever would happen later would never be as bad as this" (p. 176). Nearly forty years later, at the conclusion of his essay "The Making of a First Novel," in the new edition of *Satan in Goray* (1981b), Bashevis dedicated the book to his brother, "My literary father and master," echoing the dedication of the English version of *The Family Moskat*: "I dedicate this to the memory of my late brother, I.J. Singer, author of *The Brothers Ashkenazi*. To me he was not only the older brother, but a spiritual father and master as well. I looked up to him always as to a model of high

[3] These parallels are quite different, psychologically, from those in the lives of William and Henry James, discussed under Twins. James Strachey's *The Autobiography of a Hebephrenic*, has been withdrawn from Columbia University's Oral History Library and is thus currently unavailable for study.

morality and literary honesty. Although a modern man, he had all the qualities of our pious ancestors." Yet the shock of that passing seemed somehow to galvanize Isaac, to free him to develop his powers as an author. Could it be that awe of Joshua's success had constricted him? And now, with the death of the (surrogate) father—"the most important event, the most poignant loss, of a man's life" (Freud, 1908, p. xxvi)—was he free to speak, was he rid of the inhibiting yoke?

It is Buchen's opinion (1968) that Singer's preoccupation in his work with the

> supplanting of Esau by Jacob and his equally strong determination to persist in his demonic work and appear in translation suggest the possibility that Singer was working in the shadow, not in the light of his older brother. To be sure, the influences were there, and without I. J. Singer, Singer probably would have remained in Warsaw and, like Asa Heshel in *The Family Moskat*, perished in the Warsaw ghetto. Still, a strong brother and his influence may obscure more than it nourishes. Besides, by coming into his own literary birthright, Singer has been able to pay his brother the most lasting tribute. [pp. 176–177]

The Brothers Ashkenazi (1936), considered to be Joshua's masterpiece, shows in grim, perceptive detail the life of the Jewish population in Lodz at the turn of the twentieth century. The central characters are the twin Ashkenazi brothers, who resemble one another not in the slightest. Physically, one is frail, the other athletic; one is sadistic, clever, Machiavellian, bitter and friendless, the other outgoing, loving and lovable, giving and friendly. Could Joshua have been relying on life for his fiction? To a degree, Simcha is Isaac, and Jacob, the other twin, is Joshua. "We have met these brothers before," writes Kresh. "They are Cain and Abel. . . . They are Shem and Shaun, the eternal Janus-faced dream-world pair of brothers in *Finnegans Wake*. And they embody certain traits of Isaac Bashevis and Israel Joshua . . ." (p. 144). Joseph Singer, Joshua's son and Isaac's nephew and translator, was clearly aware of these contrasts in personality. According to him, writes Kresh, Joshua was "a gregarious type, outgoing, social. Isaac is more withdrawn, always has been" (p. 146). A nephew to both men, Carr (1975), son of Hinde Esther Singer Kreitman, was quoted in a Jerusalem newspaper to the effect that "if Isaac had had his way he would not be anybody's uncle, brother, son, husband, father or grandfather." He describes the character of Yasha Mazur in his uncle's *The Magician of Lublin* as a variant of Isaac himself, a genius, an agonized prankster, tricky and fickle. He quotes Isaac as saying, "If a father wants to sleep with his daughter, why shouldn't he? We are all governed by our passions."

So much space has been devoted to the Singer brothers because they exemplify the supporting, mediating, and restitutional functions of siblings. Their abiding love, their hidden rivalry, the overt succorance, sense of loss, sibling identification—i.e., the panoply of sibling affect—is reflected in their lives. They show how pervasive, complex, and dynamic these relations can be, and how enduring.

Although Israel Joshua Singer readily showed his manuscripts to Isaac Bashevis, the latter never repaid the courtesy. When Alec Waugh sent his brother Evelyn a copy of his best-selling *Island in the Sun*, Evelyn wrote his son Auberon that "it's rather good if you think of it as being by an American which he really is" (E. Waugh, 1980, p. 468). As Robert Kloss informs us in his chapter on the Waughs, this was a contemptuous comment, for Evelyn detested Americans. To Alec, he wrote snidely, "Thank you very much for sending me *Island in the Sun* which I have read with keen pleasure. It is very encouraging that you have the power to complete so large a composition. I must soon get the name of your rejuvenation injections" (p. 464). By comparison, Evelyn's letter to Graham Greene after having read *The End of the Affair* is sincere and generous. He expresses his "very warm admiration. . . . I hope it has a huge success. I am sure it will" (p. 352). Most revealing, perhaps, is an undated letter, probably written some time late in 1928 or early 1929, to his agent and lifelong friend, A.D. Peters. Evelyn wrote of his plans for two books, one of which would be "a detective serial about the murder of an author rather like Alec Waugh" (p. 30). This pathological ideation seems to indicate that sibling rivalry is sometimes not satisfied by vanquishing the rival in any area of life. It demands not simply that the rival be killed, but rather that he should never even have existed (Kernberg and Richards, 1982, p. 46). Throughout Evelyn's letters, whether addressed to his son Auberon, his wife, other relatives, or close friends, he refers to his brother as "Alec Waugh," never as "Uncle," or just plain "Alec" or "my brother," as though Alec were a casual acquaintance whose full name had to be written out to insure proper identification. What Evelyn was trying to accomplish, of course, was dis-identification. However, in his letters to Alec himself, there are the customary signs of polite fraternal attention.

Politeness and diplomacy were never William James's forte. In an extended footnote in her biography of Alice James, Strouse (1980) writes of William's ex cathedra and gratuitous suggestions to brother Henry:

William's constant advice to his younger brothers and sister was often aggressive and not always welcome. He freely criticized Henry's writing, for instance. In the summer of 1872, he told Henry that the letters to *The Nation* showed a tendency to "over-refinement" and suggested that a broader treatment would hit a broader mark. Two months later, he confessed that he was surprised at the numbers of people who were enjoying the pieces in *The Nation*, "as I thought the style ran a little more to curliness than suited the average mind. . . . In my opinion what you should cultivate is directness of style. Delicacy, subtlety and ingenuity will take care of themselves." He protested against his brother's "constant use of french phrases. There is an order of taste—and certainly a respectable one—to which they are simply maddening," and he found in certain phrases "something cold, thin blooded & priggish suddenly popping in and freezing the genial current."

Throughout the brothers' lives, William offered this kind of pronouncement on Henry's work—not as a question of *taste* (many have agreed with William's objections to Henry's ornate style), but as if the novelist did not quite know what he was doing. Henry, for the most part, listened, offered polite thanks, and ignored the advice. He never made similar criticism of William's work, though he did read it, and usually responded with warm, if vague praise. Finally, when William urged Henry to write a book with no "twilight or mustiness" in the plot, with straightforward action, "no fencing in the dialogue," and "no psychological commentaries," the younger brother hit back—softly. He offered to write such a book—"but let me say, dear William, that I shall be greatly humiliated if you *do* like it, and thereby lump it, in your affection, with things of the current age, that I have heard you express admiration for and that I would sooner descend to a dishonoured grave than have written. . . ." And, he concluded, "I'm always sorry to hear of your reading anything of mine, and always hope you won't—you seem to me so constitutionally unable to 'enjoy' it." [p. 152]

But Henry, ever deferential to William's primogeniture, felt it necessary to apologize to him for what was then thought to be the blatant sexuality of his female protagonist in *The Bostonians*: the lesbian Olive Chancellor. In a letter to William, he expressed regret for putting so much "descriptive psychology" into the book. Yet Henry's early short novel, *Confidence*, is heavily charged with autobiographical content. The two male protagonists show themselves to be Henry and William, one an accepting figure, the other rejecting. "In giving the William character the name 'Wright' Henry revealed his long-seated fraternal acceptance of his elder brother as always in the 'right'. But he also manipulates his own hurt feelings . . ." (Edel, 1979). The characters representing the brothers in *Confidence* show how much William's criticism of Henry's novels could embarrass Henry. The rivalry can also be seen in "The Jolly Corner"; Henry was much more careful and aware in his *Notes of a Son and Brother*, which did not afford the cloak of fiction.

Both brothers were elected to the National Institute of Arts and Letters when it was founded in 1898. Seven years later, the Institute established the more elite Academy of Arts and Letters. Henry was chosen in 1905 and on the second ballot; William was elected three months later, on the fourth ballot. In an extraordinarily revealing letter explaining why he would not accept membership in the Academy, William gave among his reasons his brother's presence: "I am the more encouraged to this course by the fact that my younger and shallower and vainer brother is already in the Academy and that if I were there too, the other families represented might think the James influence too rank and strong" (Strouse, 1980, p. 29).

A little more than a decade later, Thomas Mann found himself in a nearly parallel predicament: he was invited to accept a place on the Berlin Academy of Arts Literary Section. Like his American counterpart, he refused—but for the opposite reason from the one given by William James: brother Heinrich had not been asked. Yet Thomas, like William, was consumed by the strongest of fratricidal feelings. Unlike William, Thomas pretended to the public an equality with Heinrich, even toying with the idea of refusing the Nobel Prize unless Heinrich were to share it. Both William and Thomas were on the rack, with comparable motivations for their behavior, but had different methods of expressing their feelings.

In 1906, as he was plotting his novel *Royal Highness*, Thomas wrote Heinrich, "To portray a hero humanly, all too humanly, with scepticism, with *malice*, with psychological radicalism; and yet positively, lyrically, out of my own experience: it seems to me that no one has ever done this before. . . . The counter-figure would be his brother, the Prince of Prussia (*the fraternal problem still preoccupies me*), a dreamer, who goes to bits because of his 'feelings'. . . . Am I up to such a task? I am thirty now. It is time to start thinking of a masterpiece" (Hamilton, 1978, p. 124). The italics are Mann's. Three years later, Thomas learned that Heinrich was reading the serialized version in the *Rundschau* and wrote him:

> I am not happy at the news that you are reading *Royal Highness* in the *Rundschau*. I fear you are not in the right frame of mind to take the play on our brotherly relationship in the way it ought to be taken. If only the tone I adopted in the book weren't so accurate! What if you had said to Lula at the time: 'Listen, Lula, Ines expects

you to return her visit, you must go over'? Don't you think she would have gone? A little less stiffness and distance! A little more robustness and brotherly feeling. I always feel brothers and sisters should not allow themselves to be knocked down. They can laugh at each other or scream at each other, but they should not take shuddering leave from one another. Farewell, dear Heinrich, I hope to hear from you soon, in friendly terms. . . . [Hamilton, 1978, p. 135]

In Thomas Mann's foreword to the first edition of his Joseph quartet, *Joseph and His Brothers* (1948), he uses the phrase "brother monsters." It is a unique juxtaposition, particularly in context:

When I see this pyramidlike piece of work, which differs from its brother monsters at the edge of the Libyan Desert only in the fact that no hetacombs of scourged and panting slaves fell victim to its erection but that it is the product of years of patient labor on the part of *one* man—when I see this quadpartite work united as a proper entity between the two covers of a single volume, I am filled not only with justifiable astonishment at an almost incredible achievement in the art of book-making, but also with memories, with a kind of autobiographical pensiveness. [p. v]

Did the "memories" and the "autobiographical pensiveness" unconsciously summon up a "brother monster" among his earliest recollections? It is also notable that in Heinrich Mann's long historical novel, *Young Henry of Navarre* (1937), he writes that in sixteenth-century France, the Kingdom was so riven everywhere between Catholics and Protestants "that brother was no longer understood of brother, and became alien blood" (p. 6). The use of such bareboned, dire reference to brothers, in the circumstance of Heinrich and Thomas's relationship, becomes understandable.

James Joyce made unconscionable use of his brother as a model for numerous characters in his fiction. Stanislaus is the original model for Stephen Hero and his last flamboyant break with his family: Stanislaus-Stephen denies his father completely. Stanislaus was the

first living version of Bloom at his most paralyzed, inhibited and unfortunate. . . . Joyce immortalized Stannie as Mr. Duffy, a rather unsympathetic character in *Dubliners*, though having the politeness to christen him James. Not only is Mr. Duffy's personality created from a number of Stannie's little idiosyncrasies, but also the moment of revelation when he discovers that he is nothing more than a dead man is adapted from a moving incident in Stannie's life, taken over, disfigured and desecrated by the unscrupulous Joyce. [Cixous, 1972, pp. 148–149]

Jean Kimball's chapter on the Joyces shows how Stanislaus justifiably took credit for being the steady rock on which James's precarious existence teetered, and how without him, James might not have produced *Chamber Music, Dubliners, A Portrait of the Artist as a Young Man*, and *Ulysses*. Stanislaus acknowledged his "vicarious ambition," projected through his older brother's genius, but when James wrote *Finnegans Wake* (after the two had separated in 1919), Stanislaus's criticism of it was harsh: "If I had been at his elbow, *Finnegans Wake* would never have been written in its present form" (1949, p. 897). His criticism, states Kimball, made no difference to James.

In an article on Otto Rank and James Joyce, Kimball (1976) refers to the novelist's treatment of male relatives in his work, in which he relegates his father to the status of a minor character and reduces his son to a ghost. But what, she asks, of "that other male of his blood, so prominently featured, and in person so conspicuously absent from *Ulysses*?"

What of the brother, given a name in *Stephen Hero*, banished from *A Portrait of the Artist As a Young Man*, and briefly mentioned in *Ulysses*? "Where is your brother?" Stephen asks himself, answering, "Apothecaries' hall" (*Ulysses*, p. 211), where Stanislaus Joyce had indeed been a clerk. The question echoes God's question to Cain in Genesis 4:9, immediately after the murder of Abel, and sets the stage for Stephen's introduction of "the false or the usurping or the adulterous brother" (*Ulysses*, p. 212) as a dominant theme in Shakespeare's work. Rank, who naturally enough sees the rivalry of the brothers as a renewal of an infantile struggle over the mother (1912, p. 451), quotes a passage from Minor's biography of Schiller, which is strikingly similar to Stephen's statement and which, once again, puts a foundation under it.

"The theme of the hostile brother," Minor writes, "is the oldest tragic conflict [of] saga and poetry. . . . It stems from the Bible, and not the least part of [its] irresistible effect . . . rests on the fact *that this impression belongs to the . . . most primitive stage of our childhood. Our first love and our first hate concern the brother; our first rival is our brother*" (italics are Rank's). Rank then points out that in the Bible the first murder of all is a brother-murder (1912, p. 452), and the only acknowledgment of Joyce's brother in *Ulysses* is placed in the context of this primeval brother-murder, indicating that Joyce was aware of the significance of eliminating his brother from his "procreation," a duplication of his removal of the brother from his *A Portrait*, where, as Maurice Beebe (1964) noted, "he combined key aspects of his brother's character with his own and gave Stephen the strength of both young Joyces" (pp. 264–265).

In *Ulysses*, it is Bloom who inherits the added dimension from Stanislaus Joyce, for there is a flavor of mind in Leopold Bloom which owes much to the mind revealed in Stanislaus' *Dublin Diary* [1971]. Joyce later reproduced this flavor in the stylized pairs of brothers in *Finnegans Wake* (Schechner, 1974, p. 33) but in *Ulysses* it is personalized and goes far toward giving Bloom his distinctive character. The "prudent member" (*Ulysses*, p. 614), who remains through the day "in complete possession of his faculties . . . disgustingly sober" (*Ulysses*, p. 614) finds a model in the Stanislaus of the *Diary* (1971, pp. 36, 37, 50). This diary was an important resource for Joyce in the making of *Ulysses* [See S. Joyce, *Diary*, p. vii], and, like some exotic tropical plant, he absorbed the Stanislaus he found there into Bloom, his other self, translating the "usurping" brother into an aspect of his own image. [pp. 374–375]

If James was aware of the significance of eliminating Stanislaus from his *Portrait* and *Ulysses*, Stannie was equally conscious of the psychological nuance. Ellmann (1958) relates that when he mentioned to Stanislaus the title the latter had given his autobiography, *My Brother's Keeper*, Stanislaus replied with a smile, "You know . . . Cain." Ellmann sensed that Stanislaus said this sardonically "because the evidence would show he was not. Yet he may also have felt his own role as helper to be a little ambiguous, confused, even, by a muted struggle for mastery over the creature who so mastered him" (p. x). Joyce's impish twins, Shem and Shaun in *Finnegans Wake*, are Doppelgängers; Stanislaus undoubtedly saw himself, or parts of himself, in each twin and understandably did not like what he saw. Unlike the Shaffer twins, in whose dramas unconscious twinship themes are played out, Stanislaus could not but be aware of the portrayal—and what must have been to him, betrayal.

Although Aldous and Julian Huxley were very jealous and competitive with one another, it was always in the guise of passionate interest in what the other was doing. Literature and science link experience and discourse in surprising ways. As Philip West tells us in his chapter on the Huxleys, it is not that they ventured into each other's fields as much as that they could not keep their noses out. They supported each other in separate enterprises and were each other's best resource. Julian's seminal thoughts frequently found their way into Aldous's writing. The polymathic erudition of the two brothers covered ornithology, semantics, topology, mysticism, crystallography, love, doxology, diet, and theology. It is a fascinating, pyrotechnical literary deployment that West leads us into, a kind of psycholinguistic-cognitive rationale of the relationship enjoyed by Aldous and Julian. To describe the brothers as polar opposites would be artificial, despite their divergent tendencies. Just as the mind appears to have two cognitive strategies for memory—psycholinguistics inelegantly refers to them as "chunking" and "unpacking"—so Aldous tends to the former, Julian to the latter. Their mature relationship was one of mutual support and succorance; they complemented each other, not only intellectually, but emotionally—Julian supportive of Aldous's blindness, Aldous of Julian's depressive cycle.

Like the Huxleys, the Durrells enjoyed each other's ventures, reveling in their successes, proud of their accomplishments. Gerald tended to "borrow" from his older, more literary brother Lawrence, as Jane Lagoudis Pinchin relates in her chapter, but they did not care: "Neither would mind hearing echoes of his own images in his brother's prose." By contrast, Dante Gabriel Rossetti patiently listened to William Rossetti's dilettantish poetry at the early pre-Raphaelite readings, but then William financed the Brotherhood almost on his own, so attention had to be paid. On the other hand, William was Dante's foremost fan and booster, basking in the reflected glory of his brother's fame.

So far we have dealt exclusively with the reactions of these men to their own brothers. But there exists also an interesting pattern of comment that crosses family lines and suggests that they were in varying degrees and styles sensitive to other men in their roles as brothers and were in fact prone to form quasi-fraternal relationships to them, whether real or imagined, positive or negative. For instance, when *Eminent Victorians* appeared in April 1918, Max Beerbohm was so taken by the revolutionary style of the Strachey biographies that he "felt to him as to a younger brother. He sat down and wrote him a warm letter of congratulations. Strachey, who had long been an admirer of Max's, replied with an equally warm letter of thanks. This interchange led to what was to be the most significant new literary relationship of Max's later life" (Cecil, 1965, p. 350). Evelyn Waugh (whose first published book was a 1928 biography of Dante Gabriel Rossetti) wrote a critical article on Max Beerbohm which appeared in the London *Sunday Times* of November 8, 1964. Oscar Wilde, a contemporary of Rossetti's, thought little of him. In a review of Joseph Knight's biography, titled after its subject, which appeared in *The Pall Mall Gazette* in April 1887, Wilde flayed it mercilessly: "Personalities such as [Rossetti's] do not easily survive shilling primers." Beerbohm did caricatures of the Rossetti and Wilde brothers, which are reproduced in this book, as well as drawings of his own brother and of James Joyce.

However genteel his caricatures may appear, the stiletto is used with relish. Was it contempt or anger that powered Beerbohm's pen? The plate of the Beerbohm brothers, also reproduced here, shows a powerful Herbert dominating a rather insignificant Max. Was this how the latter felt when he compared himself with his brother?

Ailments: Physical/Psychological

What does one make of the vast number of ailments, both organic and functional, that most of the twenty-four brothers suffered? Does it merely show how mortal man is, how we are all susceptible to the ravages of time and the aging process? Or are there perhaps synergistic forces at work, a syncretism that somehow pervades fraternal relations?

For instance, both William and Henry James were tormented by constipation for years, commiserating with one another even transatlantically, and relishing one another's surcease from its miseries. When Henry and William came together, "Henry nearly always developed headaches, and William ran away as quickly as possible" (Anderson, 1979, p. 17). This polarity is confirmed by Strouse (1980): "Henry and William were for years on opposite ends of a scale: when one was healthy and productive, the other floundered in illness and a sense of uselessness" (p. 112). Henry's chronic constipation was accompanied by a mysterious back ailment, never adequately explained either in Henry's autobiography or by the critics. In battling a fire, Henry had tried to start up an old water engine and in so doing had been "jammed into the acute angle between two high fences and had done myself a horrid if an obscure hurt" (H. James, 1914, pp. 114–115). Speculation over the nature of this "hurt" is rife, as might be expected. "Henry's language intimates that it was sexual, and several commentators have assumed it was a groin injury, in their rather mechanical attempts to explain the writer's identification with women, his celibacy, and his literary indirection with regard to sex. Leon Edel argues convincingly, however, that the injury was done to Henry's back" (Strouse, 1980, p. 72). Yet *The Spoils of Poynton* reveals Henry's castration anxieties, for in it he alludes to the permanence of a legless state. From their earliest years, Henry and William knew their father had only one leg (lost, too, in an attempt to extinguish a fire!) and saw him as an incomplete man.

William James was also plagued by invalidism (Feinstein, 1979). His depressions recurred intermittently throughout his life. He suffered terribly from insomnia (like Dante Gabriel Rossetti, James Joyce, Heinrich Mann, Aldous Huxley, and Evelyn Waugh), and from eye trouble. In the illness-prone James household, mother Mary James called William's temperament "morbidly hopeless. By contrast, to William she praised Henry's 'angelic patience' in his periods of ill health" (Strouse, 1980, p. 25). Not to be outdone by Henry, William too had back troubles. His hypochondriasis prolonged his engagement to Alice Gibbens for two long, difficult years. (*Her* father was a physician, an alcoholic, and a suicide.)

In addition to William James, at least four other brothers in this study were afflicted with serious eye trouble: James Joyce, Aldous Huxley, James Strachey, and Dante Gabriel Rossetti. Joyce was nearly blind from 1907 on, undergoing ten major eye operations, all without anaesthesia. Correcting proofs in Paris in his middle years, he would lay his head sideways on the page to achieve the only angle at which he still had some vision. In addition, his teeth were neglected from childhood, leaving him with lifelong painful toothaches. Joyce's anguish over these toothaches enters *Finnegans Wake*. Glugg (Shem), Joyce's dream-self as a young poet, recites his "mouthful of ecstasy" and then suffers a toothache "pinging up through the errorooth of his wisdom" as "though it had been zawhen intwo" (p. 231). The "German *Zahn*," explains Phul (1974, pp. 355, 360), is "tooth, *Zaum* is separation. The root of his error is arrowroot, source for babies and invalids, its label contains two phallic symbols." Joyce omitted little from his autobiographical novels.

One of the reasons Joyce left Ireland was to escape malnutrition at the hands of a sadistic, alcoholic father. Like his father, James had a drinking habit but, unlike him, did not act out, and was able to maintain a discipline about his work. In 1907, he was hospitalized for rheumatic fever at the same time Nora gave birth to their daughter, Lucia. There is correspondence from Paul Léon to Harriet Shaw Weaver in 1933 (J. Joyce, 1966b, pp. 269–279) which refers to Joyce's "recent second breakdown," "the collapse the other day," "lachrymose fits," and "a very acute attack of colitis." Miss Weaver indicates that there is a touch of hypochondria here too. In addition to suffering his own personal hells, which included fear of thunder, dogs, and noisy waters, as well as insomnia, Joyce was frustrated by his fruitless efforts to shore up the sanity of Lucia. After years of "melodramatically bad health," as Kimball puts it, Joyce died at the age of fifty-nine, following an operation for a malignant duodenal ulcer. Stanislaus, the healthy one, the survivor, died fourteen years after his brother, in Trieste, on June 16—ironically on Bloomsday—1955.

At the age of sixteen, Aldous Huxley was threatened by near blindness; by eighteen he was blind for all practical purposes. A former pupil remembers him as his schoolmaster at Eton: "that long, thin body with a face that was far younger than most of our masters' and yet seemed somehow ageless—and, usually, hidden by an infinite variety of spectacles, eyes that were almost sightless and yet almost uncomfortably observant" (J. Huxley, 1965, p. 27). Huxley has also been described as "a very distinguished, very long, tall, pale piece of macaroni" (Cecil, 1970, p. 868). Max Beerbohm's caricature of him emphasizes his abnormal height as well as his weak vision. He was also, like Rossetti, Joyce, and Waugh, an insomniac. In 1960, a major tumor of the tongue was discovered which metastasized to the lymph glands of his neck. He died of the cancer in 1963. His older brother, Julian, had his own range of serious problems, extending from chronic sinusitis to jaundice, hepatitis, and severe bouts of depression.

It is difficult to ascertain the etiology of Dante Gabriel Rossetti's functional eye problem. When he was thirty, Bragman (1936) relates, "Sunlight and artificial light became increasingly painful, producing sensations of giddiness. . . . He was confused in dim light, was bothered by afterimages, stumbled against objects. Despite these symptoms . . . oculists . . . said the eyes were not organically affected, attributing the trouble to weakness, overstrain and nervousness" (p. 1114). A chronic ailment from which he suffered suggests gonorrheal urethritis. His insomnia, reflected in his poems "Sleepless Dreams" and "Insomnia," turned him to large quantities of chloral and to whiskey. He hallucinated; he was a hypochondriac and suicidal, at one time taking a near-fatal overdose of chloral. And he was obese.

So was Oscar Fingal O'Flahertie Wills Wilde. His obesity was symptomatic, perhaps, of separation anxiety, accompanied by feelings of abandonment and rejection. Then, too, his mother was obese, as was his brother—not to be outdone quinquenominally—William Charles Kingsbury Wills Wilde, so that genetic factors, as well as psychological variables, may have played a part. The grotesque mind-body relationship is obvious in the caricature of the Wilde brothers by Max Beerbohm (see figure), who said of Oscar, "He felt himself omnipotent [as do many obese people] and became gross not in body only . . . but in his relations with people" (Behrman, 1960, p. 85). Beerbohm made notes of his subjects in order to keep his memory fresh and accurate. About Oscar he wrote: "Wax statue—huge rings—fat white hands—feather bed—pointed fingers—cat-like tread—heavy shoulders—enormous dowager" (Feaver, 1981, p. 125). Willie Wilde, who suffered from depressive reactions and was impotent, died from acute alcoholism in 1899 at the age of forty-six.

The Mann brothers also had their problems, physical and psychological. Thomas had such extreme intestinal pains as to make him suicidal. The animosity Thomas felt toward Heinrich translated itself into hypochon-

driacal pain, prompted by his virulent objections to Heinrich's Francophile stance as the prophet of German Republicanism and Socialism.
Thomas was aware of this link, writing in his diary that the mere mention
of a lecture given by Heinrich "pains me each time to a hypochondriacal
degree" (Hamilton, 1978).

A review of Thomas Mann's work reveals a major preoccupation with
bodily ills. In *The Black Swan*, a widow of fifty falls in love with a younger
man. She experiences a return to menstruation which is really cancer of
the womb and which is described in repulsive detail. In *Doctor Faustus*,
creativity is bought at the price of syphilis, accompanied by a manic-
depressive personality. That epic of a pathological universe, *The Magic
Mountain*, provides with Teutonic thoroughness a clinical picture of the
tubercular patient and his treatment. In *Death in Venice*, there is the
plague. The protagonist in *The Holy Sinner* is born out of incest, marries
his "sister," who is his mother, and becomes Pope so that his mother can
call him "father."

Heinrich, too, was a hypochondriac, a symptom which began when he
was four years old, with the birth of Thomas. He was often ill in childhood,
missing school; in young adulthood he spent long periods at various health
spas. Mysophobic, he was said to have been asthmatic and to have had
a weak heart. "Perhaps illness brought a certain security, the attention
of his mother," Hamilton (1978, p. 21) suggests. In 1922, Heinrich was
hospitalized with acute appendicitis which a bout of flu was masking;
peritonitis developed, to which he nearly succumbed. It was at this near-
terminal juncture that Thomas and Heinrich were reconciled—to a degree. "As moved, as overwhelmed as I am," Thomas wrote to a friend on
January 31, 1922, anticipating the reunion,

> I have no illusions about the fragility and difficulty of the renewed
> relationship. A decent, human *modus vivendi* will be about all it
> can come to. The monuments of our rift still stand—incidentally,
> I am assured he has never read the *Reflections* [*of a Non-Political
> Man*]. That is a help—and yet it is not, for all that I went through
> he can have no idea. It wrenches my heart to hear that after reading
> a few sentences in the "Berliner Tageblatt"—in which I spoke of
> those who proclaim their love of God while hating their brother—he
> sat down and wept. But the years of struggle for everything I believe
> in, which I had to conduct half-starving, left me no time for tears.
> Of that, of how the times made me into a man, how I grew and
> became a leader and shepherd for others, of all that he knows noth-
> ing. Perhaps he will sense it somehow when we meet—for the
> moment he is allowed to see no one. [Hamilton, 1978, pp. 202–203]

In his declining years, with failing health, Heinrich complained of little sleep and fits of fear, undoubtedly brought about by angina pectoris. In 1950, at the age of seventy-nine, he died of a brain hemorrhage.

Stanley Weintraub's chapter on the Rossettis reverses the expected, for it is largely the story of William, his brother Dante Gabriel's keeper. It is another tale of the Doppelgänger, the straight and the addict, the wage-earner and the leech, the critic and the creator, the hale and the ill. The stellar attraction is Gabriel, but William upstages him, emerging as the force which kept Gabriel functioning, physically and psychologically, throughout their lives. It was, moreover, a symbiotic relationship, for it was Gabriel and his friends who kept William intellectually stimulated, a far remove from the dull ambience of the Excise Office where he labored for nearly fifty tiresome years. William put up with Gabriel's financial dependency on him over a lifetime, and also endured his brother's paranoid delusional system, his kidney and liver ailments (which were complicated by chloral addiction and alcoholism), his eye problems, agoraphobia, partial paralysis, and suicidal ideation. William bore this cross dutifully and, for the most part, uncomplainingly; it was a remarkably forbearing sibship. As Weintraub reminds us, this neglected brother of the more famous Dante Gabriel was "instrumental in rescuing Blake from neglect, Whitman from opprobrium, [and] Shelley from textual emasculation. Posterity has looked kindly on men for much less."

The great psychological influence on Lawrence Durrell's work was Georg Groddeck. Groddeck's *The Book of the It* (1923) carries an effusive introduction by Durrell, in which he lays special emphasis on Groddeck's conception and treatment of disease and the nature of health. "The causes of sickness or health," Durrell explains, Groddeck "decided were unknown. . . . Disease as an entity did not exist, except inasmuch as it was an expression of man's total personality, his It, expressing itself through him. Disease was a form of self-expression. . . . Thus while Freud speaks of cure, Groddeck is really talking of something else—liberation through self-knowledge; and his conception of disease is philosophical rather than rational" (Durrell, 1961, p. ix). Two quotations from Unterecker (1964) give expression to Lawrence Durrell's concern for the body; and a reading of his novels, particularly *The Alexandria Quartet*, shows how disease and illness are expressions of a man's personal identity.

> The theme of the quest . . . is at the core of most of Durrell's serious work. . . . Durrell's quest involves almost always a ritual journey across water to and from a sick land ruled by an ailing monarch. In many variants of the myth, the sickness is both physical and spiritual. When Durrell sets up his parallel designs, we should therefore

expect him to fill out his picture with a whole host of wounded men and women, with medical doctors, with psychologically twisted characters, and with psychoanalysts. And, of course, he does. Wounds, in fact, both spiritual wounds and physical ones, bulk almost as large in Durrell's scheme of things as mountains, islands, and roads. [p. 30]

In one way or another, hardly a character in [*The Alexandria Quartet*] escapes disfigurement or death. Think of crowds of blind or half-blind figures alone: from one-eyed Hamid, through one-eyed Scobie, one-eyed Capodistria, and one-eyed Nessim, to totally blind Liza and the whole host of minor figures—blind servants, sheiks, and priests—who fumble through the novel. [p. 40]

Lawrence Durrell, like his brother Gerald, wrote a number of books dealing with islands. He called his own "disease" *islomania*, an ailment "as yet unclassified by medical science. . . . [A] rare but by no means unknown affliction of the spirit," it causes its victims to "find islands somehow irresistible" (Friedman, 1970, p. 48). In *Reflections on a Marine Venus* (1953), an autobiographical-fictional account of the island of Rhodes, one of the characters, Mills, demonstrates the relationship of disease and personality and would appear to anticipate Durrell's later involvement with Groddeck.

His diagnosis of disease seemed somehow to be a criticism, not of the functioning of one specific organ, but of the whole man. Like all born healers he had realised, without formulating the idea, that disease has its roots in a faulty metaphysic, in a way of life. And the patient who took him a cyst to lance or a wheezing lung to think about, was always disturbed by the deliberate careful scrutiny of those clear blue eyes. One felt slightly ashamed of being ill in the presence of Mills. It was as if, staring at you as you stood there, he were waiting for you to justify your illness, to deliver yourself in some way of the hidden causes of it. [p. 35]

The critical crankiness of Evelyn Waugh, seen in his journals (1980) and in his satirical work, is perhaps a reflection of the escalating series of painful physical and emotional ailments which ravaged him during his life. The corrosive words flowing from his pen reveal a dyspeptic, iconoclastic, irascible, mean-spirited writer.

Waugh was an ambulatory biological disaster, full of corrupting symptoms and held together by a ganglia of perverse, agonizing motivations.

He lived in queasy visceral terror of his ailments and yet was held in thrall by them, bringing him close to paranoia. He had all his teeth extracted as well as a totally unnecessary hemorrhoidectomy, thus in two fell swoops extirpating both ends of his alimentary canal, the anal and oral roots of his paranoid fears.

Evelyn's personality was marked by bitterness, as evidenced by his perception that it was bad luck to be born a second son; by aggression, as seen in his comic cruelty; by boredom, as reflected in his depression; by offensive rudeness to friends and foe alike; and by pervasive irritability. Perhaps these traits were caused by his bad teeth, his hemorrhoids, his fibrositis, his rheumatism, and his failing memory. He perseverated his obsessions and torments in his fiction, giving it a smell of death. Evelyn's lifelong insomnia led to phenobarbital addiction and to drink, much like Rossetti. He suffered from a tenacious depression. Robert Kloss, in his chapter, describes the delusionary and hallucinatory system of Evelyn's paranoia. Evelyn's contemporary, J.B. Priestley (1957), judged him schizophrenic and pointed to the mirroring of his psychotic state in the character of Gilbert Pinfold. Through it all he maintained an unswervingly orthodox and devout religious affiliation.

Max Beerbohm, nineteen years younger than his half-brother Herbert Beerbohm Tree, lived for thirty-nine years after Herbert's death in 1917. Robert Viscusi, in his chapter on the brothers, tells us that Max's victory of survival over Herbert led only to creative sterility. Although heaped with honors by Oxford and knighted by the King (as Herbert had been), Max's productivity ceased with Herbert's death. His only book to appear after 1917, a novella, *The Dreadful Dragon of Hay Hill* (1928), was as awful as the title sounds and the one real failure of his career. He retired to Rapallo with his wife and lived out his remaining years in an "ease and boredom and 'awful cosiness' that must at times have worn the color of an appropriate purgatory," according to Viscusi. For many creative individuals (like Picasso and Casals), there is a second wind in growing old. But for Max Beerbohm, life became a long complaint. His purgatory makes depressing reading.

> Altogether Max's personal life during these years stagnated as much as his creative did. . . . What was true of him as a boy was true of him in middle life: he was at once older and younger than the average man of his years. Low vitality had combined with extreme sensitiveness to age him prematurely. . . . He tired very easily; to feel well he had to lead a quiet life. His fatigue was nervous rather than physical. . . . In order not to overtax his frail vitality or overstrain his hypersensitive nerves, from the age of fifty onwards he lived the life of a retired elderly man. [Cecil, 1965, p. 362]

After Max's wife died in 1951, Elisabeth Jungmann took care of him, watching as depressive moods followed periods of gaiety.

> He began to suffer from asthma, indigestion, anemia, gout. Physical ills reacted on his nerves, particularly at night. . . . He suffered frequently from nightmares. . . . His days were far better than his nights, but they were not always free from nervous troubles. . . . Loud noises like the telephone bell startled him violently: he was disturbed by any alteration in routine, a stranger arriving unexpectedly or a guest at the wrong time. He got confused and could not remember things. . . . He was liable to sudden fits of acute groundless apprehension. . . . His childishness was not mental—Max's mind had not deteriorated—but emotional; it showed itself in irrational fears and agitations, and on the way he oscillated between high spirits and dependency. . . . In some respects Max had never grown up; now he was old and weak he found no difficulty in resuming the role of a child again. [Cecil, 1965, pp. 487–489]

The low vitality characteristic of Beerbohm's last decades was also to be seen in his contemporaries, the two Strachey brothers. Lytton and James were both plagued by an array of physical ills, and Murray Sherman in his chapter recites the litany. In addition to physical frailty, which in both brothers was marked by an alarming appearance of lassitude and lethargy, Lytton suffered from indigestion, heart palpitations, high fevers, and hemorrhoids. He developed a fetish for men's ears which accompanied his lifelong homosexual behavior. At fifty-one, he died of cancer of the bowel, the ultimate ironic twist indeed, since he was on a careful and limited diet for a great many years of his life. James was little better off than his older brother, at least until his marriage. During his student career at Cambridge, he was depressed, he too had a delicate constitution, his homosexual activities became pronounced, and he was perhaps as hypochondriacal as his brother. In later life a retinal detachment necessitated a series of operations.

Depression and Suicidal Ideation

At least eight of the twenty-four brothers were depressed and had deeply felt suicidal feelings, some making actual attempts at suicide. Robert Kloss relates Evelyn Waugh's aborted suicide effort in 1925, when, after resigning his schoolmaster's job and seeing his hopes of becoming secretary to Scott-Moncrieff dashed, Waugh swam out to sea. Stung by a jellyfish, he retreated to shore, a damp if dubious flirtation with death.

In the second volume of his memoirs, Isaac Bashevis Singer (1978) brings up the subject of suicide on five separate occasions. He made a "firm resolution" that if he were conscripted into the Polish army, he would commit suicide "despite the fact that this would forever darken my mother's years, she whose bashfulness, pride, and rebelliousness against the laws of life I had inherited. I also toyed with the notion of killing her first before putting an end to myself" (p. 5), typical of the suicide's unconscious yearning to return to the womb.[4] In early adulthood, pangs of the flesh tormented Isaac. Bedeviled by three streetwalkers, sorely tempted and finally giving way, he ruminated, "If I catch syphilis, my inner enemy went on, you'll have to commit suicide and that will put an end to all the foolishness" (p. 50). When the Palestine Bureau had withdrawn his immigration certificate and it appeared that he was fated to serve in the army or else die by his own hand, he lived in "a state of suspension" (p. 129). And rather than precipitate his brother's anger, Isaac stayed away from him: "I spoke like a nihilist and a suicide and more than once I evoked his anger" (p. 132).

It may be of some import that Evelyn Waugh's first published book, as noted earlier, was a biography of Dante Gabriel Rossetti. Perhaps Waugh's identification with his subject, however unconscious, enabled him to empathize with the pre-Raphaelite poet, for neither writer was able to escape pathological ailments, many of which they shared (insomnia, hypochondria, paranoid delusions, drug addiction, alcoholism, and depression). Dante Gabriel never ceased to reproach himself for the suicide of his wife, Elizabeth Siddal (one year after the birth of a stillborn child), from an overdose of laudanum. His insomnia worsened; to counteract it, he took large doses of chloral and drank heavily. He talked daily of suicide. His morbidity prevented creative effort. Secretly he had prescriptions for chloral filled in a number of different apothecaries. At one point in 1879 he was believed to be dying of an overdose but survived for three more years, supported by frequent hypodermic and oral intake of morphine until his death.

William James suffered from a lifelong depression. During the winter

[4] Ozick (1982) raises a number of pertinent oedipal questions: "what are we to think of the goblin cunning of a man who has taken his mother's name—Bashevis (i.e., Bathsheba)—to mark out the middle of his own? Singer's readers in Yiddish call him, simply, 'Bashevis.' A sentimental nom de plume? His is anything but a nostalgic imagination. Does the taking on of 'Bashevis' imply a man wishing to be a woman? Or does Singer hope somehow to entangle his own passions in one of literature's lewdest and nastiest plots: King David's crafty devisings concerning the original Bathsheba? Or does he dream of attracting to himself the engendering powers of his mother's soul through the assumption of her name? Given the witness of the tales themselves, we are obliged to suspect any or all of these notions, as well as others we have not the wit or fantasy to conjure up" (p. 1).

of 1867, while a medical student at Harvard, he had trouble with insomnia, his back, his digestion, and his eyes. He wrote to his friend Tom Ward that he had been "on the verge of suicide. . . . Restless and depressed, he could neither resolve his conflicts nor ignore them" (Strouse, 1980, p. 110). Julian Huxley's depression was cyclical, frequent, and apparently particularly severe while he was working at the London Zoo and during his tenure as Director of UNESCO. He was hospitalized for depression at least twice, in 1912 and again in 1944. Willie Wilde, too, had depressive reactions, drowning his problems in drink, much like Rossetti. Thomas Mann's abdominal pains were of such intensity as to make him ponder the alternative of suicide. As Max Beerbohm grew old, his moods, as noted, oscillated between depression and gaiety. James Strachey's university days, it will be remembered, were markedly depressed. Thus, more than a third of these twenty-four brothers evinced suicidal ideation, pseudosuicidal attempts, or depression.

Homosexual Themes

Nigel Hamilton's chapter on the Mann brothers points out that in his review of Thomas's *Death in Venice* Heinrich makes no reference to the homosexual theme of the story and "depicted instead an aging man's seduction not by the image of a beautiful Polish boy, but by the corrupt and glorious concubine, Venice." Hamilton surmises that the homosexual theme of the novel reflects the homoerotic yearnings of its author, as well as his growing sexual frustration. "Homosexuality or at least homoerotism had characterised almost every story Thomas Mann had written. . . ."

Winston (1981) has candidly examined Thomas Mann's homoerotic tendencies. "Never in his whole life was he to admit openly to that defect except in the deep privacy of his diaries. Yet he nursed his secret as a source of pleasure, of interest, of creative power" (pp. 273–274). Fascinatingly, Mann recorded in his diaries that his early conservatism was "an expression of my sexual inversion," by which he possibly meant that the writing of *Reflections of a Non-Political Man* was influenced by his deep relationship with a homosexual friend.

The special organization of love and hate evident in many twins includes forbidden elements and intense drives that require discharge, as Jules Glenn notes in his chapter on the twin playwrights Anthony and Peter Shaffer. The love is often taboo in that it contains a strong homosexual component and a powerful narcissistic core. The latent homosexual attachment of the Doppelgänger characters in Anthony Shaffer's *Sleuth* "is more than hinted at in the relationship between Andrew and Milo, especially in Andrew's attempt to exclude women from their lives. Andrew unquestionably prefers the male Milo to women in general and to Marguerite in particular. He explicitly asks Milo to stay with him rather than run off with his wife. . . ." The love/hate relationships seen in *Sleuth* and *Murderer* exemplify the feelings between siblings, experienced perhaps more poignantly in twins.

The special love apparent in the Shaffer dramas is also seen in the lives of William and Henry James and in the latter's fiction. Howard Feinstein's chapter gives evidence of a strong homosexual strand between the two, as marked, for example, in their exchange of letters at the time of William's marriage. There is more. The theme of male and female homosexuality runs throughout Henry's novels and short stories, symbolically and realistically; orgiastic homosexual eroticism is not uncommon in Henry's work. And Henry's own homosexual proclivities are noted by Feinstein.

Both Waugh brothers engaged in discrete homosexual activity. *The Loom of Youth*, Alec's fictional account of homosexual experiences in the famous Sherbourne school incident, bemoans his bad luck in being found out and expelled. Later on, Evelyn was denied admission because of Alec. The latter's preoccupation with homosexuality as a theme is found in many of his novels, including *The Mule on the Minaret* and *A Spy in the Family*. Robert Kloss discusses Alec's headlong rush into three marriages (the first never consummated) and his frequent sexual involvement with women. This turbulent behavior was, perhaps, a declaration of his masculinity as well as a defense against further homosexual activity.

There are two periods in Evelyn Waugh's life in which he is known to have had overt homosexual experiences: at Lancing and at Oxford. His diaries are dotted with homosexual references—as lively a preoccupation as is found in Alec's novels. Evelyn saw "pansies" and "queers" everywhere and tried to sublimate his homosexuality in voyeuristic adventures as well as in his fiction. In the latter, an esthetic homosexual aura surrounds his male protagonists: Anthony Blanche, Ambrose Silk, and Sebastian Marchmain. Kloss concludes that Evelyn's work "is a repository which shows clearly the relationship between [his] paranoia and his homosexual impulses."

Oscar Wilde's homosexual escapades have been well noted and need little elaboration here. Oscar could have escaped from England to avoid a two-year jail sentence—the unfortunate result of his liaison with Lord Alfred Douglas—but chose instead to remain. Was the need to be punished so overwhelming that Oscar elected to stay? Karl Beckson's revelation, in his chapter, of Willie's role during Oscar's ordeal shows Willie's naked hostility toward his brother. Willie urged Oscar to stay, perhaps indicating a repressed wish to witness his punishment and destruction. Though Willie appeared every day in court during Oscar's trial, he was not present when his brother was released from Reading Gaol in 1897.

Like the Waughs, both Stracheys had homosexual inclinations, but unlike them, Lytton remained constant to this preference while James was bisexual. Further, their homosexual activities were of a coordinate nature, unlike the Waughs. James, according to Murray Sherman's account, was Lytton's confidant for many of his homosexual affairs and to some extent shared partners with him. It was at an English public school that Lytton developed crushes on older boys who impressed him physically. At Cambridge, his homosexual involvement with classmates was imitated by James when he entered the university some time later. Lytton was caught up in the homosexual world with a continuous series of affairs which inevitably led to disillusionment and promiscuity. His relationship with the bisexual Ralph Partridge and the doomed Dora Carrington led to a curious *ménage à trois*, with Lytton and Ralph reciprocally in love, Carrington unrequitedly in love with Lytton (who regarded her platonically), and Ralph in love with Carrington, whom he eventually married.

James Strachey's sexual life was almost as bizarre as his brother's. Madly in love with the poet Rupert Brooke, an old school chum, James pursued him doggedly only to be rebuffed and humiliated; undaunted, he redoubled his efforts. It would seem that James's affection for Rupert was a displaced, sublimated love for the idealized brother, which was too threatening ever to be consummated but could be acted out—up to a point—with a nonincestuous object. Implicit in his feelings in the triangular relationship with Lytton and Brooke were, in all probability, primary masochism, death wishes, and unconscious guilt. The thrust and parry of their neurotic relationship persisted until Brooke's death in World War I. Lytton was perhaps less intimidated by the incest taboo than was James. His affair with his cousin Duncan Grant (whose portrait of James precedes the chapter on the Stracheys) gave him unqualified joy, a joy which turned to ashes when Duncan became the lover of their mutual good friend, John Maynard Keynes. It was one of the most painful episodes in Lytton's painful life.

Financial Dependence

Heinrich Mann arrived in New York City on October 13, 1940, a refugee from Nazi Germany. He was to remain in the United States for ten years. A series of blunders, many of his own making, left him destitute. His wife's jewelry had to be sold; they were forced to move to cheaper living quarters. "In March 1941," Hamilton (1978, p. 321) reports, "Heinrich and Nelly had had to travel to Mexico to conform to official immigration rules, and Thomas had signed an affidavit agreeing to take care of or finance his brother should he ever fail to be able to support himself [even as I.J. Singer did for his brother Isaac]. 'I ask you unwillingly,' Heinrich wrote to Thomas on February 23, 1941, 'since I do not know whether it is merely a question of form or entails serious contractual responsibilities for you.' By the end of 1941 Thomas was, in fact, having to help. The story of Joseph had come true."

Thomas was his brother's financial mainstay for the next eight years, until Heinrich's death in 1950. Thomas could probably afford to care for Heinrich financially, for his books sold well in the United States, he lectured widely, and he was visiting professor at two great universities. His support of Heinrich shows a monumental role reversal, for while the two brothers were growing up, and particularly after their father's death in their formative years, Thomas looked up to Heinrich as a surrogate father. Now, in Heinrich's last years, it was Thomas who served as the nurturing parent, sustaining the destitute and ailing Heinrich.

Whether or not Willie Wilde was ever truly self-supporting is an open question. As late as 1893, when Willie was forty years old and living with Lily Lees, who later became his second wife, Oscar sent him a check, "as I don't want you to die." Willie's earlier marriage, to the wealthy American publisher Mrs. Leslie, sixteen years his senior and an obvious nurturing mother surrogate, lasted but two years. It began and ended disastrously, with Willie impotent and drunk. Disgusted by his idleness, profligacy, and parasitism, Mrs. Leslie divorced him; even as a kept man, he was a failure. Not only did Willie cadge from Oscar, Mrs. Leslie, and Miss Lees's mother, but even his own widowed mother was not exempt. Karl Beckson's chapter includes a plaintive letter from Lady Wilde to Oscar about Willie: "Just when my income has fallen so low, he announces the marriage and the whole burden of the household to fall upon me. . . . Miss Lees has but £50 a year . . . and Willie is always in a state of utter poverty." For some time thereafter, Lady Wilde housed and supported Willie and his wife. Beckson searched out the original version of *The Importance of Being Earnest*, in which Algy says to Jack, "Of course, I'm your brother. And that is why you should pay this bill for me. What is the use of having a brother if he doesn't pay the bills for one?" Jack demurs initially but then agrees to pay, the stage conversation becoming an accurate replication of life.

Of the twenty-four men studied, none relied more on a sibling for financial aid, and none took greater advantage of a brother's willingness to help, than Dante Gabriel Rossetti and James Joyce. William Rossetti was bewitched into Gabriel's service by the idea that he was succoring genius: not merely genius but family genius. Gabriel lived largely on "loans" from William and gifts from his aunts Charlotte and Margaret, as well as contributions from his mother. Only one day of his fifty-four years of troubled life did he bestir himself to seek employment, and this he peremptorily rejected. When Gabriel married the beautiful Lizzy Siddal, William assumed she would be no added drain on his own finances, limited as they were by his salaried position with the Inland Revenue. It was William who signed, falsely, as cotenant for Gabriel and Lizzy's house and guaranteed their debts. Gabriel's charismatic personality also beguiled compliant friends into subsidizing his living expenses; all were more than happy to participate in the honor. Gabriel badgered William shamelessly for money, even though at times his income as an artist was greater than William's entire salary. In the best of times, Gabriel's finances were chaotic and debt-burdened. Decades after his death, William was still settling the estate, even taking on Gabriel's moral obligations. As Gabriel's executor, the symbiotic relationship persisted, holding William in its clutches some thirty years after Dante was in his grave.

Genius, like brotherhood, has it perquisites, as James Joyce was to impress on Stanislaus. Joyce, like Gabriel Rossetti, had both genius and a supportive brother—but there was a difference. Joyce lived a hand-to-mouth existence for too many years, barely able to support his wife and two children. He eked out a living by teaching at the Berlitz School in Trieste. There he "began the series of madcap schemes [to make money] which he was to continue sporadically for many years" (Ellmann, 1959, p. 206). Joyce moved from crisis to crisis—emotional, familial, physical, and economic. At James's insistence, Stanislaus left Dublin in 1905 for Trieste, virtually starving himself en route. When he arrived, James asked whether any money was left from the trip. Five years later, his resentment festering, Stanislaus wrote his father that James "asked me very few other questions of importance concerning myself since I came here" (Ellmann, 1959, p. 220). James's narcissism was typical. While William Rossetti basked in his brother's accomplishments and enjoyed the heady experience of the company of celebrities, the reward for Stanislaus Joyce's abnegation was inward growth—at the cost of being swallowed up by his older brother. Sharing James's intellectual life, Stanislaus's contribution was insuring his brother's productivity.

Hired as an English teacher at the Scuola Berlitz, as was his brother, Stanislaus agreed to use his weekly salary of eight dollars to pay their joint household expenses. Combined with James's pay of nine dollars, it was ample to cover expenses if they managed sensibly. [But] such 'necessities' as dining out every night . . . kept them in the vestibule of poverty. . . . James borrowed a pair of Stanislaus's trousers and kept them, and trivial exploitations of this kind, to which Stanislaus consented at first cordially, later more slowly, and finally with the utmost reluctance, marked their relationship from the start. James saw no reason to limit his brother's sacrifice to genius, especially when genius had a family to support. Stanislaus was bound to James by affection and respect, but also by indignity and pain. [Ellmann, 1959, p. 221]

But Stanislaus was not as forbearing as William Rossetti. He was disgusted with his brother's drinking, loathed his life style, and was disconcerted by James's growing silences.

Throughout his life, James was pinched for money; it became a central preoccupation for him. It was Stanislaus who invariably stepped in to rescue James and his family to the extent that his own meager resources permitted (Ellmann, 1959, pp. 221, 223, 231, 235, 236). It was Stanislaus who was dunned by James's creditors in Trieste when the latter had moved to Rome in 1906. It was Stanislaus who had to rescue James in Rome. While James was drinking and dining well there, Stanislaus was eating bread and ham in Trieste in order to make ends meet. When he learned of Joyce's high living, he stopped sending money.

James's importunities increased in skill; he pictured his starving wife and child. . . . James offered intricate budgets of his expenditures to justify his being allowed to continue them with Stanislaus's help. Stanislaus did not give up without a struggle. . . . He yielded at last and sent his available money. . . . [But] James continued to implore Stanislaus for help, promising that each month would see the end of his desperation, but finding a new cause for being desperate as each month went by. [Ellmann, 1959, pp. 235–236]

Joyce was an accomplished "con" man at writing letters pleading for money. During his first stay in Paris in 1902 as a would-be medical student, he wrote his mother cash-wringing accounts of his empty stomach, just as he did not too long afterwards with Stanislaus.

Though James's exploitation of Stanislaus was a continuing aspect of their brotherhood, it was not their only significant contact. On the contrary, James felt that their relationship was the most rewarding of all he had (Ellmann, 1959, p. 245). He relied on Stanislaus for literary advice and suggestions for publication. He depended on his emotional strength. It was, altogether, a most striking bond that these two brothers, so different from one another, maintained. Sober Stanislaus, soused James; the

one penny-watching, careful, responsible, the other gratuitously profligate, a bon vivant, a narcissistic manipulator. This makes for an interesting contrast with the Rossettis, for while Stanislaus rebelled frequently
and vociferously against being held in bondage by James, William Rossetti
was the quintessential succoring brother. The claims enforced by Dante
Gabriel on William seem exorbitant, but apparently William did not
object; if he did, it was muted almost beyond human understanding.

On the other hand, Herbert Beerbohm Tree was a good-natured
brother to sponge off, and his younger half-brother, looking to him as a
surrogate father, accepted help unthinkingly from him. When Max Beerbohm quit Oxford University in June 1894, he returned to his mother's
pleasant house in London, expenses for which were paid by Herbert.
"There was enough money so that Max felt no pressure to contribute to
the household expenses. . . . It was a pleasant life with little responsibility" (McElderry, 1972, p. 35). Six months after Max left Oxford, Herbert sailed for the United States with his acting company, taking Max
along as his private secretary. "But because he composed letters with
such care that he got far behind, he was soon relieved of his duties;
Herbert good-naturedly continued his salary" (p. 36).

Twins

Psychological studies of identical twins have shown that twinship can be
a burden and that it can interfere with evolving identity, for the pair see
each other as continuing mirrors or as the same person twice. A twin has
the problem of individuating himself not only from his mother but also
from the other twin (Demarest and Winestine, 1955). John Barth (1982),
writing about his twin sister and himself as a writer, said: "I have sometimes felt that a twin who happens to be a writer, or a writer who happens
to be a twin . . . might use schizophrenia, say, as an image for what he
knows to be his literal case: that he once was more than one person and
somehow now is less. I am the least psychological of storytellers; yet even
to me it is apparent that I write these words, and all the others, in part
because I no longer have my twin to be wordless with, even when I'm
with her. Less and less, as twins go along, goes without saying. One is
in the world, talking to Others, talking to oneself" (p. 3).

Jules Glenn's chapter on the Shaffer fraternal twins and Howard Feinstein's on the James "psychological twins" cast light not only on twinship
itself but on how twinship affects work. Through analysis of four of the
Shaffers' major dramas, *Sleuth*, *Murderer*, *Equus*, and *Amadeus*, Glenn
demonstrates how twin identification can be a reflection of poor distinction

between self- and object-representations, of libidinal and defensive elements, and of pleasurable union which may succeed in quelling hostility through the triumph of affection. Identification may also diminish the twins' mutual antagonism through keeping things equal. The Doppelgänger effect becomes readily noticeable once called to attention, as does the way in which twinship is often disguised through double imagery. And importantly, Glenn shows the defenses aroused in the audience by the Shaffers' work.

In an article on the psychology of twins, Glenn and Glenn (1968) state that twins of all kinds

> often imagine unconsciously or consciously that they are half persons divided after full growth in the womb or after birth. As Plato suggested, they feel deficient and seek for their other half. Often they feel not like a half person but like less than half persons and imagine that their twin has got more than his share. They seek union with the twin lovingly and sexually, as Plato said, but also they seek union aggressively, with hostility, intending to get back the missing part in an angry and vengeful way. Often twins picture the world as full of twins that they have to cope with. Feeling like half a person similar to or identical with their twin involves other traits as well. Twins have a strong tendency to imitate others and use identification as a defense for the attainment of self-satisfaction. As a result twins may reverse roles; first one may be dominant and the other submissive and then change their relationship to the diametric opposite. In addition they may each supplement the other in regard to some aspect of their personality: one may display superego characteristics prominently and the other may be more drive oriented. [pp. 3–4]

William and Henry James, as Feinstein shows, functioned astonishingly like fraternal twins, though they were not. Their almost identical behavior patterns well exemplify the fusion in twins described by Glenn. Feinstein notes that William, after "the twinship of their youth had been largely dissolved," could see "that something was missing, some vital part that made Henry seem there only by half."

William and Henry, according to Feinstein, saw illness as a confirmation of their brotherly attachment. If Henry developed a back problem, so did William; if William became constipated, Henry also endured; they acknowledged common symptoms of heart disease, although physicians could find no organic evidence for Henry's complaints. William went to Harvard; so did Henry. If William tried his hand at art, Henry followed; when Henry became successful at writing, William took a stab at that.

Henry himself characterized his relationship with William as a mythological twinship. They were, in his own words, as Feinstein reminds us, "a defeated Romulus, a prematurely sacrificed Remus." Feinstein's emphasis, however, is not on the rivalrous aspects of the twinship theme but on the problem of individuation for William and Henry. Henry was the first to recognize it and try to work it through; William found it more difficult to accept. They met with a degree of success, but in their final years, regressed to their more formative twinship period. Unlike the Jameses, Lawrence Durrell, as Jane Pinchin notes in her chapter, understood what it meant "to be the first son expecting to be followed, wounded by the separate self your brother becomes."

The theme of fraternal twins runs throughout James Joyce's *Finnegans Wake* (Tindall, 1971). Shem and Shaun's incompatibility

> produces conflict to end all conflict: those of Jacob and Esau (or "castor and porridge," . . .), of Cain and Abel ("I cain but are you able?" . . .; am I "your bloater's kipper?" . . .), of Mutt and Jeff, and of the ant and the grasshopper. Mark that these twain are Tom Sawyer and Huck Finn, Michael and Satan (or Mick and Nick), Peter and Paul, Tweedledum and Tweedledee, Romulus and Remus, St. Thomas Beckett and St. Lawrence O'Toole, St. Patrick and Bishop Berkeley. [p. 247]

Joyce, says Tindall, applies his own career to Shem; he associates Shaun with his brother Stanislaus, as well as a composite of contemporary and literary figures.

> Shem is outsider, introvert, artist, and failure. Shaun is insider, extravert, bourgeois, and success. Shem is tree and Shaun is stone. Shem is baker, Shaun butcher. Shem drinks, Shaun eats. . . . That Joyce used details of his own life for Shem, and sometimes Shaun, is far from odd. . . . But details of Joyce's life do not make Shem Joyce. Shem is that side of Joyce which must unite with his Shaun side. . . . [pp. 246–247, 278]

Shem and Shaun are striking examples of the difficulties twins have with the problem of individuation. Joyce, using the artist's perceptual genius, portrays them to their psychologically ambivalent hilt. Evidently, Joyce perceived his relationship with Stanislaus to be as close and as confusedly undifferentiated as if they were twins.

Oddly enough, this was to some extent true, too, of Herbert Beerbohm Tree and Max Beerbohm, although Herbert was Max's elder by nineteen years. Tree was the outstanding actor of his day, achieving this reputation long before Max arrived at puberty. But Max's fame in writing and caricature began to outpace Herbert's fame. Max had repeatedly written that the printed word and the drawn figure would outlive an actor's day on the stage. He was right. In what seems to have been a desperate effort to outflank Max, Herbert began to write, but with little success. One of his short fantasy pieces is described by Robert Viscusi in his chapter on the brothers. Its title is "The Lament of a Lilliputian Twin" (1917), a story in which Tree confesses that his brother usurped him and in which he reveals his anguished fantasy life. His insights lay bare the bitter rivalry that existed beneath the polite veneer they maintained. That Herbert should view his much younger brother—a whole generation removed—as his twin is remarkable in itself. Peers of the realm they both were, but Herbert's acting legacy barely survives despite his desperate effort to surpass his rival, while Max still lives in caricature and prose.

Marie Lehning, the young peasant heroine of Heinrich Mann's *Hill of Lies* (1935), once acted as nursemaid to a brother and sister—twins. When she comes into contact with them some years later, the twins, neurotic and perverted members of a lost generation, exert a baleful influence on her. How the tale symbolically represents Heinrich's obsessional preoccupation with his brother Thomas and their influence on German politics is an interesting speculation. Equally intriguing is I.J. Singer's *The Brothers Ashkenazi*, in which unlikely twins, as different as Joseph and Esau, are the protagonists.

On the basis of empirical evaluation, Farber (1981) suggests that the intrapsychic environment of identical twins may be as important as observable external influences. Her study points to a genetic blueprint that determines both the individual's physical traits and the fundamental structure of the personaliy. Monozygotic twins, separated in early life and reared apart, show striking uniformity in such physical traits as height and weight, age of onset of numerous somatic complaints, shape of teeth and location of cavities, and mentrual cramps, and such behavioral characteristics as tone of voice and tilt of head. Further, their basic personality style is virtually the same—temperament, emotional lability, and impulsivity. However, in traits such as I.Q. and symptom choice in psychopathology, environmental effects become significant. Farber's findings are relevant for the fraternal twins found in this book, and for brothers too, as the testimony of Jane Pinchin, in her chapter on the Durrells, seems to suggest. In separate personal interviews with Lawrence and Gerald, she was intrigued to find both "greeted a stranger with the same gestures, the same drinks, and . . . magnanimity. . . ."

Expatriates and Exiles

The material provided by the contributors to this volume reveals some curious similarities among the twenty-four subjects. For example, half were at some point expatriates or exiles. The expatriate life was played out, for many, not in traditional European literary haunts à la Hemingway and Fitzgerald, but almost the reverse: in the United States, on the Mediterranean shores, or in the Caribbean. Coming to America were the Singers from Poland, the Manns via France and Portugal, and Aldous Huxley from England; from the United States to London went Henry James; from London to Corfu, Paris, Cairo, Cyprus, Argentina, and points in between went Lawrence and Gerald Durrell; from Dublin to Trieste, Rome, Paris, and Zurich went James and Stanislaus Joyce; also from Dublin but fleeing to Paris was Oscar Wilde; Max Beerbohm left London for Rapallo; and Alec Waugh lived in Tangiers and died in Tampa.

What does it all mean? Lawrence Durrell said that the only satisfactory way to deal with England was to escape it long enough to observe it dispassionately: "In order to rescue what is best in his country, the artist must subject the country to the scorching analysis of satirical rejection." According to Friedman (1970), the central impetus in Durrell's work is his

> inherent sense of deracination and his concomitant need to belong somewhere. Indeed, he would seem to embody the very pattern of the rootless wanderer imbued with a highly developed sense of roots; for like most placeless men, Durrell worships place. . . . All of Durrell's major themes and motifs are expressed as interrelationships of character and place: alienation, non-communication, a condition Durrell expresses in terms of illness, result when the individual clashes with a place of negative influence; if the dominance is overwhelming, the individual becomes will-less, passive, fails totally at art and love; if he manages to escape a landscape fertile for him, he becomes cured, attains a new sense of selfhood usually expressed metaphorically as spiritual regeneration, begins to create, and becomes capable of love. [pp. xiv–xv]

James Joyce, like Durrell, has been characterized as rootless, and his rejection of his native Ireland is ringing and vehement. According to Nabokov (1980), "In composing the figure of Bloom, Joyce's intention was to place among endemic Irishmen in his native Dublin someone who was as Irish as he, Joyce, was, but who also was an exile, a black sheep in the fold, as Joyce was. Joyce evolved the rational plan, therefore, of selecting for the type an outsider, the type of the Wandering Jew, the type of the exile" (p. 287). Joyce himself once wrote, "There was an English queen who said that when she died the word 'Calais' would be written on her heart. 'Dublin' will be found on mine." Joyce left his native city at the age of twenty-two to go into voluntary exile, as did his brother Stanislaus, but it was no more than a physical leave-taking. An intellectual and spiritual attachment, a love-hate obsession, remained to the end.

In addition to the physical exile Isaac Bashevis Singer experienced, there was another kind of exile in store for him, which Joseph Landis tells about in his chapter: "War with God and war with the moderns who rejected Him created a predicament that left Isaac the Yiddish writer in almost total isolation, an exile from two worlds, forever caught between them, caught like a typical Singer character, in a mirror, a Prometheus chained and fighting a private war with God and man."

While Max Beerbohm, Alec Waugh, Aldous Huxley, the Durrells, and the Joyces all voluntarily left their native Britain for personal reasons, the Singers, Oscar Wilde, and the Manns exiled themselves for causes that relate to man's persistent search for freedom.

Conclusion

Sibling rivalry has had a bad name, associated as it is with ambivalence and guilt, with blood chemistries and environments that frequently create a love-hate relationship. When siblings look at each other, do they see a monster winking back at them as if from a mirror? The symbolic baggage of their unconscious is burdened in later life with meanings foretold in the earlier one, despite the reduction in sibling conflict which frequently occurs with the passage of time.

The chemistry of the relationship depends on a number of variables, as the chapters show: the luck of birth order, gender, age differential, and so on. The tales of Cain and Abel, Isaac and Ishmael, Esau and Jacob, Joseph and his brothers, and the entire panoply of siblings have done less for the image of brotherly love than they might have. *Genesis* is full of stories of hatred and rivalry between brothers.

> In every instance the father is spared, and rage is turned against the brother. Jacob, with the connivance of his mother, Rebekah, steals by trickery his older brother's birthright and his blessing. The paternal blessing not only passes in the goods and power of the father, it also confers the privilege of carrying on the Covenant with God—that special relationship with God the Father (the primal parent) which led to Cain's murder of Abel. . . . If, as Freud hypothesized, and work with patients suggests, the primal crime is

parricide, the biblical myth portrays a displacement in the murder of Abel by Cain. The father is defied in the eating of the forbidden fruit, but the first murder is that of brother by brother, out of jealousy for the father's love: 'The Lord paid heed to Abel and his offering, but to Cain and his offering he paid no heed' (*Genesis*, 4:45). [Shengold, 1971, p. 475]

Blood Brothers: Siblings As Writers is not intended as a jeremiad of sibling rivalry but rather as a celebration of brotherhood; of affection, competition, natural angers, piqued feelings, bizarre behavior due to intended or unintended hurts; of pride, jealousy, bitterness, ambitions, disappointments, excesses and timidities, selflessness and narcissism. In other words, these biographies of writer-brothers resemble the lives of all of us who have siblings. We share in their ambivalent love-hate feelings, for they are all our own. *Odi et amo*: I love and I hate, said Catullus. The polarities represent a universal, because of the very nature of the kinship.

Our twenty-four subjects, like all men, are entangled in their birth. Our purpose is to search the events of their lives for meanings perhaps not hitherto realized. None of these men is apotheosized; their mortality is all too evident: raging jealousy, financial dependency, regenerated love, transparent symbiosis, psychosomatic disablements. Truth is not always coordinate with fact, and what facts the contributors have gleaned about their subjects may not always jibe with truth. Perception is a subjective variable, brought about by life experience. The inner life of people is more often than not hidden to others, unless put on the analyst's couch or subjected to the scrutiny of the psychohistorian or the literary critic. How can an experience in the world be organized to reveal hidden meanings? There is nothing more easily falsified than the unconscious.

It is impossible to calibrate closely the emotional life of individuals long since gone; an approximate assessment is the best to be hoped for. But data are often sufficiently generated by diaries, autobiographies, journals, letters, and recollections, and these can be distilled and verified. Clues can be traced, examined from various vantage points, and a thesis established. This is particularly true when such evidence is abundant. Thus when documents serve as raw material for the biographer, and patterns are revealed whose significance can be reliably interpreted (Mack, 1980), new material may illuminate what previously was dim. The two disciplines most concerned with man in his totality are psychoanalysis and biography. Psychoanalysis' debt to biography, especially to its autobiographical sources, is readily acknowledged, as seen in Freud's *Three Essays on the Theory of Sex* (1905) and the frequent passages in the four-volume *Minutes of the Vienna Psychoanalytic Society* (Nunberg and Federn, 1962, 1967, 1974, 1975) that refer to the work and behavior of great men.

The biographical sketches in this volume are exciting, if cerebral, psychological detective stories which reveal how sibship has affected brothers' creative work, whether they lived their lives apart or in close proximity. The appeal of this genre is that it edifies while indulging our insatiable appetite for news of other peoples' lives. There is nothing like a good story well told; and a well-told biography of an intriguing personality can make the most interesting story of all.

REFERENCES

Acton, H. (1928), Golden youth, doomed. *The Dial*, 3(1):46–47.

Adams, V. (1981), The sibling bond: a lifelong love/hate dialectic. *Psychology Today*, 15(6):32–47.

Anderson, J.W. (1979), An interview with Leon Edel on the James family. *Psychohistory Review*, 8(1–2):15–22.

Bank, S., & Kahn, M.D. (1982), *The Sibling Bond*. New York: Basic Books.

Barth, J. (1982), Some reasons why I tell the stories I tell the way I tell them rather than some other sort of stories some other way. *New York Times Book Review*, May 9, p. 3.

Bayer, A.E., & Folger, J.K. (1967), The current state of birth order research. *Internat. J. Psychiat.*, 3:37–39.

Beebe, M. (1964), *Ivory Towers and Sacred Founts: The Artist As Hero from Goethe to Joyce*. New York: New York University Press.

Behrman, S.N. (1960), *Portrait of Max: An Intimate Portrait of Sir Max Beerbohm*. New York: Random House.

Bragman, L.J. (1936), The case of Dante Gabriel Rossetti: a psychological study of a chloral addict. *Amer. J. Psychiat.*, 92:1111–1122.

Buchen, I. (1968), *Isaac Bashevis Singer and the Eternal Past*. New York: New York University Press.

Carr, M. (1975), An intimate pen-portrait of Isaac Bashevis Singer. *Jerusalem Post*, March.

Cattell, J.M. (1917), Families of American men of science. *Scientific Monthly*, 5:368–377.

Cecil, D. (1965), *Max: a Biography*. Boston: Houghton Mifflin.

——— (1970), The strong earth of ordinary delight. *The Listener*, 84(2178):867–869.

Cicerelli, V.G. (1981), Adult relationships of sisters and brothers. In: *The Parents' Guide to Teenagers*, ed. L.H. Gross. New York: Collier, p. 23.

Cixous, H. (1972), *The Exile of James Joyce*, trans. S.A.J. Purcell. New York: David Lewis.

Coles, R. (1972), *Farewell to the South*. Boston: Little, Brown.

——— (1980), Commentary on 'Psychology and Literature.' *New Literary History*, 12:207–211.

Demarest, E.W., & Winestine, M.C. (1955), The initial phase of concomitant treatment of twins. *The Psychoanalytic Study of the Child*, 10:336–352. New York: International Universities Press.

Durrell, L. (1953), *Reflections on a Marine Venus: A Companion to the Landscape of Rhodes*. New York: Dutton, 1962.

––––––– (1961), Introduction to Georg Groddeck, *The Book of the It*. New York: Viking Press, pp. viii–ix.

Edel, L. (1957), *Literary Biography*. Garden City, N.Y.: Doubleday Anchor, 1959.

––––––– (1969), *Henry James: The Treacherous Years (1895–1901)*. New York: Avon Discus, 1978.

––––––– (1979), Revision of a chapter in the life of Henry James. *Psychohistory Review*, 8(1–2):24–25.

––––––– (1981), The nature of literary psychology. *J. Amer. Psychoanal. Assn.*, 29:447–467.

Eliot, T.S. (1958), Preface to S. Joyce, *My Brother's Keeper*. New York: Viking Press, p. ix.

Ellis, H. (1904), *A Study in Genius*, rev. ed. Boston: Houghton Mifflin, 1926.

Ellmann, R. (1958), Introduction to S. Joyce, *My Brother's Keeper*. New York: Viking Press, pp. x–xxii.

––––––– (1959), *James Joyce*. New York: Oxford University Press.

Farber, S.L. (1981), *Identical Twins Reared Apart: A Reanalysis*. New York: Basic Books.

Feaver, W. (1981), Introduction to *Masters of Caricature: From Hogarth and Gillray to Scarfe and Levine*, ed. A. Gould. New York: Knopf.

Feinstein, H.M. (1979), The use and abuse of illness in the James family circle: a view of neurasthenia. *Psychohistory Review*, 8(1–2):6–14.

Freud, S. (1905), Three Essays on the Theory of Sex. *Standard Edition*, 7:123–245. London: Hogarth Press, 1953.

––––––– (1907), Delusions and dreams in Jensen's *Gradiva*. *Standard Edition*, 9:1–95. London: Hogarth Press, 1953.

––––––– (1908), Preface to the second edition, The Interpretation of Dreams. *Standard Edition*, 4:xxvi. London: Hogarth Press, 1953.

––––––– (1930), Address delivered in the Goethe House at Frankfort. *Standard Edition*, 21:208–212. London: Hogarth Press, 1961.

Friedman, A.W. (1970), *Lawrence Durrell and the Alexandria Quartet: Art for Love's Sake*. Norman: University of Oklahoma Press.

Galton, F. (1869), *Hereditary Genius*. New York: St. Martin's Press, 1979.

Glenn, J., & Glenn, S. (1968), The psychology of twins. In: *Dynamics in Psychiatry*, ed. S.A. Karger. Athens, Greece.

Groddeck, G. (1923), *The Book of the It*. New York: Viking, 1961.

Hamilton, N. (1978), *The Brothers Mann: The Lives of Heinrich and Thomas Mann, 1871–1950 and 1875–1955*. London: Secker & Warburg; New Haven: Yale University Press, 1979.

Harris, I.D. (1964), *The Promised Seed: A Comparative Study of Eminent and Later Sons*. Glencoe, Ill.: Free Press, p. 171.

Harrison, S.I., & Harrison, R.L. (1981), Love between squabbling siblings. In: *The Parents' Guide to Teenagers*, ed. L.H. Gross. New York: Collier, pp. 29–30.

Hinchcliffe, P. (1966), Fathers and children in the novels of Evelyn Waugh. *University of Toronto Quarterly*, 35:293–310.

Huxley, J., ed. (1965), *Aldous Huxley, 1894–1963: A Memorial Volume*. London: Chatto & Windus.

James, H. (1914), Notes of a son and brother. In: *Henry James: Autobiography*, ed. F.W. Dupee. New York: Criterion Books, 1956.

Jones, H. (1933), Order of birth in relation to the development of the child. In: *Handbook of Child Psychology*, ed. C. Murchison. Worcester, Mass.: Clark University Press.

Joyce, J. (1922), *Ulysses*. New York: Random House, 1934, edition reset and corrected, 1961.

—— (1966a), *Letters of James Joyce*, Vol. II, ed. R. Ellmann. New York: Viking Press.

—— (1966b), *Letters of James Joyce*, Vol. III, ed. R. Ellmann. New York: Viking Press.

Joyce, S. (1949), Early memories of James Joyce. *The Listener*, 41:896–897.

—— (1958), *My Brother's Keeper: James Joyce's Early Years*, ed. R. Ellmann. New York: Viking Press.

—— (1971), *The Complete Dublin Diary of Stanislaus Joyce*, ed. G.H. Healey. Ithaca: Cornell University Press.

Kernberg, P.F., & Richards, A.K. (1982), Sibling: the role and the development. Unpublished paper.

Kimball, J. (1976), James Joyce and Otto Rank: the incest motif in *Ulysses*. *James Joyce Quarterly*, 13:366–382.

Kresh, P. (1979), *Isaac Bashevis Singer, the Magician of West 86th Street. A Biography*. New York: Dial Press.

Lamb, M.E., & Sutton-Smith, B., eds. (1982), *Sibling Relationships: Their Nature and Significance Across the Lifespan*. Hillsdale, N.J.: Erlbaum Associates.

Lelchuk, A. (1978), *Shrinking*. Boston: Atlantic/Little Brown.

Leverson, A. (1895), A few words with Mr Max Beerbohm. *The Sketch* (London), 8:439, January 2.

McElderry, B.R., Jr. (1972), *Max Beerbohm*. New York: Twayne.

Mack, J.E. (1980), Psychoanalysis and biography: aspects of a developing affinity. *J. Amer. Psychoanal. Assn.*, 28:543–562.

Mann, H. (1935), *Hill of Lies*. New York: Dutton,

—— (1937), *Young Henry of Navarre*. New York: Knopf, 1935.

Mann, T. (1948), *Joseph and His Brothers*. New York: Knopf.

Markus, H. (1981), Sibling personalities: the luck of the draw. *Psychology Today*, 15(6):35–37.

Milgram, J.I., & Ross, H.G. (1982), Effects of fame in adult sibling relationships. *Journal of Individual Psychology*, 38:72–79.

Nabokov, V. (1980), *Lectures on Literature*, ed. F. Bowers. New York: Harcourt Brace Jovanovich.

Nunberg, H., & Federn, E., eds. (1962, 1967, 1974, 1975), *Minutes of the Vienna Psychoanalytic Society*. Vol. 1, 1906–1908; Vol. 2, 1908–1910; Vol. 3, 1910–1911; Vol. 4, 1912–1918. New York: International Universities Press.

Ozick, C. (1982), Fistful of masterpieces. Review of *The Collected Stories of Isaac Bashevis Singer*. *New York Times Book Review*, March 21, pp. 1, 14–17.

Pearson, H. (1950), *Beerbohm Tree: His Life and Laughter*. New York: Harper & Brothers.

Phul, R.V. (1974), *Chamber Music* at the *Wake. James Joyce Quarterly,* 11:355–367.

Priestley, J.B. (1957), What was wrong with Pinfold? *New Statesman,* August 31.

Rank, O. (1912), *Das Inzest-motiv.* Vienna: Franz Deuticke, 1926.

Schechner, M. (1974), *Joyce in Nighttown: A Psychoanalytic Inquiry into 'Ulysses.'* Berkeley: University of California Press.

Shengold, L. (1971), Freud and Joseph. In: *The Unconscious Today: Essays in Honor of Max Schur,* ed. M. Kanzer. New York: International Universities Press.

Singer, I.B. (1965), Introduction to I.J. Singer, *Yoshe Kalb.* New York: Harper & Row.

———— (1966), *In My Father's Court.* New York: Farrar, Straus & Giroux.

———— (1969), *A Day of Pleasure.* New York: Farrar, Straus & Giroux.

———— (1976), *A Little Boy in Search of God.* Garden City, N.Y.: Doubleday.

———— (1978), *A Young Man in Search of Love.* Garden City, N.Y.: Doubleday.

———— (1981a), *Lost in America.* Garden City, N.Y.: Doubleday.

———— (1981b), The making of a first novel. In: *Satan in Goray.* New York: Sweetwater Editions, 1935.

Singer, I.J. (1936), *The Brothers Ashkenazi.* New York: Knopf; New York: Atheneum, 1980.

Skura, M.A. (1981), *The Literary Use of the Psychoanalytic Process.* New Haven: Yale University Press.

Strouse, J. (1980), *Alice James: A Biography.* Boston: Houghton Mifflin.

Sutton-Smith, B., & Rosenberg, B.G. (1970), *The Sibling.* New York: Holt, Rinehart & Winston.

Thomas, D.H. (1981), *The White Hotel.* New York: Viking Press.

Tindall, W.Y. (1971), *A Reader's Guide to James Joyce.* New York: Farrar, Straus & Giroux, 1951.

Unterecker, J. (1964), *Lawrence Durrell.* New York: Columbia University Press.

Waugh, A. (1967), *My Brother Evelyn and Other Portraits.* New York: Farrar, Straus & Giroux.

Waugh, E. (1977), *A Little Order: A Selection of His Journals,* ed. D. Gallagher. Boston: Little, Brown.

———— (1980), *The Letters of Evelyn Waugh,* ed. M. Amory. New York: Ticknor & Fields.

Winston, R. (1981), *Thomas Mann: The Making of an Artist, 1875–1911.* New York: Knopf.

Long Beach, N.Y.
February 4, 1983

It is surprising how little the influence of siblings is appreciated in literary history. Generally, this is because only one brother or sister becomes celebrated as an artist, the role of the artist's brothers or sisters then being considered in a subordinate context—as say in the case of van Gogh.

Where, however, two siblings become writers we are afforded a much deeper insight into their relationship and motivating interaction. Moreover, such an insight is double-sided: not only are we able to perceive intimately the conflicting emotions that propel—and repel—the two siblings as artists, but we are given, so to speak, a heightened insight into *all* sibling relationships. Thus, just as the works of Dostoevski present some of the most telling portraits and insights for psychologists, so an investigation into some of the more outstanding creative brotherhoods ought to be of value to the psychologist.

Let us consider the example of Heinrich and Thomas Mann in this light, for there can have been few cases of brothers so distinguished as writers, so close to one another throughout their long lives (the 1870s to the 1950s), or so representative of the course of their country's fateful history. This latter dimension adds a third facet to our prism: for if the life of a single great artist can be perceived as representative of his epoch or country-

1

A Case of Literary Fratricide: The Brüderzwist Between Heinrich and Thomas Mann

NIGEL HAMILTON

49

men, then the lives of two great sibling artists may provide a key to the unlocking of an even more representative historical cabinet.

The birthplace of the Mann brothers was Lübeck, a historic Hanseatic seaport on the Baltic: Heinrich was born March 27, 1871, Thomas some four years later, on June 6, 1875. Two sisters followed, and another brother, the "Benjamin" of the family, in 1890. Both sisters were eventually to commit suicide, and the third brother became a Nazi, so we should beware of forgetting these other siblings: they too have their representative part in the Mann saga, however subordinate.

The children's father was a third-generation Hanseatic merchant, a Senator of the Republic of Lübeck: a rich and important dignitary in a city steeped in history and the Protestant ethic. Their mother was by contrast South American, Catholic by upbringing, who had lived in Lübeck only a few years when, at the age of sixteen, she was picked out by Consul Mann at a ball and soon became his bride.

Consul Mann—who became a Senator of Lübeck at the age of only thirty-six—was eleven years older than his bride. The two eldest sons seem to have seen in their father the rather forbidding symbol of patrician authority and in their mother the latently wayward, youthful symbol of love.[1] Indeed, so great was the boys' antipathy to the world of their hardworking father that as children neither could recite the names of his great warehouses in the city, though the rhymes and stories their mother read to them, as well as the music she played, they soon learned by heart.

Without exaggerating the psychological impact of their parents, one may say that Heinrich and Thomas quickly began to compete for their mother's attention and love. For a year, it is claimed, they refused to speak to one another, though occupying the same room. And when they did speak, the sharp tongue of the elder often "cut me to the quick," as Thomas later revealed. "Heinrich could be so hurtful," he once told his daughter, but Heinrich, for his part, resented the "soft" life of a second-born, as becomes clear in a symbolic short story he later wrote about two brothers. The elder owns a violin; while he is at school, his younger brother unlocks his desk and plays with the instrument (which the elder has not even had time to master), breaking it in the process. No punishment is meted out; their mother merely tells the elder to swallow his anger, for whoever the rightful owner, the violin is broken.

Here indeed was the kernel of their turbulent creativity: Heinrich

---

[1] "I sat in a corner and watched my father and mother," Thomas later recalled, "as though I were choosing between them, deciding whether life would be best spent in the dreamworld of the senses or in deed and power." (Unless otherwise specified, all quotations are from Hamilton's *The Brothers Mann*.)

proud yet unable to prevent himself from looking over his shoulder at a
brother who stayed at home and monopolized the attention of their beautiful, young, musical, and passionate mother—a fact of which Thomas was
well aware. "Of the five children it was I who was closest to my mother,"
he later boasted.

Had Heinrich only looked ahead and found a modus vivendi with his
father, he might well have become the apple of his eye, the inheritor of
his hundred-year-old commercial empire. Instead he was dutifully sullen,
and his extant letters from Russia—where his father sent him at the age
of thirteen—betray an emotional dissociation from what he was supposed
to be witnessing.

The role of first-born, of heir to the Mann dynasty, was thus rejected
by Heinrich from the moment in his early teens when he became aware
of his father's expectations. Instead he applied himself passionately to the
reading of French and German literature, and somehow convinced his
reluctant father, in 1889, that further propulsion toward a career in the
merchant house of J.S. Mann & Son was fruitless: he wished to devote
himself to literature. Reluctantly the Senator accepted this dash to his
hopes, but he insisted that, if literature was to be Heinrich's career, he
should "learn the trade"—and in the innocent eyes of the Senator of
Lübeck this meant not university study, but an apprenticeship in book-
selling!

Nothing could have been more humiliating to the proud, shy young
Senator's son than to have to soil his immaculately clean fingers dusting
the shelves of a Dresden bookstore, Messrs. Zahn and Jaensch. He spent
his father's monthly allowance on "inessentials" such as the theater, magazines, and books, and drove his father to distraction in Lübeck by begging
always for more. This the Senator would gladly have paid if he had received encouraging reports from Heinrich's employers. However the opposite was the case, and as the Senator's health began to deteriorate in
the summer of 1891, he realized that his eldest son was going to end up
a failure, being devoid of any sense of financial self-discipline or realism
in terms of his apprenticeship. In October Heinrich was recalled to
Lübeck by telegram. In his memoirs (1947) Heinrich claimed that his
father understood him, indeed gave him his blessing in his literary ambition; but it is clear from Thomas Mann's recollection that his father—who
was dying of septicemia after an operation—was in the direst pain, and
even waved away the attendant priest (1931).

The Senator's last Will and Testament had decreed that his merchant
house be liquidated on his death. There was no prospect in his mind that
his wife would be able to oversee the company's fortunes until Thomas,

the second-born, came of age—nor had Thomas shown any more inclination than Heinrich to take up a commercial career. The brief hope that
the two-year-old Viktor might prove an adequate heir was never serious,
given his ill health and premonition of death. Whether the Senator really
despaired of his offspring, or whether he simply recognized that the future
of the ancient Hanseatic entrepôt was—by virtue of the Kiel Canal (built
in 1887) and the rise of Hamburg—doomed in any case, need not detain
us; the fact remains that the Senator left a sizeable fortune to his wife and
children, enabling them to remove from the stifling confines of the little
Baltic city to the healthier cultural air of Munich, and his elder sons to
pursue literary careers upon a private income.

This they proceeded to do with a mixture of relief, excitement, and fin
de siècle bravado. Heinrich may well have suffered a nervous breakdown
at this time. At any rate his mother paid for him to go to a rest home in
Switzerland, and his hypochondria[2] thereafter remained a vital force in
his artistic makeup—as it would also in Thomas's.

It is quite clear from the letters, documents, and early stories and
essays written by Heinrich Mann that, like his sister Carla, he possessed
no natural or precocious writing talent. Rather, his early work seemed
more a product of will than of natural predisposition.[3] Indeed, Heinrich's
first full-length novel was turned down by the publishers who saw it, and
was in the end printed privately in Munich at his mother's expense, a
fact which rankled Heinrich to the end of his life. His short stories fared
better, being more suited to his unhappy, caustic wit; yet even when, in
1900, he wrote his first satirical novel (translated in 1929 as *Berlin: The
Land of Cockaigne*), he was unable to think of a suitable ending, and so
offered the book without one—traveling himself to a sanatorium at Bad
Brunnthal to recuperate from his efforts. The book caused something of
a stir, but it promised more than it delivered, in its cynical, racy account
of a young man's rise to financial success in Berlin. It was a promise that
would not be fulfilled for more than a decade, as Heinrich led the unhappy, solitary life of a quasi-exile, running away from a German impe-
rialist-capitalist culture he detested, but in which he was too steeped to
find freedom. Nothing worked; his great love affair with a South American
girl (shades of his mother?) came to grief (she was a neurotic feminist),
his novels never sold more than a few thousand copies, and as he became
more and more alienated from his roots, his family, and his society, so

[2] Until the advent of World War I Heinrich spent part of every year in Riva at the clinic
of Dr. von Hartungen. He was said to be asthmatic, suffer from catarrh, and have a weak
heart, but his "illness" was never really diagnosed.

[3] "There was no inner compulsion either—only the will was there" (Letter to Karl Lemke,
January 29, 1947).

he developed an idealistic democratic and socialist stance in both his books and his journalism.

It is not difficult to understand, then, that his relationship with his younger brother Thomas became fraught with envy, love, admiration, and dependence. For Thomas's life was very different. Thomas had never borne the brunt of his father's wrath, had been shielded by Heinrich—indeed had looked up to Heinrich with awe. It was Heinrich who had dared confound their father's commercial expectations; Heinrich who declared that only literary pursuit mattered; Heinrich who traveled to Italy and brought back tales of an arcadian, Renaissance civilization. . . . In 1897 Thomas spent the whole summer with Heinrich. Heinrich suggested they write a chronicle of their family as an interesting example of Nietzsche's theory of the decline of dynasties, generation by generation, into neurasthenia. Thomas seized upon the idea, began writing to his family for details of relatives, household stories, even Lübeck recipes. Out of this he constructed—without Heinrich's help—one of the most precocious masterpieces of modern world literature: *Buddenbrooks*.

The story of the fortunes of Thomas's manuscript (rejected as overlong, reconsidered, and finally published in 1901 in two volumes in a tiny printing succeeded by larger and larger ones in subsequent years) is a lyrical story of success—a success matched too in the young novelist's private life as he met and married a princess of his dreams, the teenage daughter of a Jewish millionaire, Katja Pringsheim. And although it was to take Thomas more than two decades to produce another novel of *Buddenbrooks'* proportion and quality, he nonetheless managed to produce a series of novellas which remain probably the best loved of their genre in this century, in particular *Tonio Kröger* in 1903, and *Death in Venice* in 1913.

Sensitive, lucid, with a limpid style of narration at once deeply realistic and yet heavy with philosophical, cultural, and literary overtones, Thomas was well aware of the irony of his easy success when placed against Heinrich's struggles; indeed Thomas mirrored this relationship in his popular novel *Royal Highness*, published in 1909, in which the slower-witted younger Prince (one of whose hands is shriveled) succeeds his abdicating, proud, and distant elder brother on the throne of the little kingdom.

Privately, however, Thomas often experienced profound torment over Heinrich. Though he might depict him as a noble, ascetic Prince, too pure to cope with the practical duties of everyday power and representative rule, Thomas in fact was often incensed by Heinrich's haughtiness, his caustic judgments of people (particularly their bourgeois sister Lulu), and his utter disregard for the most basic rules of art. Far from being too pure, Heinrich was to Thomas painfully imperfect, both in his writing and in his life. His pathetic, lingering affair with Ines Schmied created family quarrel after quarrel, and it was not surprising when, in the aftermath of the outbreak of World War I, the two brothers began a personal feud whose symbolic significance was not lost on Thomas. The latter was to spend almost two years laboring on a 650-page self-justification, *Betrachtungen eines Unpolitischen (Reflections of a Non-Political Man)* (1918), considered so chauvinistically German and so embarrassingly venomous toward the image of Heinrich that it has only recently been translated into English.

Thomas had greeted the war in August 1914 as a welcome relief. It is in this sense that the prewar story of Gustav von Aschenbach in *Death in Venice* is a work of autobiographical projection. The mood of Europe hung heavy on a spirit as sensitive and refined as Thomas's. Katja Mann's autobiography (1975) makes quite clear that the homosexual theme reflected latent homoerotic yearnings in its author—"my sexual inversion" as he later called it (Winston, 1981). He was thirty-six, well-married, with four children, was building a stately new home in Munich, and owned a large summer residence in the Bavarian hills. Already acknowledged a master of modern fictional narrative, he nonetheless found it increasingly difficult to write the great novels which the example of *Buddenbrooks* seemed to portend. He envied Heinrich's growing political leanings; he himself felt nothing but foreboding at the rise of socialism in Germany and in Europe, threatening both German bourgeois culture and its comfortable young bourgeois doyen: himself. He suffered not so much writer's cramp as genuine intestinal pains that made him at times suicidal. Heinrich's torrential output of bad books, which deservedly sold poorly, as well as his ridiculously naive and idealistic political posturing—he had never gone without a starched collar or a three-course lunch in his life—only irked Thomas the more.

The war put an end to all this. "Shouldn't one be thankful for such a completely unexpected opportunity to witness such great things?" Thomas wrote in excitement to Heinrich as the curtain went up. It was indeed a drama for him, protected by a corrupt doctor's signature from call-up,[4] avid for distraction and other people's destruction. Flushed with enthusiasm, he saw it as his writer's task to give moral support to the brave

---

[4] Thomas Mann reported for voluntary military service on October 1, 1899 in Munich. Although pronounced fit by the army doctors, he appealed to his mother's own doctor, Hofrat May, who by negotiation with the chief medical officer of the regiment obtained his discharge before Christmas that year.

German troops fighting in the innocent countries they had occupied. He not only wrote newspaper articles, jingoistic essays, and even a book about Frederick the Great, but he accepted invitations to visit German army staff officers in occupied Belgium.

To Heinrich the war, from the very beginning, was anathema. His political concern with democracy in Germany went far deeper than Thomas gave him credit for, and it is in this light that Heinrich's contribution to German letters may be judged as transcending the flaws of any of his individual works. To his brother Thomas, Heinrich's posturings seemed irritatingly high-minded, a Francophile myth, but to the impartial chronicler there is indeed something noble in the openly pacifist stance Heinrich took, his refusal to indulge himself in late romantic or self-deceptive patriotism. Small wonder then that the quarrel which broke out between the brothers in 1915 became a cause célèbre in Germany. Never in literature had two such distinguished writers collided with such bitterness and ill feeling in the midst of a national war. Was the quarrel simply exacerbated by brotherly envy, or did the fact of their brotherhood lend a deeper, symbolic note to a rift that divided one German, one European from another?

The feud began with an essay by Heinrich (1915) in a literary magazine, depicting the stand of Emile Zola in the Dreyfus case: Heinrich had already published in serial form part of a satirical novel on the life of a typically chauvinistic Wilhelmine bourgeois, *The Man of Straw*. Serialization and publication in book format had been halted by the outbreak of war in August 1914, and Heinrich's indirect *J'accuse* against German hostilities in November 1915 came like the considered blow of an executioner's ax. Word soon spread. Thomas in fact heard of it through his brother's solicitor. Obtaining a copy of the offending article, he immediately identified himself with the establishment figures who had eschewed all moral principles in order to join the popular cry of death to the traitor Dreyfus; every line, every adjective used by Heinrich in the Zola essay seemed to Thomas a thinly veiled attack upon himself. There later followed an amazing correspondence between the brothers (Wysling, 1968) in which they tormented each other's conscience as only brothers can. Lifelong feelings of repressed envy and even hate poured out, fashioned in the distinctive prose styles they had made their own: Heinrich's now increasingly simple and direct, using short, sharp sentences pivoting on forceful verbs, in contrast to Thomas's mastery of nuance and innuendo, his love of psychological penetration and caricature—now focused on the image of his elder brother.

Like boxers who withdraw to their corners after an opening round,

Heinrich and Thomas withdrew to their desks in Munich, the one in the Leopoldstrasse, the other in the Poschingerstrasse, a scant mile apart. Thomas severed all personal contact with Heinrich; henceforth they would not speak to each other for seven years—until, in fact, Heinrich lay in a hospital with peritonitis, near death.

Severance of verbal communication, however, did not restore peace of mind to either brother. Thomas's riposte to Heinrich's Zola article began as an essay, but soon turned into a gigantic tract, a self-apologia and an assault upon all the ideas and postures he identified with Heinrich. Rarely can an artist—and Thomas Mann was nothing if not that—have labored so intently to produce such a vitriolic and mean denunciation of his own brother. *Reflections of a Non-Political Man* was monstrously ignoble and must cause us to question the balance of Thomas's mind at this point in his life. His son Klaus later recalled (1942) that this wartime father, who even stopped shaving for a while and grew a "prickly" beard, was nothing like the father he otherwise knew; locked in his study day after day, month after month, year after year, he worked out his spleen against Heinrich, an exercise in invective with no parallel in European literature. Even Thomas himself likened his three-year stint to slave labor in a medieval galley.

Here surely is the critical moment in the respective careers of Heinrich and Thomas Mann, as well as the psychological catharsis. In a sense one may justifiably consider the two essays, *Zola* by Heinrich and *Reflections of a Non-Political Man* by Thomas, an act of mutual literary fratricide—a fact not lost on the hypersensitive Thomas, who, in response to the request for an article on "World Peace" at the end of 1917, accused Heinrich of spouting love of God while hating his own brother.

Such a consideration leads us to ask how, in fact, two siblings can reasonably be expected to assert their individual identities through their work and yet not harbor jealousies or feelings of competitiveness toward one another. Thomas, certainly, kept using the word *doomed*, and even Heinrich traced back his brother's hostility to a declaration of incompatibility made by Thomas when they lived together in Rome as far back as 1897. The two essays thus became final gestures, gauntlets flung down by two brothers who for too long had attempted to repress natural feelings of rivalry and who now wished to go their own way, regardless of one another.

If Thomas's crisis was deeper and more excruciating than Heinrich's, this was perhaps to be expected in a younger brother who had for so many years been accustomed to his brother shielding him and standing up for him. "It is like old times: someone attacks me, and my elder brother comes and avenges me," he wrote when Heinrich defended him against a silly but venomous critic in 1906. The feud between Heinrich and Thomas was therefore much more than an expression at last of hitherto latent rivalry and hostility: it was a belated realization by Thomas that he could no longer take shelter behind the armor of Heinrich as elder brother. There can be little doubt that, since the death of Senator Mann in 1891, Thomas had looked upon Heinrich as a substitute father; indeed, given the Senator's preoccupation with his merchant house, as well as the affairs of state of the little Republic of Lübeck (of whose finances and taxes he was for many years the chief arbiter, as Committee Chairman), it is more than likely that Thomas's admiration for his elder brother went back even further into their childhood.

Reflections of a Non-Political Man was not then simply the literary murder of a hitherto esteemed father-figure; it was as well an important step in a psychological adjustment to adult life for Thomas. The longing for death which had been such an integral theme of *Buddenbrooks, Tonio Kröger*, and *Death in Venice* was, as Heinrich sagely observed in his vain attempts at a reconciliation at the end of 1917, a fear of life, an unwillingness to grow up. Heinrich refused to read the *Reflections* when they were published at the end of 1918, nor (if he is to be believed) did he read them later.

His own test had come when the Senator died and he suffered his own form of breakdown. It had come also in the early years of the new century, as he recognized the central importance of the writer in a corrupt, imperialistic society heading inexorably for war. His fatherly concern for the future fortunes of his country is attested in his copious writings before World War I. Even the style of his handwriting changed as he switched to an almost childlike orthographic simplicity. Moreover, opposition to the trends of his own nation sharpened his perception and gave a new maturity to his judgments. His "hymn of democracy," *Die Kleine Stadt*, was an artistic and commercial failure,[5] but his Wilhemine satire, *The Man of Straw*, remains a masterpiece of its kind. The very fact that Heinrich had been rejected by his country—in the sense that his novels didn't sell—as well as by his lover, Ines Schmied, served to give greater depth to his work and to his vision of the writer's role in society—a vision which seemed, however, to exclude his brother Thomas.

It was not that Heinrich deliberately denied Thomas a place on his idealistic, democratic galleon; indeed, to the very eve of war Heinrich still vacationed regularly with his brother. They journeyed together to

[5] The word *democracy* was not permitted by the publisher in any advertisement or announcement of publication.

Italy and Venice on the fateful spring holiday that inspired *Death in Venice*; and when it was published Heinrich was the first to write an enthusiastic review. Rather, the problem was in according a place to a younger brother who, living on fat advances from an admiring publisher and married to the daughter of a millionaire, seemed not only unwilling to help counter the ominous imperialistic tide sweeping Germany toward war, but was intent on driving his late-romantic pessimistic and narcissistic self over the precipice. Heinrich genuinely admired his brother's gifts of narrative skill and symbolic imagery; but even in his enthusiastic review of *Death in Venice* Heinrich chose to ignore the homoerotic theme of the story and depicted instead an aging man's seduction not by the image of a beautiful Polish boy, but by the corrupt and glorious concubine, Venice.

This heterosexualization of a homosexual story reveals a vital distinction between the brothers Mann at this period of their lives, before the Great War. Many psychiatrists consider homosexuality a form of arrested ego development, reflecting a preoedipal level of gratification needs vis-à-vis the mother. This being so, we may perhaps see in Thomas Mann's homoerotic obsession (it must be remembered that *Death in Venice* was founded on the true story of the author's homoerotic infatuation) the very stunted emotional growth that precluded him from joining Heinrich's ship. His life and art were locked on a different course, one which, as in its homosexual dimension, led to a dead end.

Homosexuality or at least homoerotism had characterized almost every story Thomas Mann had written since the final tale of Hanno Buddenbrook in his first novel. Tonio Kröger's infatuation with Hans Hansen, the incestuous pairing of the twins in *The Blood of the Walsungs*, and the fatal yearnings of Gustav von Aschenbach for Tadzio all point to a repression of homosexual feelings, and one is entitled to ask whether, if Heinrich played the role of substitute father to Thomas, Thomas entertained oedipal guilt feelings of some kind toward Heinrich. Both men adored their mother, and it is not altogether fanciful to suppose that unconsciously both were rivals for her love. The reader may object that psychological speculation of this sort is highly dangerous and that if pursued would lead toward a sanatorium rather than fratricidal war. This, however, is a significant point, since Thomas Mann was increasingly attacked by psychosomatic illnesses—chiefly intestinal—and was frequently incarcerated in a sanatorium or health spa during this prewar period. Indeed one cannot but come to the conclusion that here was a great artist at war with himself. Even when actual war was declared, he chose a homosexual king to extol—Frederick the Great, who as soon as he became king banished his wife and all women from the palace of Sans Souci.

The crisis induced by Heinrich's fratricidal gauntlet—the story of the deeply heterosexual Zola—may justly be seen, then, as the turning point of Thomas Mann's life. Like a tobacco addict who is told to give up the fatal habit, he withdrew into his study to smoke himself sick in defiance. Borrowing books from friends and libraries, he clothed his invective against Heinrich in an immense and culturally sophisticated smoke screen, one so elaborate and weblike in its construction that he was actually awarded an honorary doctorate upon the strength of it in 1919! Germany, he claimed, had the right to go her own way, following her own historic path, obeying her own gods and an instinct deeper than any constructed by the apostles of French or European "civilization." Germany, for good or ill, would do as she was historically destined to do, regardless of "Boulevard moralists," "oaf-psychologists," "political New-wavers," and "civilization-littérateurs" like Heinrich.

Congratulations poured in from Thomas's more chauvinistic—and homosexual—friends when the book was published. Curiously, Thomas himself virtually washed his hands of it, even though he rejected Heinrich's peace offering. "As soon as our thoughts have found their way into words, they are no longer heart-felt. . . . The essayistic expression of my thoughts is much more the only safe way of getting rid of them, of getting beyond them to other, new, better and where possible completely oppositional ones—sans remords!" he warned one overenthusiastic correspondent. Heinrich, his substitute father, had after almost two decades of adult life chided him, and Thomas had reacted with all the scorn, all the talent for self-justification he could as a great writer muster. But having grappled with his brother; having not only defended himself but swiped and lunged; having cut his elder brother's body into a thousand pieces; having mutilated his corpse in every conceivable way, desecrating their relationship and insisting on his right to a romantic, even homosexual self . . . he realized he had changed.

This transformation from infantile self-preoccupation toward adult self-recognition and self-acceptance is all the more interesting in that it was not mirrored—yet—in the course of German history. It led in fact to furious condemnation by those who identified Thomas with his old persona, and who thenceforth accused him of being a turncoat. But to Thomas's eternal credit, he never looked back or regretted his conversion, though it would in time lead him into exile and vilification. Not one story, novella, or full-scale novel of his ever again exalted the homosexual, death-desiring cultural narcissist.[6] Instead, the struggle between morality and

[6] He still "fell for" handsome, lithe young men, as his diaries record, just as he would walk out of oppressively female company—but such experiences merely amused him (see T. Mann, 1979).

instinct became the mainspring of his creative output, winning him the
Nobel Prize as well as recognition, in his own lifetime, as one of the
greatest novelists of this century.

Was there any particular experience or causal trigger for this conversion? None is known, but in 1979 Thomas Mann's diaries from the years
1918 to 1921 were published in Germany, and they provide a new insight
into what may have happened. First, it would appear that the birth of his
fifth child, Elisabeth, in April 1918 came as something of a shock to him.
His next youngest had been born eight years previous, and in his diary
entry of January 20, 1918 Thomas confessed that "someone like me 'ought'
never to bring children into the world"; nevertheless he found himself
carrying the new baby when it cried and experiencing a strange sense of
rebirth. On September 14, 1918—only weeks before the Armistice—he
noted:

> . . . survey of my own life. Death—melancholy. During my midday
> walk I thought again how appropriate it would be if I were to die
> now. Then a feeling of love for the baby and turning over the
> hexameter-poem in my mind. Also had an insight into the thematic
> connections between the works I'm planning with the current at-
> mosphere surrounding me as I read [about Nietzsche]: the death-
> romanticism and yes-to-life in the *Magic Mountain*, the Protes-
> tantism [Felix Krull] of the Confidence Man. Self-confidence.

He had already begun, upon ending the *Reflections of a Non-Political
Man*, a new novella and a new poem in hexameters—both loving idylls:
the first the story of a master and his dog, the second a celebration of the
birth of the new baby. He planned also to start work again on the two
novels he had put aside in order to write his massive self-justification:
the *Magic Mountain* and *Felix Krull*. His three years of slave labor on
the *Reflections* had in fact brought him to the very opposite of the patriotic
romantic fatalism with which he had begun the work. Though it brought
him first to the verge of suicide, certainly of serious death-wishes, he
stepped back from the brink of self-immolation, from flailing vindictively
at Heinrich and those who "knew better," and miraculously found himself
suffused with love for the new baby, with the notion of life as an open
door beckoning toward adventure. Looking at his four older children, he
saw four lives not created because he wanted them, but living inde-
pendently of him: "Was lebt . . . hat auch sich selbst gewollt, denn es
lebt." With baby Lisa it was different, he confirmed in his diary: a difference he was forced to articulate since his wife Katja was now convinced
she was again pregnant, expecting what would be their sixth child:

A sixth child? There is no great difference between five and six, and after the war there'll be no question of whether we can support so many. The laws of inheritance will be abolished completely, so the very idea of wealth is illusory. Education is a matter of home-surroundings, nothing more. Apart from Katja's health the only thing I have against a sixth child is that the experience of "Lisa" (she is, in a sense, my *first* child) will thereby be diminished.

It seems quite clear, then, that the transformation which Thomas Mann underwent in 1918 had, at its heart, the overthrow of his narcissistic homosexual individualism in favor of a new, loving self: a self that made love to Katja not simply out of duty but as a celebration of their mature man-woman relationship and in a newly found pride and wonder at parenthood. In the case of a writer so talented and many-faceted, it would be a mistake to speculate too simplistically about Thomas Mann's homo-sexual-heterosexual conversion. Heterosexuality certainly does not guarantee greater writing, as will be seen in the case of Heinrich; moreover, homosexuality certainly does not automatically entail lesser creativity. What one can now say is that a great, precociously gifted novelist who had reached a sort of dead end in his life, who had turned more and more inward, even to the point of intestinal cramps and other physical pains, began suddenly to see a resolution. In this deeply personal resolution, the idea of heterosexual love, of children conceived and brought up in love, formed the foundation stone of an open, adventurous life—a life which in his case was to be more full of adventure, fame, humiliation, travel, challenge, tragedy, and stature than he could ever have imagined in 1918, in even his wildest dreams.

That Thomas recognized such a momentous transformation is now evidenced by his diaries; yet the recognition was not such as would enable him to accept a reconciliation with the brother he had spent three laborious years murdering. In a remarkable dream at the end of September he had projected a moment when they would have made up their quarrel:

> I dreamed I was the best of friends with Heinrich and out of sheer goodwill allowed him to consume a whole pile of cakes, little cream ones as well as two pastry gateaux, on his own, while declining my rightful share. Feeling of helplessness as to how this amity will be affected by the publication of the *Reflections*. It won't work, will put us in an impossible position. Relief when I wake up and find it was all a dream.

The dream conveys Thomas's nagging unconscious and his shame at the imminent fratricide, made worse because the collapse of the German armies in the West, and the likelihood of German defeat and the Kaiser's downfall, made his bilious condemnation of Heinrich's Francophile republican-democratic and socialistic ideal less and less sensible. Katja had always thought the book a mistake; they now discussed it and decided that on balance it would be better to suspend publication and allow it to be issued only posthumously, as a footnote for literary historians. A telegram was sent to Fischer in Berlin, asking him to consider this. But Fischer felt quite rightly that it was too late to mess about; he had some three thousand orders from bookshops, was about to send out copies from his warehouse, and recognized instinctively that, at a time of great national debate over peace proposals, the possible abdication of the Kaiser, and the future political landscape of Germany, Thomas Mann's *Reflections* was as topical as could be. He cabled back that the book had already gone out to the bookshops. Reconciliation, even by the selfless abjuration of rightful cream cakes, became an impossibility.

I must confess that when I wrote my full-length biography of the Mann brothers almost ten years ago, I assumed that Thomas, having vented his fratricidal spleen by publishing the *Reflections*, was emotionally and spiritually ready for the reunion with Heinrich that would occur four years later, in 1922.

I was wrong. It is quite clear from Thomas's diary that the figure of Heinrich as Francophile prophet of German republicanism, socialism, and democracy continued to haunt Thomas to the point of causing psychosomatic illness. He was furious to learn that Heinrich had no intention of reading the *Reflections*; and when Kurt Wolff, the publisher, issued an edition of no fewer than one hundred thousand copies of *The Man of Straw*, Heinrich's Wilhemine satire, Thomas experienced feelings of profound fraternal hate and envy—as bad or worse than any he had felt when writing the *Reflections*.

It was obvious to Thomas that, far from expiring from the many wounds inflicted in the *Reflections*, Heinrich was uncomfortably alive and well—and being feted by republicans and activists everywhere in Germany, a situation that reduced Thomas at times to apoplexy. "Unleidlich"—unbearable—was Thomas's response in the privacy of his diary. "I realized suddenly what a solitary, insulated, brooding, strange and sorry existence I lead. Heinrich's life by contrast is blooming now," he noted four days after Christmas 1918. Indeed the renewed envy, stimulated by Heinrich's apparent victory in their feud, gave a sharper edge to the novel which Thomas had resumed—*The Magic Mountain*. The celebrated Settembrini-Naphta struggle for Hans Castorp's innocent soul was without doubt Thomas's own version of his quarrel with Heinrich. "Work is the best answer," Thomas recorded in his diary, after noting the way in which mere mention of a lecture given by Heinrich "pains me each time to a hypochondriacal degree."

At a conscious level, Thomas's violent hatred for Heinrich (which even went as far as wishing Heinrich's wife[7] dead when she was reported ill in Prague) was directed against Heinrich's "stupid" rhetoric on behalf of republicanism in postwar Germany. Knowing Heinrich as deeply as he did, Thomas was able to penetrate his brother's lofty idealism, and to point out the contradiction between it and political reality in the chaos of the early years of the Weimar Republic. Yet at a more profound, unconscious level, Thomas was still determined to succeed in his fratricidal attempt on Heinrich's life; feelings of recurrent "hate" warred with tenderer, more magnanimous feelings of love.

This war, waged in his own heart, went on far longer than I, innocent biographer in my twenties, ever realized. Only the recent publication of Thomas's 1918–1921 diaries (1979) made clear its true extent. Heinrich, in an unsent letter of reconciliation early in 1918, had written of Thomas's "furious passion for your own 'I' . . . your inability ever to grasp the real seriousness of anyone's life but your own," and had prophesied that "if God wills, you will have another 40 years to prove yourself, if not to 'assert' yourself."

Did Thomas ever really "see" his brother? Innocently I assumed that with their reconciliation in 1922 he did. Now I wonder, for it seems clear that Thomas's rivalry with Heinrich, his fratricidal feelings, were psychologically the heaviest cross of his life, as well as a vital creative mainspring. To put it another way, Thomas's ambition was to triumph over Heinrich: to kill his brother/father. If anyone else declared victory—as some writers did after publication of the *Reflections*—Thomas was quick to deny it, and to picture himself and his brother as equals. This he took as far as the refusal of a place on the Berlin Academy of Arts Literary Section unless Heinrich were also elected; he even toyed with the idea of refusing the Nobel Prize if it were offered, unless he could share it with Heinrich. These were noble thoughts, but a close reading of the diaries makes it evident that such sentiments were but the reverse side of an ambition that dominated his life at this time. *The Magic Mountain* (which indeed won him the Nobel Prize) was, unlike the idylls *A Man and His Dog* or *Gesang vom Kindchen*, a direct literary challenge to Heinrich, using all the literary, psychological, philosophical, and artistic skill Thomas could command. When he heard through friends that Hein-

---

[7] In 1914 Heinrich had married his Czech mistress, Maria Kanova, an actress.

rich was writing his own large-scale novel of the period and might publish before him, his anxiety quickened: "It's clear that Heinrich is preparing a terrific broadside with his contemporary novel," he recorded on September 18, 1921, and returned with renewed frenzy to *The Magic Mountain*.

Thomas need not have worried. Since the spring of 1919 he had in fact perceived the gaps in Heinrich's shining and triumphant armor. Encouraged by vanity, his silly wife, and his aging dream of an honorable, republican Germany, Heinrich had allowed himself to become the symbolic head of republican, socialist intellectuals in Munich and beyond. This was fatal for, as Thomas wisely perceived, Germany after the Kaiser's empire was unlikely to oblige. The Soviet Republic in Munich was a short-lived fiasco, and the Weimar Republic the artificial creation of the Allies, not the end-result of an historical development within Germany. Thomas mocked Heinrich's fine oratory at the graveside of the murdered Bavarian Prime Minister, Kurt Eisner, for the Weimar Republic would never fulfill Heinrich's vague, impossibly Francophilic vision. He laughed at the story of Heinrich's cowardly "escape" from Munich during its brief communist rule, and felt contempt for his brother's 1917 novel *Die Armen* (*The Poor*); for to Thomas it was quite obvious that Heinrich was terrified of anyone who didn't wash.

However inspired by jealousy it might have been, Thomas's diagnosis of his brother's political idealism ("Of course he disapproves of Bolshevism, not only as political means to an end, but as an idea, because in fact he is nothing other than an old-style democrat of the Celtic–Romantic–Woodrow Wilson kind and simply sees the bourgeois parliamentarian Republic at heart as the framework within which mankind can continue to advance") was very close to the mark. The seeds of Heinrich's downfall were in fact sown in the very moment Wolff issued his vast popular edition of Heinrich's *Man of Straw*—the precise time of his triumph. In July 1919 Thomas remarked how strange was the case of his brother: "His hour is already over, despite his Odeon-speech to the memory of Eisner"; and by the spring of 1920 he actually felt a mixture of contempt and pity for Heinrich's pathetic Western orientation, his Francophilia, his Wilsonism, which he thought antiquated and flabby. "In truth," Thomas added with a sneer, "it is simply not worth upsetting one's digestion out of jealousy." The inference, then, was that Thomas no longer *needed* to feel jealous (though feelings of "disgust," "depression," and "hate" still punctuated his diaries on occasion, at the thought or mention of Heinrich and his latest reported political utterances.

Thomas had in reality won, and in the very moment when, it seemed,

Heinrich could not lose. While the Germany which Thomas had extolled in his *Reflections* had collapsed, the republican ideal so long espoused by Heinrich was being enacted. Yet Heinrich was creatively silenced, reduced to a sort of sham political patronage, while Thomas produced masterpiece after masterpiece (*A Man and His Dog, Gesang vom Kindchen, The Magic Mountain, Early Sorrow*)—masterpieces which enabled him to squint first contemptuously at Heinrich, then with pity. In the strangest possible manner his fratricide had succeeded: that is to say, Heinrich had not been killed by Thomas's weapon (the *Reflections*), but had, as it were, fallen upon his own sword.

It was this "death" of Heinrich which at last, in 1922, enabled Thomas to entertain the possibility of reconciliation. And when Heinrich fell ill, mortally it seemed, with peritonitis, Thomas was forced to move. For if Heinrich died, Thomas knew well enough his conscience would not be clean. He rushed flowers to the hospital together with a message of love and concern, and as soon as the doctor permitted, went to see Heinrich.

Poor Heinrich. It is impossible not to sympathize with him, dogged by a younger brother who stole his mother's love when they were children, and then his honors and prizes in later life. Heinrich had, as a stylist, introduced wholly new literary techniques to German writing—a new vibrance, a new pace, a veritable fireworks display of modern linguistic command. He was in fact a poet in novelist's clothing, and may justly be said to be the father of contemporary German prose, so much closer to its French and English counterparts than was German prose of the nineteenth century. And yet his novels had always suffered from their experimental structure; the unfinished first satirical novel was somehow symptomatic of his artistic failure. In his writing as in his life Heinrich was an alien, unable to settle with the traditional or the accepted, and doomed to unhappiness.

The wisest course Heinrich could have adopted at the end of the Kaiser's war would have been to go abroad and let the destiny of republican Germany take its course, as he had in his gypsy life abroad during the Wilhemine period. Instead he permitted himself to be caught up in the tragedy of Weimar, acting a role which Thomas correctly perceived to be ridiculous. The German people, Thomas had noted, were not fitted for political democracy; moreover, Heinrich was too alienated from the mainstream of German literature and too impractical as a personality to fit the cap of republican greatness as a writer now. The qualities Heinrich admired—concepts of honesty, nobility, humanity, justice—were qualities paradoxically more present in Wilhemine society than in the crazy attempt at social democracy after the Armistice. Catastrophic inflation, repeated putsches, the communist fiasco in Munich, the constant danger of assassination, these were hardly the virtues of republican democracy as Heinrich had envisaged them in his famous condemnation of Wilhemine Germany.

Thus Heinrich found himself locked in a charade, a general called out of retirement to fight with weapons and tactics that were quite beyond him. To his French friend Felix Bertraux he lamented: "How much happier I would be to be sitting at my novel now rather than continually interrupting it with articles, but if people like me do not do their duty, who will be left?"

Heinrich thus sustained a double defeat: he was forced to watch while his naive vision of a humanitarian social democracy in Germany failed to mature, and while his younger brother, once so determinedly steering his course toward late-Romantic self-pity and national chauvinism, now changed course with unbelievable ease and sailed toward literary, financial, and popular success. For not only did Heinrich's "contemporary novel" turn out a hopeless flop; in addition, his marriage began to founder. He separated from his wife and moved to Berlin, leaving the field of battle in Munich to his brother.

Thomas, to his credit, did not abuse this victory or betray the psychological freedom gained by his fratricide. He became a convinced social democrat, a stalwart champion of Weimar, an opponent of fascism, and in most respects a loyal brother to Heinrich.[8] His important essay *Goethe and Tolstoy* is a twentieth-century update of Schiller's *On Naive and Sentimental Poetry* in which he contrasts his own approach to creativity with that of Heinrich—the natural and the moral, respectively. In 1925 he wrote in the American literary magazine *Dial*, apropos Heinrich: "It was he who, while we still lived in splendour, suffered most deeply from the basic stagnation of our political life; and, in literary manifestoes the fulminant injustice of which sprang from a higher justice, he dragged our leaders into the forum of the intellect."

The irony was that Heinrich's real influence had been felt in the years of prewar Germany; now he had none. There is thus some ironic logic in the fact that Heinrich's greatest postwar success was the filming, in 1929, of his 1905 novel *Professor Unrat*. The novel—remarkable even today for its virtuoso modern style and breathtaking narration—had proved a commercial failure in 1905; but in the context of anarchical Weimar, at a moment when the German film industry was about to launch

---

[8] Thomas acted as personal guarantor when Heinrich formally applied for permission to live in the United States in March 1941, and thereafter had to support his elder brother financially to the end of his life.

its first talking films, the story of a tyrannical North German school teacher's infatuation with a nightclub singer had great appeal. Symbolically the *Blue Angel* was a mirror of the Weimar Republic's decline: the image of an educated, disciplined, old-fashioned Teutonic German falling madly in love with a talented tart, and abasing himself utterly to live with her. Originally conceived to represent the dirt lurking beneath Prussian standards of uprightness, the story now became the classic portrayal of Weimar shamelessness—reputedly Goebbels's favorite film—starring Emil Jannings and Marlene Dietrich. "My head—and Marlene Dietrich's legs," Heinrich remarked after the film had become a worldwide box-office success. The remark concealed a cynical truth, for Heinrich was living with a beautiful actress in Berlin when the project was first mooted, and had given his permission for filming the novel on condition that his mistress (Trude Hesterberg) be given the role of Lola-Lola.

The collapse of Heinrich's marriage, the failure of his postwar writings, and his moral dissoluteness in Berlin (Trude Hesterberg soon dropped him, and he took up with a bar-girl from the Kurfürstendamm) would paradoxically have relegated him to a very minor role in German literature after World War I had it not been for the rise of Nazism, a development which now gave the dissolute "schoolmaster" a role which surpassed even that of his anti-Wilhemine stance before World War I. It is no exaggeration to say that, between 1933 and 1939, Heinrich became the undisputed literary leader of the antifascist movement, the first German to be deprived of his citizenship in exile by Hitler, and the most admired writer among those forced to leave Germany in the years leading up to "Hitler's war." The record of his stand against Nazism, from the late 1920s, is a noble one. It may truthfully be said that in this respect he set an example for Thomas, who, though no less an opponent of Nazism, was more concerned to continue the greatest undertaking of his life, the unsurpassed tetralogy of novels depicting the life of the biblical Joseph: *Joseph and His Brothers*.

Thus, although Thomas was similarly forced into exile in the spring of 1933, before Hitler even took total power, he continued to allow his books to be published in Germany, and maintained a forced silence on political matters for some three years in order that his publisher, Fischer, could avoid running afoul of Rosenberg's Reich Office for the Furtherance of German Writing. Other emigré writers felt that this was a betrayal of the antifascist cause, but Heinrich reassured his brother repeatedly, urging him to see that continued sale of his humanistic work in Nazi Germany was more valuable than noble but vain politicking abroad.

This time, Thomas made no jealous dissections of his brother Heinrich's anti-German attitudes and sentiments. Both had seen, from the very beginning, that the rise of German fascism could only end in one thing: war. In fact Thomas had sensed this inevitability already in the chaotic days following the Armistice in 1918: "Pacifism! League of Nations!" he spat in his diary on January 8, 1919. "The next war is already at the door, one can feel it, even without knowing who is going to wage it." Moreover, Thomas had also regretted, in his diary entry for November 19, 1918, his erstwhile "wishes regarding German hegemony": "This people," he confessed, "has shown itself quite unsuited to power. I would be quite happy to see the German Empire being broken up, with possibly a collection of unpolitical, powerless republics, with Bavaria plus German Austria, being formed."

Such prophetic feelings did not, however, lessen Thomas's sense of betrayal when, after giving a sardonic lecture on Richard Wagner (1933), he was hounded out of his homeland, with even his friends—the composers Hans Pfitzner and Richard Strauss among them—signing an official, Nazi-inspired protest against him. The story of Joseph's strange exile in Egypt was already far advanced, but the extraordinary parallel in Thomas's own life gave to his burgeoning novel an uncanny veracity. Undoubtedly, too, the experience of his great quarrel with Heinrich during the First World War had helped Thomas to view their quarrel with Nazi Germany in the epic light of a brotherly quarrel—a quarrel that would one day bring reconciliation, once the forces of nationalist self-assertion had been played out. Thomas even went so far, in 1939, as to write an essay entitled "Hitler—My Brother," in which he identified the quasi-artistic concern of Hitler to "compensate" for feelings of inferiority. (Heinrich was embarrassed by the essay and advised Thomas not to publish it.)

What is certain is that Thomas Mann, so sensitive to the currents of his culture, could never have faced the extraordinary exile and vilification with which he was confronted in the 1930s and '40s unless he had already undergone an even more profound catharsis with Heinrich. Thus both writers went on writing irrespective of exile and deprivation of German citizenship—Heinrich completing his great historical novel of the life of Henri IV of France, Thomas his Joseph tetralogy (interrupted only for a brief tour de force in 1939, when he reconstructed a period of his beloved Goethe's life: Lotte in Weimar).

The advent of World War II, however, was effectively to extinguish Heinrich's light. Despite Thomas's accusations of Woodrow Wilsonism, Heinrich had never made any attempt to get to know the Anglo-Saxon world, either Britain or America. He stayed on in Vichy France long after the defeat of the Anglo-French armies at Dunkirk, and succeeded in avoiding arrest only by crossing the Pyrenees. From Portugal he managed to get the last Greek boat to New York before the Germans conquered Greece, but in New York he found himself an unknown emigré. A year's generous employment by MGM in Hollywood was the first and last American acknowledgment of his significance as a writer; thenceforth he lived on the earnings of his bar-girl second wife (who committed suicide in 1944) and monthly payments made by Thomas. He died in utter obscurity in Santa Monica in 1950, possibly the most influential but flawed German novelist of the century, a strange mixture of high German culture and profane fascination, a political and literary rebel, a shy, reserved man with few intimate friends, who never found the love or ideal society he sought.

Thomas Mann, by contrast, seemed as blessed as Joseph. Although he chose to live in Switzerland after being hounded out of Germany in 1933, and took long summer holidays in the south of France, he did not neglect the Anglo-Saxon world he had once castigated. On his fourth visit to the U.S.A. in 1937, Thomas decided to settle there, and accepted a lectureship at Princeton University for 1939–40. When war broke out in September 1939 he made straight home for the New World. There, feted as a Nobel Prizewinner (awarded in 1929), and with his books achieving considerable fame in English translation, he quickly attained the position which Heinrich had held in France in the 1930s: unofficial leader of the German antifascist emigré movement. The success of his books in America enabled him to build a villa in California, near Los Angeles, where in 1946 he finished work on his own *Man of Straw*—the biography of a fictional German composer of the twentieth century whose contract with the devil ends in the ruins of Nazi Germany: *Doctor Faustus*.

Nor was this all. While Heinrich died in penury and obscurity, Thomas enjoyed a position in the democratic postwar world that was quite unique. Without becoming a communist fellow traveler, without being a Jew, he had opposed the Nazi movement and borne, on unlikely shoulders, the greatness and tragedy of German culture into exile. To have undertaken such masterly works, to have been a beacon for German refugees in America, to have consistently broadcast, written, and lectured against the infamy of Hitler's Reich, and to have had the courage, after the war, to take a gospel of reconciliation and humanitarian hope back to Germany—East as well as West—gave him, undoubtedly, an historical stature second to none. "Il a préservé l'honneur de l'Allemagne," wrote François Mauriac as part of a tribute paid by two hundred French writers, artists, and other dignitaries on his eightieth birthday.

Thomas was by then the "grand old man" of European, of world letters, and yet his final novel, the completion of his *Confessions of Felix Krull*, demonstrated how young and humorous his approach had remained. Stung by the excesses of McCarthyism toward some of his closest emigré colleagues, he had left America and settled once again in Switzerland. He had several times considered writing a family chronicle continuing the story of the Buddenbrooks (or rather the Manns). The suicide of his two sisters, the Nazi leanings of his younger brother Viktor, would all have contributed to this epic: but its primary theme was always going to be the *Brüderzwist*, the fateful quarrel between himself and Heinrich which had been the most important motivating force in his creative, even his personal life. "If you have found me a difficult brother," he had responded to Heinrich's attempt at reconciliation in January 1918,

> I naturally found you even more so. . . . It is not true that my conduct in the war has been "extreme." Yours was, and in fact to the point of being utterly detestable. But I have not suffered and struggled for two years, neglected my dearest projects, sentenced myself to silence as an artist, probed, compared and asserted myself [in writing the *Reflections*] just to answer a letter which—understandably—exudes triumph . . . and concludes that I need not regard you as an enemy. . . . Let the tragedy of our brotherhood take its course to the bitter end. [T. Mann, 1961, pp. 88–89]

Reconciliation had, in 1922, avoided a tragic end—though the tragedy of German history took its course nonetheless. "The hour will come, I hope, in which you will see people, not shadows; and then perhaps me," Heinrich had replied—and, movingly, the hour not only came, but remained with Thomas. To the end of his life, in the summer of 1955, Thomas continued to see the "person" of Heinrich, forgiving his weaknesses (including those of his schizoid barmaid wife) and lauding his virtues. Indeed the last essay Thomas wrote was in celebration of Schiller, on the occasion of the one hundred fiftieth anniversary of the great poet's death: and the person of Heinrich spoke through every line. "My basic attitude towards him and his somewhat formidably intellectual work was always that of the little brother looking up at the elder," he confessed in a letter only six weeks before his death. "It was an incredible shock to me, and seemed like a dream," he went on, "when shortly before his death Heinrich dedicated one of his books to me with the words: 'To my great brother, who wrote Doctor Faustus.' What? How? *He* had always been the great, the big brother. And I puffed out my chest and thought of Goethe's remark about the Germans' silly bickering over who was the greater, he or Schiller: 'They ought to be glad they have two such sons.' "

Knowledge of the sibling rivalry of the Manns may not be essential to an understanding of their individual works, but it *is* essential to an understanding of their achievement. The theme of brotherly confrontation which runs through their novels and stories was not simply a haphazard ingredient in a patchwork of fictional pieces, but reflected an epic journey in their own lives, as men and artists: a story of rivalry and resolution, of human weakness and nobility as both brothers finally mastered their passionate mutual envy, and began to work together to defend what they saw as their country's humanitarian honor. They failed in that both were forced into exile by Hitler, were deprived of German citizenship in the 1930s, and yet were abused by nationalists when they "dared" to think of returning after the Second World War. Yet in a deeper sense they succeeded; their stand against fascism was exemplary, and in the most honorable way they proved bankrupt the traditional ostrichlike refusal of German artists to concern themselves with the political development of their country. Their epic development is perhaps without parallel in the annals of literature, and serves to remind us of the *moral* content of art. For in the struggle between these two great German artists is reflected not simply the problem of sibling rivalry, but its personal resolution—in two lives that will never be forgotten as long as literature and the course of modern human history is studied.

REFERENCES

Hamilton, N. (1978), *The Brothers Mann: The Lives of Heinrich and Thomas Mann, 1871–1950 and 1875–1955*. London: Secker & Warburg; New Haven: Yale University Press, 1979.

Mann, H. (1915), Zola. *Die weissen Blätter*, November; In: *Geist und Tat: Franzosen, 1780–1930*. Berlin.

————— (1929), *Berlin: The Land of Cockaigne*. London: V. Gollancz, 1900.

————— (1947), *Ein Zeitalter wird Besichtigt*. Stockholm: Neuer Verlag, 1946.

Mann, Katja (1975), *Unwritten Memories*, ed. E. Piessen and M. Mann. New York: L.B. Fischer.

Mann, Klaus (1942), *The Turning Point: Thirty-Five Years in This Century*. New York: L.B. Fischer.

Mann, T. (1918), *Betrachtungen eines Unpolitischen*. Frankfort A/M: S. Fischer.

————— (1925), Disorder and early sorrow. *Dial*, 81:269–284, 402–422, 1926.

————— (1931), Fragment über das Religiöse. In: *Dichterglaube*, ed. H. Braun. Berlin: Eckart Verlag.

————— (1933), Sufferings and greatness of Richard Wagner. In: *Freud, Goethe, Wagner*. New York: Knopf, pp. 101–121, 1937.

————— (1961), *Letters of Thomas Mann, 1889–1955*. Selected & translated by Richard & Clara Winston. New York: Knopf, 1970.

————— (1979), *Tagebücher 1918–1921*. Frankfort A/M: S. Fischer.

Winston, R. (1981), *Thomas Mann: The Making of an Artist, 1875–1911*. New
    York: Knopf.
Wysling, H., ed. (1968), *Thomas Mann–Heinrich Mann: Briefwechsel 1900–1949*.
    Frankfort A/M: S. Fischer Verlag.

As the galleys for *Blood Brothers: Siblings As Writers* were being edited, Thomas
    Mann's *Reflections of a Non-Political Man* was finally published in English
    in May 1983 by Frederick Ungar.

As the twentieth century enters its final decades, James Joyce appears assured of a significant place in its cultural history. "I want to be famous while I am alive," he told his Aunt Josephine (Ellmann, 1959, p. 147), and he was. Jung (1932b) characterized this Irishman at the height of his fame in the thirties as a "literary brother" to Picasso in his exemplification of the essential spirit of modern art (p. 135)[1] and a "literary counterpart" to Freud in his revelation to his contemporaries of "the other side of reality" (1932a, p. 121). Fifty years later, in his centennial year of 1982, James Joyce, with only a handful of published volumes to his credit, is acknowledged as one of the towering figures in modern literature.

This preeminence rests basically on three books, the autobiographical trilogy which dramatizes his personal inward journey of self-discovery and self-revelation and presents at the same time a universalized portrait of the twentieth-century artist: *A Portrait of the Artist as a Young Man*, *Ulysses*, and *Finnegans Wake*. Seldom, if ever, has a creative fiction been so apparently true to biographical fact as Joyce's *Portrait*, so compulsively

2

James and Stanislaus Joyce: A Jungian Speculation

JEAN KIMBALL

---

[1] Jung identified schizophrenic elements in the art of both Joyce and Pjcasso, though explicitly denying that he regarded either artist as psychotic (Jung, 1932a, p. 117; 1932b, p. 137). See Jung, 1975, p. 589, for further comparisons between the two, and see Prinzhorn, 1922, pp. 270–273, on the importance of schizophrenic art for our time.

accurate about historical and geographical detail as *Ulysses*, or, in contrast, so mythologized and depersonalized as *Finnegans Wake*. But at the same time, never has fiction been more literally *auto*biographical than in all three, for whatever his shifts in technique and perspective, Joyce's purpose never really deviates from the basic aim of self-definition, to which historical narrative, as well as neo-mythology, is drastically subordinated.

Thus, although both *A Portrait* and *Ulysses* are peopled with characters drawn from life, speaking lines which are often so marvelously real that they might have been transcribed from tape recordings, in both these fictions the sense of personal relationship is all but absent. The autobiographical hero, embodied in Stephen Dedalus in *A Portrait* and duplicated by a sort of cell division into Stephen and Leopold Bloom in *Ulysses*, is not truly related to any other conscious personality. Thus, although one of the central biographical facts about James Joyce is that he was the oldest of a family of ten children, nowhere in either of these autobiographical novels is there a portrayal of any significant, continuing relationship between Stephen Dedalus and any of his brothers or sisters. Not until *Finnegans Wake*, in which concrete reality and linear historicity are abandoned and conscious personality is replaced by shifting relationships between the paired opposites which people the unconscious, do we find the brother relationship as a significant feature, although here, in the night world, it is central, "one of the few immediately apprehensible aspects of the *Wake*" (O'Brien, 1966, p. 183).

To be sure, in August of 1904 the young Joyce wrote to Nora Barnacle, who was to leave Dublin with him less than two months later, that "my brothers and sisters are nothing to me," following this, however, with the curious qualification: "One brother alone is capable of understanding me" (J. Joyce, 1966a, p. 48). And this one brother, John Stanislaus Joyce, "Stannie" to his family, who was almost three years younger than James, served his older brother in an extraordinary range of capacities for over half the years of the artist's life: audience and companion; servant, messenger, and representative; literary source, advisor, and editor; guardian and provider, not only for his brother but for his brother's family as well. And after the artist's death in 1941, Stanislaus, whose life had been almost completely separated from James's for over twenty years, became curator for his brother's memory, defending, explaining, correcting, and finally providing source material of unparalleled authenticity in the letters and diaries which he made available to Richard Ellmann for the definitive biography of James Joyce.[2]

---

[2] For Herbert Gorman's difficulties with the earlier biography, written with "help" from Joyce himself, see Ellmann, 1959, pp. 644–645 and 735–738, and note Gorman's vow that "I will never write another biography of a living man" (p. 719).

James's letters to Stanislaus during the fairly brief periods of their separation in their early adulthood are, as Ellmann recognizes, as nearly a "frank expression of his intellectual position" as we have (J. Joyce, 1966a, p. li), and the diaries, which Stanislaus kept from the time of James's University College days in Dublin through the brothers' years together in Trieste, are at least as much a record and interpretation of his brother's life as of his own. Though he burned the first diary, the second, written between 1903 and 1905—the period surrounding the day memorialized in *Ulysses*—has been edited and published as *The Complete Dublin Diary of Stanislaus Joyce* (1971).[3] This diary, along with the posthumously published memoir, *My Brother's Keeper*, are the only two published volumes which bear the name of Stanislaus Joyce, so that some adjustment of our customary definitions may be required to think of Stanislaus as a writer. Still, T.S. Eliot, in his preface to the memoir, provides a rationale for this perspective. "Possessed as he was by the subject of his memoir," Eliot writes, "Stanislaus Joyce, under the exasperation of this thorn in his flesh, became himself a writer, and the author of this one book which is worthy to occupy a permanent place on the bookshelf beside the works of his brother" (S. Joyce, 1958, p. ix).

And this is where we find Stanislaus Joyce's books—shelved with his brother's, an adjunct to the works of James Joyce, even as his life, during the crucial years of Joyce's beginnings as an artist, was an adjunct to his brother's. But without his quite extraordinary contribution, both practical and psychic, to James Joyce's life, there might have been no books at all on the shelf. At the same time, had there been no separation of the brothers by the war—had Stanislaus not been interned in Austria from 1915 until the end of the war while James moved on to the special cosmopolitan atmosphere of Zurich—Joyce might not have developed and exploited those unique qualities which put the stamp of greatness on *Ulysses* and perhaps go beyond the bounds of judgment in *Finnegans Wake*, but which make both such characteristic expressions of the spirit of his age as to insure his place as one of its great artist-prophets.

Such might-have-beens are, of course, beyond proof or disproof, but they do provide a useful perspective on what was. For these two brothers, in their shared existence, present us with a relationship which in a sense follows the "law of participation" identified by Lévy-Bruhl (1922) as characteristic of primitive mentality. Indeed, James and Stanislaus Joyce re-

---

[3] The earlier *Dublin Diary of Stanislaus Joyce* (1962) was abridged to sharpen the focus on James Joyce. Stanislaus's Trieste diary, which obviously has provided Ellmann (1959) with the bulk of his source material for that period, is not, as far as I can discover, presently available in any known collection of Joyceana.

semble brothers in many primitive tribes, who according to Lévy-Bruhl (1927) appear "to consider their quasi-identity as a self-evident thing" (p. 89); in their lives, as in the primitive situation, "a very strong sense of their own personality" appears to coexist with "an idea which makes, as it were, the two brothers into one individual" (p. 90). Thus, though Stanislaus Joyce, in his service to his brother's needs, may be considered "one of the martyred siblings of literary history" by Edel (1980, p. 485) and as a "victim" of his brother's "cannibalism" by Cixous (1972, p. 120), such judgments do not apply to a relationship of participation, where there is no question of exploiter and martyr; there is no victim; there is no "theft" (Cixous, 1972, p. 129). For "the two brothers make but one person: One does not steal from oneself" (Lévy-Bruhl, 1927, p. 91).

Now the idea of two persons in one and as one is a key metaphor in Jung's model of the psyche, in which there are two personified forces in a dynamic relationship of conflict and compensation: the ego of the conscious personality opposed and complemented by the shadow, Jung's personification of the personal unconscious, which not only accumulates contents repressed by the conscious personality, but also provides the vital link to the vast resources of the collective unconscious. And the goal of this mutually compensatory relationship is the unknowable totality of the Jungian self, which embraces both conscious and unconscious. Thus the psyche is "a self-regulating system that maintains its equilibrium just as the body does" (Jung, 1934, p. 153), through a "natural, automatic function" of compensation which "is constantly present" (Jung, 1918, p. 18). Thus Jung (1918) proposes, as "a complement to the repression theory" (p. 15) of Freudian thought, a "theory of compensation," which asserts as a "basic law of psychic behaviour" that "the relation between conscious and unconscious is compensatory" (Jung, 1934, p. 153).

And it is in a frame at least analogous to this law of compensation that I am considering in this essay the relationship between James and Stanislaus Joyce, which despite its apparent one-sidedness achieved a functional reciprocity analogous to the natural, automatic interaction of conscious and unconscious in the individual psyche. This reciprocity was not dependent upon any pretense of altruism or upon good intentions on either side, qualities which seem conspicuously absent from the relationship between the Joyce brothers, but rather upon a natural complementarity of temperament and consequently of needs and contributions. Thus Stanislaus, whose great strengths lay in his relationship to external reality, appeared to take it for granted—as did James—that he should accept responsibility for the burdens of his elder brother's practical life, serving as "a kind of extra draught horse" (S. Joyce, 1941, p. 507) in the Joyce household in Trieste. But both brothers also took for granted the deeply personal nature of Stanislaus's stake in his brother's artistic achievement, an achievement which depended upon the intensity of Joyce's relationship to an inner reality as it resonated to the harmonies of his extraordinarily dominant ego.

The two brothers thus embody the fundamental opposition between the extraverted and introverted attitude-types identified and examined by Jung in his *Psychological Types*, and in this essay the way this compensatory opposition worked in their life together, in terms of both attitude-type and function-type, will be considered. For the extraordinarily close and complementary relationship between the Joyce brothers can be seen as a significant means of survival and indeed success for both. The elder brother, James Joyce, though he died before he was sixty, after years of melodramatically bad health, achieved fame while he lived and after his death the practical immortality which comes with recognition as a great writer. Stanislaus Joyce, though he was while he lived, as T.S. Eliot writes, "the brother of whose existence the world remained unaware" (S. Joyce, 1958, p. viii), and though he did not in any direct way achieve greatness, nevertheless became a respected university professor, lived for over seventy years in unusually good physical health, and appears to have achieved a psychic balance and an approach to wholeness which hardly any observer would claim for his brother.

Different as these outcomes were, both can be seen as success, and this success can be attributed in no small measure to the compensatory working of the fraternal relationship, which is not to say that it was the only significant relationship or even necessarily the most significant relationship in the life of either of these men. But it is the one being looked at here, largely to the exclusion of others. While the relationship between these brothers can obviously be viewed (and has been) from other perspectives,[4] this essay is considering it exclusively in the frame of Jung's typology. Finally, even though James Joyce's work is perhaps the only real rationale for any interest we may have in his life and personality, or that of his brother, the emphasis here is on the life and personality of each as it affected the other and only incidentally on the work itself. The basic thesis is that these brothers were opposites in personality, and the sharing of their opposite qualities made each richer than he might otherwise have been.

Since the popularization of Jung's "extraverted" and "introverted" cate-

---

[4] For two quite different approaches to the relationship, though both focus on Stanislaus's role, see Arnold Goldman (1974) and Hélène Cixous (1972), pp. 119–159.

gories, like the popularization of many Freudian terms, has led to a distorting simplification of their original meaning, the use of this Jungian scheme requires some of the same disclaimers which Jung himself repeatedly made with regard to his typology. Recognizing that far too many readers of his *Psychological Types* had taken his book as "a system of classification and a practical guide to a good judgment of human character," Jung, denying that his purpose was "to stick labels on people," described his typology as "a critical apparatus" (1921, p. xiv) through which he could "express in a comprehensible way the peculiarities of an individual psyche and the functional interplay of its elements" (1975, pp. 550–551).

If in this essay, then, I put James Joyce into the frame of Jung's introverted attitude-type in contrast to his brother Stanislaus as an exemplification of the extraverted type, my purpose is not to label or judge either of the brothers and certainly not to offer any full-scale analysis of their personalities, but rather to make use of Jung's conceptual scheme in order to examine the "functional interplay" of the elements of their relationship. For the "problem of the opposites," which Jung (1973, p. 186) considered basic to his *Psychological Types*, and which is a fundamental feature of his vision throughout his work, is also dominant in James Joyce's artistic vision and basic to the dynamics of the relationship between the Joyce brothers.

The attitude-types with which these brothers are identifiable represent real opposites; as Jung (1921) points out, they "are so different and present such a striking contrast that their existence becomes quite obvious even to the layman, once it has been pointed out." For "everyone knows those reserved, inscrutable, rather shy people who form the strongest possible contrast to the . . . approachable characters who are on good terms with everybody, or quarrel with everybody, but always relate to them in some way and in turn are affected by them" (p. 330).

This contrast is obvious in James and Stanislaus Joyce, curiously reinforced for those who saw them by a striking contrast in physical appearance. James, according to Curran (1968), was "tall, slim, and elegant" with "an erect yet loose carriage" and "light-blue eyes," which were "at times altogether expressionless," giving "an air of inscrutability and . . . lack of interest in the surroundings of the moment" (p. 4). Stanislaus Joyce, on the other hand, seemed to Fifield (1967) when he interviewed him in Trieste "more a fit brother for Buck Mulligan than Joyce," with his "thick Buck Mulligan chest" and "round, rubicund, beaming" face. In contrast to "the lean, pale man with the ashplant," Stanislaus was "rough, open, and blunt," a "squat and somehow lonely figure" (pp. 70–71).

It was doubtless this physical contrast which led their Triestine friend Italo Svevo to characterize the brothers as "Don Quixote and Sancho Panza" (S. Joyce, 1949, p. 897), but in the brothers, as in Cervantes's great archetypal double portrait of the opposites, the physical contrast was duplicated by a psychic contrast in their relations to the world of objective reality. For Jung (1921) distinguishes the two attitude-types in terms of their contrasting habitual attitudes toward the "object," which is to say, whatever is not the subject. The interest of the introvert, that is, "does not move towards the object, but withdraws from it into the subject," which is the "prime motivating factor" for the introvert, whereas the object is of "secondary importance" (pp. 452–453), representing in fact a positive threat to the introvert, "as though he had to prevent the object from gaining power over him" (p. 330). Thus, though the introvert necessarily "orients himself in accordance with the data supplied by the outside world," he habitually "holds in reserve a view which interposes itself between him and the objective data" (p. 333).

Now this analysis of the introvert fits the stance of Cervantes's hero, whether he is tilting at windmills or wooing Dulcinea, and it fits James Joyce, though the view which he interposes between himself and the "objective data" is, of course, radically different from Don Quixote's. And equally appropriate, both for Quixote's squire Sancho Panza and for Stanislaus Joyce, is Jung's characterization of the extravert, who, with his "positive relation to the object" (p. 330), "thinks, feels, acts, and actually lives in a way that is *directly* correlated with the objective conditions and their demands," allowing himself "to be oriented by the given facts" (p. 333), which have a "determining value" not accorded to any "subjective view" he may have (p. 334).

Thus, though "for the introvert the idea of the ego is the continuous and dominant note of consciousness," the extravert focuses predominantly "on the continuity of his relation to the object and less on the idea of the ego." And though the introvert is ruled by a conviction, Jung (1921) says, quoting Schiller, that "the 'person' reveals itself 'in the eternally constant ego, and in this alone,' " for the extravert "the person reveals itself simply and solely in its relatedness" (p. 90).

There is a wealth of testimony from observers of James Joyce throughout his life which affirms his identity as an introvert by Jungian definitions, starting with the testimony of Stanislaus's early diary, which is also, of course, virtually our only source of observations about Stanislaus himself. Stanislaus's estimations are confirmed, not only by others who knew Joyce as a young Dubliner and those who knew him in his maturity as a European, but also by Joyce himself in the various stages of his fictional self-portrait. Stanislaus (1971) notes, for example, his brother's "wilful, vicious selfishness," his "protestant egoism" (p. 3). This egoism rules Joyce's autobiographical artist throughout his fictional life, from the "ineradicable egoism" attributed to the unnamed subject of the unpublished 1904 "Portrait of the Artist" (Scholes and Kain, 1960, p. 361) through the final, fragmented portrait of Shem the Penman in *Finnegans Wake*, "self-exiled in upon his own ego" (J. Joyce, 1939, p. 184).

This primacy of the artist's ego is further confirmed by other observers. Curran (1968), for example, looking back at Joyce as a University College student, identified the "ineradicable egoism with which he endowed Stephen" as evident enough in Joyce himself to estrange him from his classmates (p. 21), while Oliver St. John Gogarty (1954) saw, in the "intensity, self-absorption and silence" (p. 92) of this "unlovable and lonely man," a deliberately willed detachment from humanity which was "inhuman" (1950, p. 67). Indeed Joyce, as is characteristic of an introverted personality, "lived a withdrawn life" (Curran, 1968, p. 21). Because the ego is the essential reality for the introvert, he is correspondingly removed from "relatedness or proneness to affect" (Jung, 1921, p. 90).

For Eva Joyce, her brother's detachment was simply a matter of his being "a very lonesome boy," whose loneliness "was the one thing that had been outstanding in his life" (Rodgers, 1972, pp. 35, 40). But Stanislaus (1971) pointed to an inner source of this lack of relatedness with his observation that "Jim cares nothing, he says, what others think of him," which, as a painfully self-conscious adolescent himself, he could hardly credit (p. 58), though he affirmed it in full force years later, after his brother's death. "All his life . . . my brother never cared a rap what people thought, said, or wrote about him. His indifference to obloquy surpassed belief" (1958, p. 212). In fact, his indifference to most of the world outside himself is a recurrent theme in the reminiscences about the mature James Joyce.

Nino Frank (1967), for example, who had contact with Joyce over a period of fourteen years in Paris, writing of the "anonymity" of Joyce's apartments, says it was as if "his sole place of intimacy was within himself"; he "seemed plunged in a well of thought where he could not be reached" (p. 78), creating around himself "a big zone of silence" (Rodgers, 1972, p. 48). The Danish journalist Vinding (1963), who was with the Joyces for three days in Copenhagen, reports a similar impression that "Joyce really was never aware of his surroundings, or had only one will: a will that centered on Joyce and apparently reduced the world around him to something just to be used," but "not interesting in itself" (pp. 143–144). Arthur Power (1974), Joyce's fellow expatriate, records that "the life he lived was, socially speaking, hermetically sealed" (p. 39), while the French critic Gillet (1941) saw Joyce as "not of this world . . . a stranger, a phantom whose shadow only was among us" (p. 168). This perception was echoed by Joyce's countryman, Niall Sheridan, who in a 1950 BBC broadcast about Joyce, noted that "he was a person withdrawn entirely from the real world" (Rodgers, 1972, p. 50).

This "peculiar detachment the man had, in all personal relations" may be attributable, as an anonymous friend suggested at the close of the BBC broadcast, to "theological despair" (Rodgers, 1972, p. 73). Or it may even justifiably be labeled "schizoid," as it has been by Andreasen (1973, p. 67), but certainly these impressions of James Joyce's relation to the world indicate an extremely one-sided, introverted attitude.

For his brother Stanislaus, though, the case is quite opposite, but it is a case which must depend largely on Stanislaus's own self-observation in his diary. It is an oddity of the extraverted type that because he realizes himself primarily in relationship, he is generally not an object of detached scrutiny and, as Jung (1921) points out, almost never fairly represented by "intellectual criticism." For his "specific value lies in his relation to the object," which is "one of those imponderables that an intellectual formulation can never grasp" (p. 162). Since he is, in contrast to the introvert, so continually affected by the life outside himself—people, objects, situations—the extravert may well appear to others, not as the comfortable, outgoing man of our American stereotype of the extravert, but rather as "fitful and uncertain in temper and behaviour, given to petulance, fuss, discontent and censoriousness" (p. 160).[5] It has not been difficult for others—especially his brother, who was for so many years the object of his concern—to see Stanislaus in this way.

Even the adolescent Stanislaus, who confesses in his diary to being "tormented by a longing to please and to be liked" (1971, p. 46), can see that he produces an effect which works against this. Writing of this problem, which he shares with his brother Charlie, Stanislaus perceives that "that familiar, Self-consciousness, which keeps constantly telling us what we have done and why we did it, and which does not flatter . . . induces in us a manner which our relatives mistake for pride in us" (pp. 15–16). "I stride in my walk," he writes, "but I am drooping with fatigue in my interior. I have never dared to act as I please, but think in a little way 'what will be thought of it?' 'Will so-and-so be displeased, will so-and-so despise me?' " (p. 32). When he reports his brother's declared indifference

---

[5] From Furneaux Jordan's description of "the less impassioned man," which Jung (1921) equates with the extravert, crediting Jordan with being "the first . . . to give a relatively appropriate character sketch of the emotional types" (p. 165).

to the opinion of others, it is with disbelief, for "I know his pride must suffer from being subjected to their manner as much as I do" (p. 58). On the other hand, when, in *My Brother's Keeper*, he considers the real-life background for the "religious crisis" which Joyce put at the center of *A Portrait*, he remembers no real sympathy with his brother, for "I was always more upset by a blunder or a gaffe than by sin. The offence to the Godhead never troubled me, but faults in my relations with others did" (1958, pp. 80–81).

It is excruciatingly clear in his *Dublin Diary* that this kind of awareness of others is a source of continuing distress, even real pain, to the young Stanislaus: "I have so much sympathy with people I know," he writes, "that when I am in the same room with them and silent, everything that happens [to] them seems to happen [to] me and I pass through every mood of theirs." He then asks himself, "How can I believe, then, that I have a mind of my own?" (p. 175), putting his finger, young as he is, on the extravert's danger of losing himself entirely in relatedness.

For if the introvert, with his ruling assumption that the "person" is "exclusively the ego" (Jung, 1921, p. 90), courts the danger of losing himself in an inner world (pp. 133, 167), the extravert's assumption that the person "lies in his affectivity . . . i.e., his relatedness" (p. 90) exposes him to an opposite danger. That is, in his felt need to meet the demands of existing objective conditions—however abnormal—the extravert's tendency to subordinate the demands of his inner life to "external necessity" (p. 334) may actually threaten his psychic health. Jung makes a distinction between "adjustment," which is at once the extravert's greatest virtue and his greatest limitation, and "adaptation," which "requires observance of laws more universal than the immediate conditions" (p. 335). His "normality," that is, depends, not only "on his ability to fit into existing conditions," but also "essentially on whether he takes account of his subjective needs" (p. 335).

The question of balancing his subjective needs against his acute awareness of the demands of others runs through Stanislaus's diary, revealing a continuing tension between these two motivations, which focuses on his relationship with his brother Jim and gives the diary a kind of narrative suspense. In *My Brother's Keeper*, Stanislaus characterizes his youthful diary as "a record more of [my brother's] doings and comings and goings than of my own," adding, however, that "we were almost always together" (1958, p. 111). And the young Stanislaus indicates in his *Dublin Diary* that the earlier diary, which he burned, "was a journal of his life," speculating that "perhaps Jim owes something of his appearance to this mirror held constantly up to him" (1971, p. 20). But it is clear to the reader of the diary that it is a mirror also held constantly up to its author to remedy what he himself sees as a significant personal problem. "Though it is written carefully, even painfully," Stanislaus records, "I appreciate that it is badly written because I do not know myself. These are notes made for my private help" (p. 28).

He indicates that he is consciously moving toward a goal of self-knowledge by objectifying and establishing a relationship with himself. "I have a habit of listening to my thoughts" (p. 39), and "I reflect my thoughts on paper so that I may know my state," for "I must know myself and the life that fits me, and act rightly out of my true character" (p. 49). He is "oppressed by the want of understanding myself" (p. 63); "one of my chief reasons for keeping these notes," he writes, "is to prevent myself becoming stupid" (p. 57). Stanislaus, like so many adolescents, feels himself "left naked to the ridicule of the normal mind without, and my habitual self-contempt within" (p. 59), and his vulnerability is heightened by the nature of the "normal mind without" whose opinion means most to him—his brother Jim. "Not an encouraging person in criticism" (p. 20), Jim, Stanislaus perceives, regards his younger brother "as quite commonplace and uninteresting—he makes no attempt at disguise—and though I follow him fully in this matter of opinion, I cannot be expected to like it" (p. 51).

Furthermore, because of his acute sensitivity to his brother's opinion and his habit of "follow[ing] Jim in nearly all matters of opinion" (p. 50), Stannie is never quite sure whether his judgments of himself are really his own or mere reflections of his brother's. When, for example, his Aunt Josephine tells him he underrates himself, Stannie disagrees, but reminds himself, "Yet I take myself at Jim's valuation of me," adding "because it is my own," but qualifying that with "perhaps" (p. 59). Later he suggests to himself that his opinion of himself is so low "probably because I have a very high standard," which, however, may be principally "the reflection of Jim's nature" and yet "really in the essence of my character" (p. 76). Truly, as this younger brother writes at one point, "it is terrible to have a cleverer elder brother" (p. 50).

Terrible or not, Stannie recognizes that this cleverer elder brother's example has provided him with the model for his own life (p. 50), though he also records in the diary his further recognition, almost in the nature of a revelation, that his brother is radically different from himself. He reports meeting Jim after not seeing him for a few days and realizing all at once that his own progress in life is not, as he has assumed, simply a matter of catching up with his older brother, "for it seemed to me that the difference between us was not a difference of degree but of kind" (p. 75).

This difference in kind may usefully be thought of in Jungian terms as a contrast between the brothers in function-type as well as attitude-type. Admittedly, the identification of function-type is uncertain even with living subjects, since it is often "uncommonly difficult," Jung (1921) says, "to find out which function holds prior place" (p. 149), and in actual life, as Jacobi (1942) points out in her synopsis of Jung's psychological theory, "the function types almost never appear in pure form but in a variety of mixed types" (p. 17). Furthermore, in contrast to the stability of attitude-type, "the function-type is subject to all manner of changes in the course of life" (Jung, 1973, p. 230). Clearly then, to assign a function-type to these two men, dead for a generation and more, is a speculative, not to say suspect, undertaking.

Thus, when I say that James Joyce was an introvert, whose dominant function appears to be a mix of thinking and intuition, in which it is very difficult to determine which function takes precedence, I am aware of the built-in dubiety of this identification. It is an unverifiable hypothesis, as is my assumption that Stanislaus Joyce was an extravert, whose dominant function was sensation, with well-differentiated auxiliary functions of feeling and thinking. But these companion assumptions have an empirical base and simply put into a Jungian frame a contrast between the temperaments of the two brothers which was apparent to those who knew them and, to some extent, to the brothers themselves, and which may be considered a significant factor in the compensatory nature of their relationship, in which their individual strengths and weaknesses achieved a kind of working balance.

In this discussion I am not attempting to fine-tune the contrast I am suggesting to harmonize with all the nuances which have built up around Jung's definitions of the types. Rather, I am using Jung's "almost colloquial terms," based as he says "on rules of thumb" (1975, p. 552), in the spirit in which he proposed them: to provide "a terminology in which at least the crassest differences between individuals can be formulated" (1973, p. 130). Since Jung's terms are being used, the broad outlines of the terminology of his theory of function-types[6] should at least be briefly reviewed.

Jung (1921) identifies four psychic functions, dividing them into two pairs of opposites. Thinking and feeling, the rational functions, represent

---

[6] While Jung (1921) provides descriptions of the types in Chapter X (pp. 330–407) and definitions in Chapter XI (pp. 408–486), many important qualifications and elucidations are scattered through his work and *Letters* (1973, 1975). A useful condensed discussion of the functions is found in Jacobi, 1942, pp. 10–26. See also von Franz, 1971, pp. 1–18.

opposite ways of judging, which may be employed alternately but not at the same time. Both are "decisively influenced by *reflection*" and accord with "the laws of reason" (p. 459), but thinking judges according to "conceptual relations" while feeling, by contrast, aims at judgment in accordance with "a definite *value* in the sense of acceptance or rejection" (p. 434). Sensation and intuition, irrational functions in the sense of being "*beyond* reason" rather than "*contrary* to reason" (p. 454), represent opposite ways of perceiving, sensation being "conscious" perception and intuition "unconscious perception" (p. 463).

The preference for one function, which ordinarily appears to be inborn, results in its being regularly favored in dealing with life, so that it becomes dominant at the expense of the other three functions, which are correspondingly neglected and undeveloped. Of this "inferior function triad" (Jung, 1948, p. 244), one or two functions may be partially differentiated, that is, made conscious and accessible to the will. These auxiliary functions, though not equal in power to the dominant function, nevertheless exert a "co-determining influence" (1921, p. 405) on the individual's attitude, "affording welcome assistance" to the dominant function (p. 406).

But the function which is the polar opposite of the dominant function cannot be brought sufficiently under the control of the conscious will as to be useful and remains attached to the unconscious, "inaccessible to our will," coming and going "of its own volition" (1948, p. 238). And this is the inferior function, which, Jung (1921) says, is "in no way morbid but merely backward as compared with the favoured function" (p. 450). Like a backward child, however, the inferior function, particularly when it has been severely repressed or neglected, often manifests itself in infantile, uncontrolled ways.

My basic assumption is that James and Stanislaus, in their dominant and inferior functions, present almost perfect mirror images of one another, a psychic situation which is represented in the diagrammatic circles in Figure 1. Adapted from the explanatory circles provided by Jacobi (1942) in her synopsis of Jung's theory of the functions (pp. 11–18), these circles show the dominant and auxiliary functions for each brother at the top, unshaded to indicate the accessibility of these functions to consciousness. At the bottom of each circle, then, is the inferior function, the shading indicating its entrapment in the unconscious. In the circle representing Stanislaus's psyche, the auxiliary functions of feeling and thinking on either side of the dominant sensation function are partially unshaded to indicate his considerable differentiation of both, whereas a greater portion of James's circle is shaded to represent his considerably less balanced development of the functions.

FIGURE 1

James and Stanislaus Joyce
Attitudes and Functions

STANISLAUS
Extraverted
Sensation Type

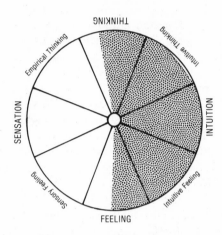

JAMES
Introverted
Intuitive-Thinking Type

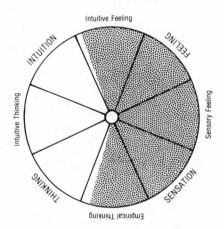

For if, as I assume, James Joyce was an intuitive-thinking type, both these functions—the one perceiving and the other judging—would have been highly developed at the expense of their opposites, so that his inferior function could be expected to be a mix of sensation and feeling, a "characteristic fusion," Jung (1921) says, in the introverted thinking type (p. 98).[7] And in the psychic picture I am suggesting for the two brothers, Stanislaus, a sensation type with feeling as one of his auxiliary functions, was equipped to provide compensation for his brother's one-sidedness in both perception and judgment. For sensation "perceives things as they are and not otherwise"; it is "the sense of reality, par excellence—what the French call the 'fonction du réel' " (Jacobi, 1942, p. 12). In Stanislaus this perceiving function was assisted by a highly differentiated feeling function, which judges perceptions according to value, an activity which is a dominant note of his diary and compensates for his brother's inability or refusal to make value judgments.

To be sure, with his dominant development of the sensation function, Stanislaus could be expected to be correspondingly deficient in intuition, that "unconscious 'inner perception' of the inherent potentialities of things" (Jacobi, 1942, p. 12), which is "neither sense perception, nor feeling, nor intellectual inference, although it may also appear in these forms," and which grasps a content "whole and complete, without our being able to explain or discover how this content came into existence" (Jung, 1921, p. 453). This mysterious function was extraordinarily developed in James Joyce, who, Stanislaus (1958) writes, "used to say that he didn't see things, that he absorbed them" (p. 120). For Stanislaus, however, intuition is the inferior function, and he admits that though "I see the road I go plainly . . . I do not see one step before or after. But for the light of the conscious glass my mind is dark" (1971, p. 173).

Thus, the two brothers, taken together, have a combined command of all the psychic functions, and if each compensated for the other and used the other's skills, this is not an unheard-of phenomenon. In fact, as Franz (1971) points out, there is a common tendency in families to "distribute the functions," one member giving up what another can do better and in turn "relying on the superior function of the other" (p. 4). If James could write of the youthful subject of his 1904 "Portrait of the Artist" that

[7] Nowhere is this fusion more strikingly displayed than in the notorious pornographic letters which Joyce wrote to Nora in 1909 and 1912 (J. Joyce, 1975, pp. 157–196). The combination of mawkish sentimentality in the expression of feeling for Nora—very nearly incredible in so gifted a master of the language—and the astonishing recital of polymorphous-perverse sexual practices, with the accompanying infantile fixation on the bodily functions, is truly a demonstration of Jung's comment about the inferior function: "You do not have it under your thumb; it has you" (Jacobi, 1942, p. 17).

"his training had early developed a very lively sense of spiritual obligation at the expense of what is called 'common sense' " (Scholes and Kain, 1960, p. 360), there is every indication that this early imbalance was Joyce's own and that it continued throughout his life. It never became necessary for him to develop "common sense," the *fonction du réel*, because there was always someone else to deal with the facts for him, to soften the real.

This service, which later fell so heavily on Stanislaus, surely began with the older brother's sheltered position in the large Joyce family, where the reality of life for the children was harsh. These brothers did not, like William and Henry James or Heinrich and Thomas Mann, come out of a solid, supportive family background, but rather struggled to survive despite the peculiarly Irish misery of their family: an unemployed, alcoholic father; too many children; and a "priest-ridden" mother, "a naked nerve" according to Gogarty (1954, p. 90), who could understandably never quite cope with the conflicting demands of husband, children, and Church. But in the midst of the "progressive disintegration" of this "lower-middle-class" family (S. Joyce, 1941, p. 486), James had the most of whatever there was. To begin with, he was born into relatively comfortable circumstances and started his schooling with the Jesuits at Clongowes Wood during the "interlude between relative prosperity and real poverty" (S. Joyce, 1958, p. 47). It was not until his father lost his government job and began his permanent retirement in 1891 that James was withdrawn from Clongowes (Ellmann, 1959, p. 34) and returned to the realities of home life.

Added to this advantage of birth rank and circumstances was the fact that he was the favorite, not only of his mother, which Freud felt was so auspicious a circumstance, but of everyone in the family, as Eva Joyce remembered it in 1950: "Father and mother idolised him, and all the brothers and sisters seemed to be quite happy that he was the one that got the most attention" (Rodgers, 1972, p. 35). Though her sister Eileen remembered that her brother's favored position, particularly with their father, was not so readily accepted, in fact "used to drive the others mad," she agreed with Eva about the favoritism and detailed its very real benefits.

"There was no money at all, and all the relatives were saying that Jim should get a job and help with the big family—he being the eldest, but Mother never took that point of view. She always did everything in her power to help him follow his bent" (Curtayne, 1963, p. 44), which required that *he* be taken care of first. As for their father, "From boyhood he gave him everything—absolutely everything. He deprived the rest of the family to give to Jim" (Rodgers, 1972, p. 35), including, of course, the University education which none of the others had and even money to buy books for his self-education, "whether or not his family had enough to eat" (Ellmann, 1959, p. 78). If Gogarty's characterization of Joyce as "torn between a miserable background and a sumptuous education" (1954, p. 90) may overstate the quality of the education provided by University College, this education was nevertheless well beyond Joyce's means and provided the base at least for the development of his quite extraordinary erudition.

Thus, his favored position with both parents shielded him to a great degree from the necessity of dealing with "common sense" realities in the larger picture of his expectations of life, but he was also able to avoid dealing with many of the details because he had Stanislaus, who in their life together in Dublin served him in minor ways—exchanging books for him at the library, carrying messages to his brother's friends, borrowing money from them for Jim and repaying his debts[8]—faithfully, though not always cheerfully, as indicated by his complaint in his diary about his brother's borrowing his clothes: "It is really unfair when I need so little and keep my things so long, that that little should not be left with me. . . . Jim [has] my rain cloak and this morning wanted my hat" (1971, p. 30). For Stanislaus took care of things, even when there was little to take care of, and he notes in his diary that he is "considered hardier and healthier than either Jim or Charlie" because "I take care of myself and watch my body almost as carefully as I watch my mind" (p. 173).

Certainly James used this practical superiority of his brother's, for Stanislaus's Dublin service prefigured his major contribution of "common sense" and practical service in his brother's life after James left Dublin. Even in the period of James's first brief flight to Paris during the winter of 1902–1903, his letters home were sprinkled with imperatives directed to Stanislaus: "Tell Stannie to go to Eason's. . . ." "Tell Stannie to send me the December no of S. Stephen's and to write to the Unicorn Press. . . ." "Please ask Stannie to go to Hodges, Figgis . . . [and] order 'A Book of British Song'. . . ." "Tell Stannie to send me *at once* . . . my copy of Wagner's operas" and also take care of "a pawn-ticket for two books" (J. Joyce, 1966a, pp. 20, 21, 25).

By the time James left Dublin with Nora in October of 1904, this time for good, his mother was dead, the family in a shambles, and nineteen-year-old Stanislaus his only reliable source of support. So when the young couple arrived in Zurich to find that the expected position with Berlitz

---

[8] See S. Joyce, 1958, pp. 210–211; Curran, 1968, p. 75; letter of October 11, 1904, J. Joyce, 1966a, p. 66.

was nonexistent, it was Stannie who was directed to "make up" a pound and send it "before Saturday" (J. Joyce, 1966a, p. 66). During the year James was separated from his brother, living first in Pola and later in Trieste, the demands on Stannie were a persistent refrain in his letters to Dublin. Many were missions of the same order as those he had delegated to his brother in his letters from Paris: "Send BA and birth and medical certificates—also no of Irish Homestead containing my 'After the Race' " (p. 67). "Send on the key [to my trunk] at once" (p. 68). "Send on by *return* my music" (p. 74). "I send you the fourth story of 'Dubliners'—'Hallow Eve'—which I want you to offer at once to the Editor of the Irish Homestead" (p. 77). A new dimension of service is suggested in his request to his brother "to study by yourself or with Cosgrave some midwifery and embryology and send me the results of your study" (p. 73), a preface to his later announcement that "Nora has conceived, I think" (p. 75), but for the most part what he was requiring of Stanislaus was messenger service.

Along with the often peremptory requests to run this errand, carry that message, or send something *at once*, there is another kind of demand in the letters, a call on Stanislaus for a critical response to what Joyce is writing—the stories for *Dubliners* and chapters of the first version of his autobiographical novel as he completed them. On January 19, 1905, he demands more frequent letters, since "you know I have no-one to talk to," and a week later, complaining of the dullness of his brother's letter, he demands that Stanislaus "send criticisms of my chapters and story." On February 7 he writes that he expects "dilated reference" to a story Stanislaus has received and assures him that "your criticism of my novel is always interesting" (J. Joyce, 1966a, pp. 78–79). He tells his brother that he intends to dedicate *Dubliners* to him "because you seem to find the stories to your taste. Do you think they are good? . . . You must know I can't answer such questions in my worse than solitude" (p. 80).

"Such questions" of taste and value are, of course, answered by the exercise of the feeling function, which judges according to value—accepting or rejecting, liking or disliking, approving or disapproving—and in the "distribution of the functions" between the brothers, it is Stanislaus who carries the burden of this function. He writes in his diary that though "Jim says that my mind secretes bile and that the brilliancy of my mind is mechanical . . . he tells people also that my literary judgments are better than his own" (1971, p. 84), for, he continues, "of prose style I know really very little but my taste is, I think, good" (p. 85). His brother's taste, on the other hand, has been questioned more than once, though not by Stanislaus. His Triestine friend, Francini Bruni (1922), for example, found Joyce's "sense of values so paradoxical with respect to the work of others that you find him accepting equally eagles and rabbits, the sun and the mud puddle" (p. 34), while Dame Rebecca West (1928) began her essay on *Ulysses* with the insight that though "a writer of majestic genius" (p. 2), "Mr. James Joyce is a great man who is entirely without taste" (p. 3), an opinion echoed by a Paris friend of Joyce's: "He had not taste, only genius" (Ellmann, 1959, p. 443).

Stanislaus, who "always believed" in his brother (1958, p. 111), and "believed in genius" (p. 121), which, even as a boy in Dublin, he saw in him (1971, p. 17), put his taste, his willingness to make value judgments, at the service of his brother's art. Although James acknowledged this service only obliquely, referring to the "exaggerated notion you have of my indifference to the encouragement I receive" (J. Joyce, 1966a, p. 83), he almost literally cried out for his brother's response to his writing in his letters during the first year of his exile. "I must ask you to exert your imagination a little with regard to me" and "answer me promptly, money or no money," for "I am much obliged for your careful criticisms of my stories" (p. 106). By the end of September, he was lining up a job for Stanislaus in Trieste, but still sending him stories and complaining when Stanislaus, although copying them as directed, sent them back without criticism: "In addition to answering the letter now on its way you might send me a criticism" (p. 113). When one reads a long letter from Stanislaus (pp. 114–119), which combines careful answers to questions of fact, even-handed judgments about his brother's stories, and practical suggestions about selling his work, James's insistence on his response is understand-able. For in an important way, Stanislaus, with his judgments, completed the creative process in which his brother was engaged.

Although it is more difficult to document because it was more nearly unconscious on both sides, he also completed his brother's being-in-the-world, especially in the intimate world of the family, where it would appear that Stanislaus reacted and judged for both of them, compensating for James's habitual detachment with his own strong, judgmental re-sponses to the family situation and to individual family members. Since these brothers were in constant contact and apparently always talking, Stanislaus's judgments—communicated surely during their "endless dis-cussions" (S. Joyce, 1958, p. 131) and emphatically recorded in Stannie's diary, which his brother read—became a part of James's life as well, supplying a dimension in which he was notably deficient. The elder brother's inability or unwillingness to exercise his feeling function, to make value judgments, which became a defining characteristic of his art and a pervasive fact of his later life, was clearly evident in the Dublin years. If Stanislaus (1954) could identify "the judgment of irony" as "the only one my brother allowed himself" in his mature work (p. 49), the same refusal to make value judgments which defines irony was also characteristic of the young James Joyce's response to friends and even to family in Dublin.

Curran (1968) thus remembers that in any kind of serious discussion with his classmates at University College Joyce "did not debate. Question was turned aside by dark or gnomic answer," an evasive technique which was not given up in his maturity, for "the cryptic answer, the reticence on deep issues, which always seemed to me his dominant characteristic, never disappeared." And "irony, wry humour, grotesquerie, courteous evasion, or silence—each in turn was enlisted to build up an impregnable defence against intrusion on the inner sanctuary" (p. 35). Curran's interpretation of the Joycean irony as a defense is carried a significant step further by Giedion-Welcker (1973) when she speculates that joking for Joyce "meant release from all complications and it meant liberation from the burden of reality into the more sublime regions of the intellect and imagination" (p. 268).

Certainly James appears to have maintained a good-humored detachment from the realities of the Joyce household in Dublin, for, Stanislaus testifies (1958), "in the midst of all-pervading squalor and disintegration" (p. 85), his brother, "far less depressed by our conditions at home than I was," was "never subject to the moodiness or plain tantrums" which tormented the younger brother. Instead, he "took things as they came with good-humoured, almost gay indifference" (p. 242). Even in matters which directly involved him he maintained an "unaffected imperturbability" which suggested that "he might have been assisting at a badly rehearsed comedy that did not concern him." Indeed, the "cold lucid indifference" which Joyce later attributed to Stephen Dedalus in *A Portrait*, Stanislaus says, "seemed never to forsake him" (p. 71). When their mother's confessor accused Jim of cowardice in leaving his family "to its fate" when so much had been expected of him as the eldest, it was not Jim who reacted "with violent and bitter curses," but Stannie. "He said nothing," Stanislaus remembers. "It was I that spoke" (pp. 230–231).

It is Stanislaus who speaks and judges in his diary, where indeed he observes that the biblical injunction to "judge not" is "peddling, winking cowardice. Judge constantly, by all means, without fear and without favour, and as you hope to know yourself, apply your judgments to yourself." This he does, for "I consider it as cowardly not to condemn vice in others because we ourselves are vicious, as it is jealous not to appraise virtue in others because we wish ourselves to shine" (1971, p. 83). The *Dublin*

Diary covers the period following his mother's death in August of 1903, and in a house which "is and always has been intolerable with bickering, quarrelling and scurrillity" (p. 17); in which the three brothers take turns staying home to protect their sisters from their father's drunken attacks and Stannie does "most of the duty" (p. 24), it is not surprising that he has "moods constantly recurring in which I loathe everything and everyone near me," when "this house seems to be rotten, useless and decaying, like the hollow tooth I have my tongue in" (p. 92).

The dominant tone in the diary entries is understandably negative, though there is an occasional note of happiness to justify Stanislaus's reminder to his brother in later years that "in these same surroundings that you describe [in *Ulysses*] I have not rarely been penetrated by a keen sense of happiness" (J. Joyce, 1966b, p. 104). He notes, for example, being "quietly, observantly happy" on a day when "we have had very little food—no meal at all in fact" (S. Joyce, 1971, p. 69) and admits on another day that "I feel exhilarated sometimes without cause" (p. 77), as any nineteen-year-old might. But there was little cause for happiness, and the expressions of feeling are rejecting rather than accepting, disliking rather than liking, disapproving rather than approving.

"Hate" and "loathe" are favorite verbs, with quite a range of objects, impersonal and personal. "I hate the commonplace. I was born amongst it; I belong to it, body and blood. Therefore I hate it" (p. 110). Defining his relationship to his family as "an intimate but repugnant dependence," he asks himself, "Do I, then hate all my family?" (p. 175). Of his elder brother, he writes: "I hate to see Jim limp and pale, with shadows under his watery eyes, loose wet lips, and dank hair. I hate to see him . . . swallowing spittle in his mouth and talking in an exhausted husky voice, as if to show how well he can act when drunk" (p. 101). He "loathes" the memory of his "silly confessions," including in his loathing, himself, the priest, and "his little box, his sinnery" (pp. 102–103). But most troubling of all, "I loathe my father. I loathe him because he is himself, and I loathe him because he is Irish" (p. 23).

This feeling, modified variously in its expression and examined persistently for its implications, is a leitmotif of the young man's diary, in which he presents a powerfully documented indictment against John Stanislaus Joyce, Sr., the "Pappie" of the diary, whose namesake he is. Stanislaus tells himself that he should remember that Pappie, this "crazy drunkard," whose only concern for his children is expressed in "a peculiar sense of duty arising out of his worship of respectability" (p. 6), "is my father" (p. 15). But though he admits that "I admire those who treat their fathers with respect" (p. 135), he is nevertheless "better pleased with myself when I treat him with dislike" (p. 79). And he is "happier, happier, happier, freer and better without [Pappie's] liking," an idea which is "repugnant" to him (p. 168).

His pronouncement that he "loathes" his father is later modified to "I have absolutely no liking for him" (p. 75). And his judgment that "I have not a particle of original affection for him" is tempered in the interest of fairness with his recognition of "just a particle of admiration for a character of vitality and a judgment which is occasionally strange and his own" (p. 153). But Stanislaus's dislike for his father is a constant of his youthful diary and indeed remained a constant of his long life, an "antipathy" which, he wrote in his maturity, "seemed to have been born with me" (1958, p. 49). In the diary he presents a bill of particulars which justifies his antipathy and deepens it to condemnation.

"Domineering and quarrelsome" (p. 5), "lying and hypocritical," Pappie is "spiteful like all drunkards who are thwarted, and invents the most cowardly insults that a scandalous mind and a naturally derisive tongue can suggest" (p. 6), calling "all his children bastards as a habit" (p. 7), and going much further in personalizing his abuse as he taunts them "with their deformities. 'Ye dirty pissabed, ye bloody-looking crooked-eyed son of a bitch. Ye ugly bloody cornerboy, you've a mouth like a bloody nigger.' 'Ye black-looking mulatto. You were black the day you were born, ye bitch. Ye bloody, gummy toothless bitch. I'll get ye a set of teeth, won't I . . .' " (p. 28). Remembering in one entry that he has written of the "aggressive" injustice of his father's mind, Stanislaus reminds himself that "to call Pappie's mind unjust is as distinct a euphemism as to call a drunken fishwoman's abuse unladylike" (p. 79). To be sure, when John Stanislaus, Sr., is sober, he is "pleasant spoken," but "this phase is regrettably rare and of short duration. It comes at times of dire poverty and does not last till bedtime" (p. 7).

Though Stanislaus acknowledges that his father "has not been able to be a senseless bully," he points out that "Pappie supports us indifferently, knows practically nothing about us, shows us a low example, treats those who let him with the highest moral brutality" (p. 71). In the final entry in the diary Stanislaus presents an itemized indictment against his father, which, he writes, is "somewhat understated," for " 'moral brutality' does not convey to a stranger mind the eternity of abuse that in memory impinges monotonously on my accustomed ear at will" (p. 176). He accuses his father of undermining his children's health, handicapping their chances in life, causing his wife's "unhealth, unhappiness, weakening mind, and death," being indirectly responsible for the death of Georgie Joyce before he was fifteen, and "pulling down his children's character as he sinks lower" (pp. 175–176). The final scene of the diary features Pappie, returning home drunk and penniless to a family who have had nothing to eat for fourteen hours: "This is a true portrait of my progenitor: the leading one a dance and then the disappointing, baffling, baulking and turning up drunk—the business of breaking hearts" (p. 178).

Thus Stanislaus passes judgment on the man who was also James Joyce's progenitor and the model for the portrait of Simon Dedalus in the autobiographical fiction, "an effective and amusing literary creation," as Stanislaus (1958) himself recognized (p. 50), who is, like the rest of the world of *Ulysses*, exempt from judgment. At first glance, we might agree with George Healey, the editor of Stanislaus's *Diary*, that "it is hard to believe that the same man, the same father, stands behind both James's portrayal of Simon Dedalus and Stanislaus's portrayal of 'Pappie' " (S. Joyce, 1971, p. vii). And yet there is nothing in the portrait of Simon which really contradicts the reality described by Stanislaus.

In fact, if we look at the one scene in *Ulysses* in which Simon is shown as a father—his encounter with Dilly in "Wandering Rocks" (J. Joyce, 1922, pp. 237–239)—the whole substance of Stannie's indictment is acted out, with Simon taunting his daughter for her poor posture and publicly mimicking her; delivering an abbreviated tirade against his daughters, "insolent pack of little bitches"; and absolutely refusing to provide for his family, whose near-starvation has been dramatized pages earlier (pp. 226–227). Simon, like Pappie, is in "the business of breaking hearts," but the nonjudgmental perspective of the son-author is reinforced by the daughter in the fictional scene itself, who grins at Simon as he mocks her need and says, "You're very funny" (p. 238). He is. Even though the "battered wreck in whom even the wish to live carefree has become a vague memory," which Stanislaus (1958) could see in his brother's portrait of Simon (p. 50), may exist by implication in the fiction, what the author explicitly delivers to the reader is an Irishman of appealing energy with marvelous lines to speak. For "to his latest days," Curran (1968) says, "Joyce, like his sisters, spoke of the old man with the same despairing, humorous affection and appreciation" (p. 70).

It may indeed be true, as his sister Eileen claimed, that "Jim understood my Father even better than my Mother did. He never blamed him like the others used to," especially Stannie, who "was hard on my Father" (Curtayne, 1963, p. 44), and who thus relieved his brother of the obligation to judge. Though he did not judge, James nevertheless saw himself threatened by his father's demands in ways that never occurred to his younger brother. Stanislaus's blame was straightforward, a matter of circumstances and deeds and relationships, and he could identify his reason for disliking

Pappie as "the same reason that I do not like my country, because he has surrounded me with unhappiness and opposition from my youth continually" (1971, p. 155). This is an extravert's reason. But for his introverted brother, the problem of his father, like the problem of his country, for that matter, is related primarily to his ego; his judgment about both father and country is based, not on any assignment of value or on any empirically provable effect on his life, but on a complicated conceptualized intuition about their role in the shaping of his ego and their intentions to subject it to their own purposes.

On the one hand, as Stephen Dedalus declares to Davin in *A Portrait*, "This race and this country and this life produced me. . . . I shall express myself as I am" (J. Joyce, 1916, p. 203). The corollary of this is, as Stephen tells Bloom in *Ulysses*, "Ireland must be important because it belongs to me" (J. Joyce, 1922, p. 645), because, that is, it is an essential part of "myself as I am." The same logic obviously applies to his father; as Stanislaus points out in his diary and repeats in *My Brother's Keeper*, "Honouring one's father is a subtle way of honouring oneself" (1971, p. 135; 1958, p. 237). The young Stanislaus contrasts his own attitude toward his father with Jim's professions of respect, at least "amongst strangers" (1971, p. 152), and after his brother's death he insisted that James's "attachment to his father" remained always "one of the dominant motives in his character," explaining it in part by James's absence at school in his early years, so that he knew only "the more amiable side of my father's character, and the image of him formed in those years was never to be effaced" (S. Joyce, 1958, p. 57). Thus, "neither brawling in the home, nor tireless political ranting to cronies, nor the near imbecility of tipsiness ever spoiled his accord with his father" (p. 59). And "the two dominant passions of my brother's life were to be love of father and of fatherland" (p. 238).

But James Joyce, like his autobiographical hero Stephen Dedalus, would not serve either, a refusal which Stephen spells out to Cranly in *A Portrait*: "I will not serve that in which I no longer believe, whether it call itself my home, my fatherland, or my church." Repeating his determination to express himself "as freely as I can and as wholly as I can," he lists the now famous items in his arsenal of defense: "silence, exile, and cunning" (J. Joyce, 1916, p. 247). The father is not separated out as a threat to Stephen's freedom in *A Portrait*, but in *Stephen Hero*, where Joyce explicitly describes the family situation which is only implicit in *A Portrait*, it is the father who represents "the tyranny of the home" (J. Joyce, 1944, p. 126).

This "tyranny" is directly connected with his father's intention to shift "the burden of responsibility" for his family onto "his eldest son's shoulders" (p. 109), an intention which was recognizable in Joyce's own father and which perhaps explains Stanislaus's observation that Pappie "represents feudalism" to Jim (1971, p. 55). For primogeniture works both ways; if James, as the eldest, had been given more than the others, more was in turn expected of him. Curran (1968) points out that "with a father who even in middle years had thrown over his responsibility for a numerous family and built all his hopes for himself and them on his eldest son—the situation was quite impossible," for "Joyce was unfitted for that burden" (p. 68).

And Joyce refused it. First he removed himself through silence, as Stanislaus reveals in his diary and as Joyce himself underlines in his fictional representation of his situation in *Stephen Hero*, where the "son's distaste for responsibility" (p. 110), likened to his father's own, is communicated at first only through his "silence during the domestic battles," which, however, his father rightly comes to interpret as "a covert menace against castellar rights" (p. 111). Later, as a sort of prelude to exile, Stephen begins to avoid his father "sedulously because he now regarded his father's presumptions as the most deadly part of a tyranny, internal and external, which he determined to combat" (p. 209). For though Stephen maintains "a studious demeanour" toward his parents, he is willing to serve them only in ways that are not "spiritually dangerous" to him, which, since he has "cultivated an indpendence of the soul which could brook very few subjections," effectively "nullifie[s] his charity" (p. 111).

This insistence on "independence of soul," this typically introverted vision of the object, the relationship, as a threat to the ego, is demonstrably Joyce's own, coexisting, however, with a comparably strong "sense of filial honour," which Stanislaus (1971) found "quite humoursome" (p. 55), and which clearly involved James in an existential contradiction. For neither of these ideas had an existential outlet. In practical terms James was always dependent on others; in Dublin, Stanislaus (1971) notes, "he lives on borrowing and favours" (p. 55), as later he would live on Stanislaus and still later depend on Harriet Shaw Weaver and a shifting cadre of surrogates for Stanislaus. As for his "filial honour," there was no real possibility of his implementing it, since its object was quite as self-centered and opportunistic as he was.

His sister Eileen, noting that their father "never took much interest in us—he lived his own kind of life," indicates also that this lack of interest extended even to the works of the favored eldest son, which "he never spoke of" and in fact never read. "The bond between Jim and Pappy," Eileen concludes, "was the love between father and son. Nothing that happened could change it" (Curtayne, 1963, p. 44), perhaps because this bond, one of the greatest ideas we know, was just that for both these Joyces—an extraordinarily powerful idea, which had little to do with what happened.

Like his father before him, Joyce had a strong conceptual reverence for family; his declaration to his sister Eva when his son was born that "the most important thing that can happen to a man is the birth of a child" (Ellmann, 1959, p. 212) was reiterated to Arthur Power (1974) when his grandson was born: "It is the most important thing there is" (p. 110). All his life he "set great store" upon the set of "glazed and wooden" family portraits, "furniture pictures," according to Stanislaus (1958), which were his father's "credentials" and his own (p. 122). Hanging on the walls of Joyce's apartment, they testified, as Francini Bruni (1922) saw it, to his pride in his origins. For "Joyce is a great gentleman, a born gentleman . . . from a very noble family in the West of Ireland, a region that bears the name of his ancestors—the Joyce Country. He stinks of the gentleman a mile away, even when he is stinking drunk" (p. 33).

Despite his theoretical pride in family and his conceptualized attachment to his father, his existential relationship with his father was the negative one of avoidance. Thus, though Gillet (1941), in an extended, largely hypothetical, analysis of this father-son relationship, concludes that the "peculiar rapport with his father" was "the central factor in Joyce's life" (p. 190), he also notes that when he visited Ireland, Joyce, who sent various messages to friends through Gillet, gave him no message for his father (p. 188). And though Joyce acknowledged in a letter to T.S. Eliot his "grief and remorse" at the time of his father's death for his own failure to visit him, he admitted that "an instinct which I believed in held me back from going, much as I longed to" (J. Joyce, 1957, p. 311). Similarly, writing to Ezra Pound of his father's death as "a great blow to me," he also wrote that "in spite of my own deep feeling for him I never dared to trust myself into the power of my enemies" (J. Joyce, 1966b, p. 240).

This wariness need not refer directly to the "tyranny" of his father, which he had escaped through exile, and it does not in all probability consciously include his father, but surely, not very far below the surface, the fear of the father motivates these expressions of mistrust. At no time, though, does James Joyce's sense of the paternal threat to his personhood translate into any kind of negative judgment of this man whom his younger brother saw as such a destructive force in the Joyce children's lives. This he left to Stanislaus, who exercised his feeling function and made value judgments as a matter of course, just as through the exercise of his superior sensation function he compensated for James's deficient sense of reality.

But in these early years, which set the pattern for the Joyce brothers' lives, the compensatory contribution inherent in the fraternal relationship was by no means completely one-sided. For Stanislaus, in his conscious attempt to model his life on James's, opened himself to significant pressures for inward growth. Imitation of an elder brother seems hardly extraordinary as a family phenomenon, especially when an observer considers the flawed model provided by the Joyces' father, but this particular elder brother was himself extraordinary. He appears, in fact, to have produced on others an effect which is reminiscent of Jung's comments about "mana personalities" (1958), which, because of a special access to the unconscious, "involuntarily" produce "the kind of effect which the primitives call 'mana,' " that is, "an unintentional influence on the unconscious of others, a sort of unconscious prestige" (p. 303).

James Joyce did have such an effect on many besides his younger brother, which was, even to them, oddly inexplicable. Andreasen (1973) may explain the truly remarkable fact that "so many people were drawn to admire and assist him although they received little in return except the opportunity to associate with him" as "a tribute to his literary genius" (p. 70), but it appeared to those who met him as something more than this. For what the young Stanislaus (1971) saw as his brother's being "so much alive" that even his idleness was "of more importance" than the work of others (pp. 141, 146) is surely akin to an admiring young Frenchman's perception that Joyce, who "gave the strongest impression of human genius he had ever encountered," was able "to talk of nothing and still seem a genius" (Ellmann, 1959, p. 535). This same quality of an unexplainable power is conveyed by the observation of one of his many ophthamologists that Joyce was "a strange fellow," but "a *big boss* [using the American phrase] just the same" (p. 550), as it is by Archibald MacLeish's "sense of something vivid and maybe dangerous" under Joyce's apparent shyness, "a hard, strong actuality that, if not greatness, was at least something you were always conscious of" (p. 611).

This was the personality—as a young man, to be sure, but even then one who, his friend Gogarty (1941) remembered, "expected to be taken blindly at an undisclosed but apparently unlimited valuation" (p. 16)—who represented for Stanislaus Joyce (1971) "the individual life that has influenced me most" (p. 51). The threat of being swallowed up in such a relationship is not surprisingly very real to Stanislaus, and his diary reveals the persistence of his self-questioning about the integrity of his own identity. Nor is this exclusively a question of inner uncertainty of this identity, though this troubles him as it does most adolescents; but for Stanislaus the question is compounded by an uncertainty about making any independent impression at all upon the outer world. For in the small world of Dublin and the even smaller world of the Joyce family, there appear to have been almost no mirrors to give him a reflection of himself which was not blurred by the dominant image of his brother.

"We are, of course, constantly compared in their minds," Stanislaus writes (1971, p. 61). "Everybody who knows us is anxious to accuse me of aping Jim" (p. 93), beginning indeed with their father, who, Stanislaus (1958) reported, "called me my brother's jackal," alternating this with the taunt that "I gave no light of my own, but that I shone with borrowed light like the moon" (p. 176). Gogarty's opinion, obviously quoted to him by his brother, that he is "a 'washed-out imitation of Jim' " (1971, p. 93), Stanislaus assumes is only a particularly unkind statement of a general view among Jim's friends, among whom he was "dubiously accepted . . . as my brother's rather taciturn henchman" (1958, p. 176; cf. Curran, 1968, p. 75).

The close relationship between the brothers thus involved the younger in a continuing examination of the conflict it represented between the promise of enlargement of his world—"my intimacy with Jim brings me [sic] in ways I like" (S. Joyce, 1971, p. 72)—and the threat of diminution of his self-esteem in the face of his brother's "frankly contemptuous" attitude toward him (p. 76). The diary reveals a persistent debate with himself about the nature of his feelings for his brother. An early declaration that "there was never any friendship for Jim in my relations with him for there was never any real trust" (p. 35) is countered by his later recognition of "an appreciation in Jim of what I myself really admire and wish for most," followed, however, by the underlined statement: *"I think I may safely say I do not like Jim"* (p. 50). This judgment he partially retracts later, only to reaffirm the basic ambivalence of his feeling. Though "wrong" in "saying that I dislike Jim," he still has "no liking for him but I see that his life is interesting" (p. 75).

In the course of his attempts to evaluate his intensely ambivalent feelings about his brother, he produces an insight which defines and illuminates the role Jim played in his own development and self-definition. "Now that I think of it," he writes, "I suggest I may have been irritated by the demands which, quite unknown to me, Jim's presence made on my character" (pp. 143–144). These demands, like the proverbial sand for the oyster's pearl, irritated the younger brother productively, forcing him to grow. In terms of the Jungian functions, Stanislaus's "envy" of what he calls his brother's "state of mind" (p. 57) forced him when quite young to develop not just one auxiliary function but two. That is, in addition to the feeling function, through which he helped to compensate for his brother's inferior feeling function, he also developed the thinking function, dominant in his brother Jim.

Despite his characterization of himself and his brother as "distrustful and mutually so little affectionate," Stanislaus recognizes in his diary that his interest in Jim is "chronic" and that he has habitually tried "to live Jim's intellectual life as well as my own" (p. 144). Certainly such a participation in the intellectual life of James Joyce represented a push for growth in this young man who felt himself lacking in "strong intellectual curiosity" and indeed in "intellect" (p. 32). For Stanislaus, who observes in his diary "how cumbrously my brain works in its shell" (p. 173), was aspiring to share the intellectual life of a man who, "in the quality of pure intellect," Mary Colum wrote in her review of *Ulysses* (1922), "is probably unsurpassed by any living writer" (p. 334). Through his somewhat contradictory identification with his brother, Stanislaus used the demands of James's presence for his own growth, developing both feeling and thinking to a point of real service to his dominant sensation function and consequently becoming a more balanced, more integrated person than he could otherwise have been.

This reciprocal psychic compensation between James and Stanislaus, of course, could not have been the only division of the functions operating in the large Joyce family, although it seems probable that for Stanislaus it was more nearly exclusively determining than for James. For James's position as favorite, not only with his parents, but also with his six sisters (S. Joyce, 1958, pp. 59, 237), made it practicable for him to remain more one-sided than the others and to depend on other family members to take on the burden of solving his function problem, serving him where he was deficient.

Chief among those who gave a sense of completeness to this first-born son was his mother, who, Stanislaus (1941) wrote, had been "the companion of his boyhood devotions, when he was very religious" and, before resigning herself to his "change of belief," had entered into "bitter and painful conflict" with him (p. 491), thus giving him a personal focus for his opposition to the Church. At the same time, however, she served him faithfully in practical ways and felt for him wholeheartedly; her letters to this son during his brief stay in Paris in 1902 and 1903 (J. Joyce, 1966a, pp. 20–41) fully support his sister Eileen's judgment that he "completely depended on her" (Curtayne, 1963, p. 43) and testify also to her complete dependability. She thus provided both unwavering support and unwavering (but somewhat muted) opposition, a contradictory combination which later devolved on Stanislaus, though the opposition from Stanislaus focused on James's duty to his artistic vocation rather than to the Church.

If James depended all his life on the generosity of others simply to survive, it was also true, as Stanislaus (1941) asserted, that "opposition was necessary to Joyce; it was breath to his nostrils" (p. 513). This opposition apparently needed to be personalized; as his sister said about his need for support, "he had to have someone" (Curtayne, 1963, p. 44), and eventually it would take both Nora Barnacle and Stanislaus to fill the void in James's psychic economy left by the death of his mother.

Though the pragmatic scheme of distributing the functions among family members may indeed, as Franz (1971) points out, result in "vital groups which function well," the individual family members "get into trouble when the group falls apart" (p. 4), as the Joyce family did after the mother's death. In this period of disarray, James appears to have attempted to work out a compensatory adjustment on his own, reaching for the tie to reality and the flesh, which his mother had evidently represented for him,[9] and which Nora would later provide, through a determination "to live," in which Stanislaus (1971) found "something experimental, something aesthetical," and, more than that, a threat to his brother's artistic vocation (pp. 51–52). Indeed, he notes that "Jim says he is not an artist. I think he lives on the excitement of events" (p. 14). In *My Brother's Keeper* he quotes his brother as saying, "I don't care if I never write another line. I want to live" (p. 248). At any rate, during this "interval of loose living," which perfectly exemplified the typically distorted and inappropriate manifestation of an inferior sensation function, James's way of life was, as Curran (1968) remembers it, "startling, being lived openly and in defiance of convention, and . . . in plain contradiction with his life before and after" (p. 66).

For this brief interval, then, James temporarily abandoned a reliance on convention which was characteristic of his behavior during most of his life, and which was most immediately obvious to observers in his extreme politeness, which his brother early saw as "obviously and distressingly assumed" (S. Joyce, 1971, p. 101) and which T.S. Eliot saw as a mask for arrogance (Ellmann, 1959, p. 509). But for Paul Léon (1942), Joyce's "exquisite politeness" and "outward observance of conventions" were a defense, part of his "tendency to take infinite precautions" to distance himself from others (p. 288). Ellmann (1959) concludes that "politeness became one of Joyce's principal social defenses" (p. 509). The many descriptions of this peculiar politeness of Joyce's, his "great and watchful courtesy" (Curran, 1968, p. 88), make it recognizable as the typical "feeling mask (persona) of politeness and mannered consideration" which

[9] See Stephen's comments in *Ulysses* on "*amor matris*" as "the only true thing in life" (J. Joyce, 1922, pp. 27–28, 207) and see Kimball, 1976, p. 377, for the significance of the tie to the mother.

Hillman (1971) identifies as a common substitute for a feeling function which cannot be brought to consciousness. Though Hillman points out that "involvement with a man who is bound in this way leaves the impression that he is 'not really there' " (p. 115), an impression which the mature Joyce did leave with many, still the mask is a workable defense for someone who cannot handle feeling. During this time, which is the time dramatized by *Ulysses*, the young Joyce appeared to be without workable defenses.

He found in Nora Barnacle, ten months after his mother's death, a life partner who was strong where he was weak, for she appears to have been a clear opposite to Joyce himself, with both an unusual acceptance of sensuality, as evidenced by the letters they exchanged in 1909 (J. Joyce, 1975, pp. 157–196) and also a highly developed feeling function. According to Budgen's description (1934), "Her judgments of men and things were swift and forthright and proceeded from a scale of values entirely personal, unimitated, unmodified" (p. 36). With Nora to complete him, Joyce could feel whole enough to leave the family structure he had grown up with.

This new two-against-the-world structure was not workable for long. For if Joyce had found the "someone" he had to have in Nora—and he truly had—still, he was used to having many, and with his intuitive understanding of "the inherent potentialities in things," he sensed this and re-created at least a remnant of his family in Trieste, "the city," he reminded Stanislaus during one of their many quarrels, "discovered by my courage . . . whither you and [Eva and Eileen Joyce] came in obedience to my summons" (J. Joyce, 1966a, p. 288). Thus in 1905 he summoned Stanislaus, who accepted the call "with my eyes open," knowing that "he wanted me to remain and second him in his struggle" (Rodgers, 1972, p. 40).

The obligations that went with that second were very nearly total, including, as Ellmann (1959) reports it, James's appropriation of his brother's trousers and his salary, which he then squandered along with his own (p. 221). Along with this more or less involuntary support, Stanislaus, a boy of twenty, who "acted forty-five" (p. 220), also took on the man-sized job of curbing his brother's drinking. And when, in July of 1906, James escaped his younger brother's surveillance by taking a bank job in Rome, there was no real surcease for Stanislaus as long as mail and telegraph service operated, for James's demands for money, as well as for sympathy in his struggle with Grant Richards over the *Dubliners* stories, were constant (J. Joyce, 1966a, pp. 144–220), ending only with his wire of March 7, 1907: "arrive eight get room" (p. 220). Indeed, the quality of the relationship between the brothers during the decade of their life together in Trieste is epitomized by Jim's blithe reply to Stannie's furious questioning about how his brother planned to live when he arrived in Trieste from Rome, against Stanislaus's advice, with no money, no place to live, and no assured means of support: "Well, then, I have you" (Ellman, 1959, p. 265).

Certainly Stanislaus was the mainstay financially during the Trieste years, although James also added two of his sisters, Eva and Eileen, to the household, returning with them from a trip to Dublin in 1910, because, his sister Eva felt, "He really wanted to have as many members of the family with him out there as he could possibly manage" (Rodgers, 1972, p. 40). Though it was Stanislaus who had to come up with the money for passage for the family group (J. Joyce, 1966a, pp. 243, 260, 278), it was Jim who, in Eileen's eyes, "took me out there" and "was like a father to us," seeing to Eva's tonsils and buying both new clothes for the journey (Curtayne, 1963, p. 44). Although Eva returned to Dublin the following year, Eileen remained as a part of the household, doing "most of the housekeeping and [taking] care of Jim's two children, Giorgio and Lucia" until her marriage in 1915 (Curtayne, 1963, p. 45).

For Eileen the six years she spent in this stormy, often squalid household were "the happiest years of my life," and they appear to have been happy years for her brother Jim as well. He was, of course, in constant conflict with Stanislaus, who, Eileen said, since he was providing most of the housekeeping money, "used to get mad at Jim's extravagance and was always preaching economy" (Curtayne, 1963, p. 45). While the tensions between them made Stanislaus "miserable," as might be expected of an extravert with his sensitivity to relationships, "they made James comfortable" (Ellmann, 1959, p. 323), providing the opposition which was essential to his well-being.

This opposition was expressed not only against Jim's extravagance, which Stanislaus (1958) said "was like a hair-shirt during all our life together" (p. 231), but also against his drinking, which Stanislaus always saw as a direct threat to his artistic productivity. Thus this younger brother, forced by his brother's assumption of the Prodigal Son's role into the opposing role of Elder Brother, was constantly preaching and often physically enforcing temperance, administering a frequent "tongue-lashing or even a beating" (Ellmann, 1959, p. 277) to his brother. But his attempt to "break him" of his "intemperate habits" succeeded, for, Stanislaus (1941) writes, Joyce "became abstemious again" (p. 507).

Although "such victories are not won without bitterness," he justifies his efforts with a listing of the fruits of James's "first years of sobriety," which included *Chamber Music*, most of *Dubliners*, all of the rewritten

Portrait, and "a considerable part" of *Ulysses*. "And that," Stanislaus concludes, "is enough for me" (pp. 507–508). It is a great deal, and the list embraces all of Joyce's work which represented a satisfaction of Stanislaus's ambition for his brother as an artist, since his rejection of *Finnegans Wake* was so absolute that when his brother offered him a copy at the time of its publication, Stanislaus refused it (S. Joyce, 1941, p. 514).

This realization of his acknowledged "vicarious ambition" (S. Joyce, 1958, p. 120), considerable as the achievement is, represents by no means all that Stanislaus gained from his service to his brother in Trieste, which obviously cost him so much. For one thing, it can be assumed that as he responded to the practical demands which James made on his own dominant *fonction du réel*, he surely became more resourceful and knowledgeable than he would otherwise have needed to be. He also benefited directly and tangibly from his brother's dominant intuitive function, his sense of the inherent possibilities in situations, so that the course of his life was radically and expansively changed because of his brother's demands. When Fifield (1967) in his interview with Professor Stanislaus Joyce speculated that but for his elder brother "he would be simply an obscure Irish professor living in Trieste" (p. 70), he surely understated the effect of this elder brother. The fact is, melodramatic as it sounds in James's letter to Stanislaus, Trieste, which became the younger brother's permanent home, *was* discovered for the Joyces—all of them—through James's "courage," and he *had* summoned his brother there. If it had not been for James Joyce's sense of possibilities, coupled with his crucial need for Stanislaus's sense of the real, Stanislaus would never have been in Trieste, and it seems wildly improbable that he would have become a professor at all. One cannot imagine its happening in Dublin.

The relationship between the brothers thus achieved, because of the inherent, compensatory balance of needs and contributions of each, an odd, almost unconscious reciprocity, sustaining both brothers and preparing them in quite different ways for the separation which came in 1915. Stanislaus was arrested in January and interned for the duration of the war, while James left Trieste for Zurich in June, a separation which for all practical purposes marked the dissolution of this reciprocal relationship. By 1915, seconded in his struggle as he had been by Stanislaus, James had established his artistic direction and even the beginnings of a rationale of greatness which could attract a succession of surrogates for Stanislaus in solving the practical problems of his daily life. The services which the younger had performed, consciously and unconsciously, were never again combined in one person. Even before the brothers separated,

James had been discovered by Ezra Pound and was sliding under the wing of Harriet Shaw Weaver, whose generosity became a lifelong resource.

As for Stanislaus, just turned thirty, the age at which he had prophesied in his diary that he would "be myself" (S. Joyce, 1971, p. 33), he was apparently now equipped to fulfill the prophecy. The four years he spent in various camps firmed up the resolve he had made so many years ago in Dublin, and not yet managed to carry through, "not to put myself anymore in the way of Jim's rudenesses" (p. 76), which continued during the separation. For while Jim was in Zurich moving toward international recognition, accompanied by financial support, Stanislaus, in one or another internment camp, felt himself ignored and all but forgotten. His brother, he complained to Nora in 1916, had written him "nothing but short cards in German for the last year and a half."[10] Stanislaus should perhaps have been prepared for this kind of neglect, since he had himself noted in his diary that "at any crisis of his life, in any times of importance, in times when he has money and notoriety, Jim's life separates from mine. When these have passed after a while, we seem to come together again" (1971, p. 59). But this separation was different; Stanislaus (1941) felt his brother "had let me down" (p. 511), and when the war passed, they did not come together again.

James did move his family back to Trieste late in 1919, when the major subsidy from Edith Rockefeller McCormick was withdrawn (Ellmann, 1959, pp. 481–483), but Stanislaus had become a separate person with a separate life. He had warned his brother of his abdication in a rather bitter letter in May, notifying James that he had vacated the Trieste apartment which Joyce kept through the war:

> Some eight years ago I took the quarter for you, moved in and paid the first rent. Now I have paid the last rent for you and moved out. The packing up and moving out of a flat ankle-deep in dust has been a week's dirty work for Frank and Eileen [Joyce's sister and her husband]. It has cost me nearly three hundred lire. I have just emerged from four years of hunger and squalor, and am trying to get on my feet again. Do you think you can give me a rest? [J. Joyce, 1966a, p. 443]

The final question was in effect a declaration of intent. For "to be my brother's keeper," he later wrote, "was a whole-time job and very ex-

---

[10] Letter of July 30, 1916, to Nora, in the Cornell Joyce Collection, Cornell University. Cited with permission of Cornell University Library.

hausting," and "I had not the energy to tackle him again" (S. Joyce, 1949, p. 897). And he did not.

Thus within three months of Joyce's return he was trying to lure Frank Budgen to Trieste, in much the same way he had summoned his brother fifteen years before, promising that there would be work and complaining that there was "not a soul to talk to about Bloom," for "my brother . . . thinks it a joke, besides he was four years in internment, has a devil of a lot to do and likes a gay elegant life in his own set" (J. Joyce, 1957, p. 134). But Budgen did not come, and in July, James and his family left Trieste for Paris and Ezra Pound. Joyce formally marked the finality of this parting in a footnote which he added to Gorman's biography: "The relations between the brothers practically end here" (Ellmann, 1959, p. 496).

Certainly the continuity of the relationship, broken by the wartime separation, was never resumed. The brothers met only three times in the next twenty years, and correspondence between them was sporadic. Stanislaus took over his brother's position at the University and married at forty-three. James finished *Ulysses* and turned to *Finnegans Wake*, making sure that Stanislaus received copies of his work as it was produced, to which Stanislaus responded with unwaveringly harsh criticism, taking, he said, "so little pleasure" in what he had to say that "I cannot bring myself to write to you" (J. Joyce, 1966b, p. 103). His criticism appeared to make no difference to Joyce, who in the interval between the two wars was surrounded by an ever-increasing number of others at an ever-increasing personal distance from him, who provided most of the services Stanislaus had formerly taken care of. Stanislaus did indeed disappear as a significant presence in his brother's life.

With Joyce's death in 1941, however, he again took up his role as representative for his brother and became in this way a writer, although his entire output was as a brother about a brother. Because of his solid grasp of the real, his reliable memory, and his habit of recording facts and feelings, his writing helped significantly to make possible a trustworthy biography of his legendary brother, which, in turn, since Joyce's writing is so connected with the facts of his life, has added an important dimension to the understanding of his works. The same qualities which Stanislaus brought to the recording of his brother's life also underlie the direct contribution he made to the work itself.

For during the years when his life was in effect combined with his brother's, Stanislaus inevitably contributed heavily to the literal substratum of the work through his diaries, letters, and daily conversations with his brother, combined with his role as a continuously available audience and a continuously vocal critic of the work in progress—"probably his harshest critic," he says (S. Joyce, 1949, p. 897). Specific instances of Joyce's appropriation of material from his brother have been identified by Stanislaus and others. But these isolated, provable instances of appropriation do not compare in significance with the ongoing process they exemplify. It was during these years that Stanislaus provided his artist-brother with a continuing reflection of the outer world of facts and things and people in relationship, which Stanislaus in his extraverted fashion was so embroiled with and which complemented Joyce's own sure grasp of the inner reality he was determined to exploit. Because this was his brother's view of the external reality of his own life, and because his fiction was autobiographical in intent, the material was perfectly suited to his artistic purposes.

This is particularly true of Stanislaus's portrait of Jim in the *Dublin Diary*, which provides the solid external reality of the young artist who appears as Stephen Dedalus in *A Portrait* and *Ulysses*. In his carefully detailed analysis of the effect produced by Jim on others, most notably himself, he could give Joyce the other side of the character which the artist himself knew so well from inside; he could give him his shadow, himself seen from the outside, with a completeness and a truth otherwise inaccessible to him, for, as Jung (1921) points out, "the introvert cannot possibly know or imagine how he appears to his opposite type unless he allows the extravert to tell him to his face" (p. 164).

We really cannot know, of course, the extent of Joyce's use of Stanislaus's portrait of Jim or any of the other material provided by Stanislaus, nor can we know the degree of consciousness with which he used it. Furthermore, we cannot with certainty judge the effectiveness of Stanislaus's conscious influence, "sometimes amounting to pressure," which, he says, was "always deliberately towards the beaten track, because I felt that he ought not to leave it too easily" (S. Joyce, 1958, p. 121). What we do know is that the sense of the real, the fact, the person placed in an identifiable environment, which is a part of the characteristic texture of the work Joyce produced while his life was combined with his brother's, progressively fades out of the fiction produced after their separation, as James turned more and more toward the exploitation of an exclusively inner reality. And we can speculate that the compensatory interaction between the opposing dominant attitudes of the brothers when they were in constant contact helped to produce in the fiction a balance between the facts of external reality on the one hand and the symbols of the inner world on the other. Even in *Ulysses*, though much of the last half leaves the beaten track of the conscious world for excursions into the trackless wilds of the unconscious, so that the connections between Joyce's text and outer reality become difficult to keep track of, the balance holds.

With *Finnegans Wake*, however, written during the last years in Paris, Joyce deserted the conscious world entirely for the world of the dream, but a dream without a clearly identifiable dreamer, which makes a problem for interpretation. As Jung (1934) points out about any dream, "Without a knowledge of the conscious situation, the meaning of the dream [remains] in doubt" (p. 155). It is probably safe to say that there is general agreement that this magnificent oddity is a work of genius, and there is no question that Joyce is playing some fascinating games with the connections between language and the unconscious. Jung (1921) has observed that "the more deeply the vision of the creative mind penetrates [into the collective unconscious], the stranger it becomes to mankind in the mass," until it reaches a depth where "it is difficult to decide whether it is a morbid product or whether it is incomprehensible because of its extraordinary profundity" (p. 192). While we have at least one medical opinion that Joyce's art in the final years did represent a morbid product, became in fact "psychotic" (Andreasen, 1973, p. 71), the verdict on *Finnegans Wake*, by and large, is still out after more than forty years.

Stanislaus's negative verdict, however, was immediate and never withdrawn, and his conviction was firm that "if I had been at his elbow, *Finnegans Wake* would never have been written in its present form" (S. Joyce, 1949, p. 897). Perhaps he was right, and perhaps the world would be poorer for that. But Stanislaus cannot dissociate himself from this final work, for with his disappearance from his brother's life, he reappeared as an identifiable fictional presence in the work, reversing a process which started in *A Portrait*.

For although Stanislaus was solidly present as a character in *Stephen Hero*, and as "transcriptive Maurice," Stephen's younger brother, filled the role which Stanislaus filled in James's life, this character completely disappeared from the rewritten *Portrait*, which presented Stephen in isolation, though a Stephen who, as Beebe (1958, p. 70) and Cixous (1972, pp. 145–148) have noted, incorporates a number of Stanislaus's attitudes as they are expressed in his diary. In *Ulysses*, however, though a brother identifiable with Stanislaus is briefly mentioned by Stephen, it is as an eminently forgettable factor in the artist's life (J. Joyce, 1922, p. 211). But in Leopold Bloom, who, as I have elsewhere argued,[11] emerges from the

---

[11] See Kimball (1982) on Bloom as the Jungian shadow; Kimball (1973) on Stephen and Bloom as the divided self of the artist; and Kimball, 1976, pp. 374–375, on features of Stanislaus in Bloom. See also Cixous, 1972, pp. 148–149, on connections between Stanislaus and Bloom.

unconscious as the Jungian shadow to complete Stephen so that he may become a productive artist, Joyce merged essential features of his brother with his own features. In doing so, he repeated the process of absorption which gave Stephen in *A Portrait* "the strength of the two young Joyces" (Beebe, 1958, p. 70), except that in the mature figure of Bloom in *Ulysses*, the brother-pair combine in another self, separated from the ego personality Stephen. And again in *Finnegans Wake*, Joyce has in Shaun—named for (John) Stanislaus as Shem is named for Jim, and even further identified as "Stainusless"—merged features identifiably linked to his brother with his own features, although the autobiographical intent remains pure and exclusive.

It thus seems clear that while Stanislaus was a part of his life, Joyce projected much of his own shadow side on his brother, and in the final work, as he projected this shadow into his art, it is still identified with Stanislaus. Thus, the symbolic purpose of the brother-pair in the final work is self-analysis and self-revelation, and what we are dealing with again is two opposing tendencies in the artist's own psyche, a further abstraction of the opposition embodied in Stephen and Bloom, which, though very tenuously, resolve into an identity of the opposites.[12] Even though these fictional oppositions are by no means a direct translation of James Joyce's relationship with his brother, they are to a significant degree influenced, if not determined, by the nature of that relationship, which was in life a kind of *participation mystique* and which is reduplicated and given immortality in the fiction.

REFERENCES

Andreasen, N. (1973), A portrait of the artist as a schizoid. *J. Amer. Med. Assn.*, 224:67–71.

Beebe, M. (1958), Joyce and Stephen Dedalus: the problem of autobiography. In: *A James Joyce Miscellany: Second Series*, ed. M. Magalaner. Carbondale: University of Southern Illinois Press, 1959.

Benstock, B. (1965), *Joyce-Again's Wake: An Analysis of "Finnegans Wake."* Seattle: University of Washington Press.

Budgen, F. (1934), *James Joyce and the Making of Ulysses*. New York: Harrison Smith and Robert Haas.

Cixous, H. (1972), *The Exile of James Joyce*, trans. S.A.J. Purcell. New York: David Lewis.

Colum, M. (1922), The confessions of James Joyce. In: *The Freeman Book, 1920–1924*. New York: B.W. Huebsch, 1924, pp. 327–355.

[12] See Benstock, 1965, pp. 216–246, for a detailed analysis of the relationship between the twins as a synthesis of opposites. See also DiBernard, 1980, pp. 73–74, on the alchemical implications of the mingling of identities between Shem and Shaun; and see Norris, 1976, pp. 50–51, on the "Wakean twins" as a divided self.

Curran, C.P. (1968), *James Joyce Remembered*. New York: Oxford University Press.

Curtayne, A. (1963), Portrait of the artist as brother: an interview with James Joyce's sister. *Critic*, 21:43–47.

DiBernard, B. (1980), *Alchemy and Finnegans Wake*. Albany: State University of New York Press.

Edel, L. (1980), The genius and the injustice collector. *American Scholar*, 49:467–487.

Ellmann, R. (1959), *James Joyce*. New York: Oxford University Press.

Fifield, W. (1967), Joyce's brother, Lawrence's wife, Wolfe's mother, Twain's daughter. *Texas Quarterly*, 10:69–87.

Francini Bruni, A. (1922), Joyce stripped naked in the piazza. In: *Portraits of the Artist in Exile*, ed. W. Potts. Seattle: University of Washington Press, 1979, pp. 7–46.

Frank, N. (1967), The shadow that had lost its man. In: *Portraits of the Artist in Exile*, ed. W. Potts. Seattle: University of Washington Press, 1979, pp. 74–105.

Franz, M.L. von (1971), The inferior function. In: Franz, M.L. von, and Hillman, J., *Lectures on Jung's Typology*. Irving, Texas: Spring Publications, 1979, pp. 1–72.

Giedion-Welcker, C. (1973), Meetings with James Joyce. In: *Portraits of the Artist in Exile*, ed. W. Potts. Seattle: University of Washington Press, 1979, pp. 256–280.

Gillet, L. (1941), Farewell to Joyce; The living Joyce. In: *Portraits of the Artist in Exile*, ed. W. Potts. Seattle: University of Washington Press, 1979, pp. 165–169; pp. 170–204.

Gogarty, O. (1941), The Joyce I knew. *Saturday Review of Literature*, January 25, pp. 3–4; 15–16.

——— (1950), *Intimations*. New York: Abelard Press.

——— (1954), *It Isn't This Time of Year at All!* Garden City, N.Y.: Doubleday.

Goldman, A. (1974), Stanislaus, James and the politics of family. *Atti del Third International James Joyce Symposium*. Trieste: Universita degli Studi, pp. 60–75.

Hillman, J. (1971), The feeling function. In: Franz, M.L. von, and Hillman, J., *Lectures on Jung's Typology*. Irving, Texas: Spring Publications, 1979, pp. 75–146.

Jacobi, J. (1942), *The Psychology of C.G. Jung: An Introduction with Illustrations*. New Haven: Yale University Press, 1973.

Joyce, J. (1916), *A Portrait of the Artist as a Young Man*, ed. C.G. Anderson and R. Ellmann. New York: Viking Press, 1964.

——— (1922), *Ulysses*. New York: Random House, 1934, edition reset and corrected, 1961.

——— (1939), *Finnegans Wake*. New York: Viking Press.

——— (1944), *Stephen Hero*, ed. J.J. Slocum and H. Cahoon. New York: New Directions, 1963.

——— (1957), *Letters of James Joyce*, Vol. I, ed. S. Gilbert. New York: Viking Press.

——— (1966a), *Letters of James Joyce*, Vol. II, ed. R. Ellmann. New York: Viking Press.

—— (1966b), *Letters of James Joyce*, Vol. III, ed. R. Ellmann. New York: Viking Press.

—— (1975), *Selected Letters of James Joyce*, ed. R. Ellmann. New York: Viking Press.

Joyce, S. (1941), James Joyce: a memoir. *Hudson Review*, 2:487–514; 1949.

—— (1949), Early memories of James Joyce. *The Listener*, 41:896–897.

—— (1954), An open letter to Dr. Oliver Gogarty. *Interim*, 4:49–56.

—— (1958), *My Brother's Keeper: James Joyce's Early Years*, ed. R. Ellmann. New York: Viking Press.

—— (1971), *The Complete Dublin Diary of Stanislaus Joyce*, ed. G.H. Healey. Ithaca: Cornell University Press.

Jung, C.G. (1918), The role of the unconscious. *Civilization in Transition. Collected Works*, 10:3–28.[13] New York: Bollingen Foundation, 1964.

—— (1921), *Psychological Types. Collected Works*, 6. Princeton: Princeton University Press, 1971.

—— (1932a), *Ulysses*: A monologue. *The Spirit in Man, Art, and Literature. Collected Works*, 15:109–134. New York: Bollingen Foundation, 1966.

—— (1932b), Picasso. *The Spirit in Man, Art, and Literature. Collected Works*, 15:135–141. New York: Bollingen Foundation, 1966.

—— (1934), The practical use of dream analysis. *The Practice of Psychotherapy. Collected Works*, 16:139–161. New York: Pantheon Books, 1954.

—— (1948), The phenomenology of the spirit in fairytales. *The Archetypes and the Collective Unconscious*, 2nd ed. *Collected Works*, 9:207–254. New York: Bollingen Foundation, 1966.

—— (1958), The undiscovered self (present and future). *Civilization in Transition. Collected Works*, 10:245–305. New York: Bollingen Foundation, 1964.

—— (1973), *Letters of C.G. Jung: 1906–1950*, Vol. I, ed. G. Adler and A. Jaffe. Bollingen Series XCV:1. Princeton, N.J.: Princeton University Press.

—— (1975), *Letters of C.G. Jung: 1951–1961*, Vol. II, ed. G. Adler and A. Jaffe. Bollingen Series XCV:2. Princeton, N.J.: Princeton University Press.

Kimball, J. (1973), The hypostasis in *Ulysses*. *James Joyce Quarterly*, 10:422–438.

—— (1976), James Joyce and Otto Rank: the incest motif in *Ulysses*. *James Joyce Quarterly*, 13:366–382.

—— (1982), A Jungian scenario for *Ulysses*. *Comparative Literature Studies*, 19:195–207.

Léon, P. (1942), In memory of Joyce. In: *Portraits of the Artist in Exile*, ed. W. Potts. Seattle: University of Washington Press, 1979, pp. 286–291.

Lévy-Bruhl, L. (1922), *How Natives Think*, trans. L.A. Clare. New York: Knopf, 1925.

—— (1927), *The "Soul" of the Primitive*, trans. L.A. Clare. Chicago: Regnery, 1966.

Norris, M. (1976), *The Decentered Universe of Finnegans Wake: A Structuralist Analysis*. Baltimore: Johns Hopkins Press.

---

[13] *The Collected Works of C.G. Jung*, 18 Vols., ed. H. Read, M. Fordham, and G. Adler; executive editor (from 1967), W. McGuire. Translated by R.F.C. Hull, except as otherwise noted. New York: Pantheon Books for Bollingen Foundation, 1953–1960; Bollingen Foundation, 1961–1967. Princeton, N.J.: Princeton University Press, 1967–1978.

O'Brien, D. (1966), The twins that tick *homo vulgaris*: a study of Shem and Shaun. *Modern Fiction Studies*, 12:183–199.

Power, A. (1974), *Conversations with James Joyce*, ed. Clive Hart. New York: Barnes & Noble.

Prinzhorn, H. (1922), *Artistry of the Mentally Ill: A Contribution to the Psychology and Psychopathology of Configuration*, trans. E. von Brockdorff. New York: Springer Verlag, 1972.

Rodgers, W.R., ed. (1972), James Joyce: a portrait of Joyce as a young man; James Joyce: a portrait of the artist in maturity. In: *Irish Literary Portraits*. New York: Taplinger, 1973, pp. 22–47; 48–74.

Scholes, R.E., and Kain, R.M. (1960), The first version of "A Portrait." *Yale Review*, 49:355–369.

Vinding, O. (1963), James Joyce in Copenhagen. In: *Portraits of the Artist in Exile*, ed. W. Potts. Seattle: University of Washington Press, 1979, pp. 139–152.

West, R. (1928), The strange necessity. In: *The Strange Necessity: Essays by Rebecca West*. Garden City, N.Y.: Doubleday, pp. 1–213.

3

The Importance of Being Angry: The Mutual Antagonism of Oscar and Willie Wilde

KARL BECKSON

The Importance of Being Earnest, Oscar Wilde's theatrical masterpiece, involves a relationship between brothers who are, for most of the play, unaware of their true kinship. The plot draws its strength, in part, from the actual relationship that existed between Oscar and his brother Willie, the prototypes of the play's main characters: Jack, the concerned, protective guardian; and Algy, the idle, irresponsible spendthrift. The progressive mutual antagonism between Oscar and Willie that forms the basis for the plot is not uncommon, to be sure, between siblings, but in the lives of these two writers (one major, the other quite minor), it was accompanied by an awesome self-destructiveness. Oscar's indiscreet homosexual liaisons with "renters" (male prostitutes) at a time when he was easily recognized in hotels and restaurants and when homosexuality was a crime, and Willie's extravagance, idleness, and alcoholism, undoubtedly the result of periodic depression, reveal uncontrollable impulses acted out in the context of a restrictive Victorian morality. The models for such behavior, however, had been readily at hand in the lives of their brilliant parents, at once distinguished and notorious in mid-nineteenth-century Dublin.

Sir William Wilde, an eye and ear surgeon of international repute, was also a man of letters, archeologist, folklorist, and editor of the

Dublin Quarterly Journal of Medical Science. In 1853, after he had
founded a hospital in Dublin, Queen Victoria appointed him Surgeon
Oculist in Ordinary to Her Majesty. In 1864 he was knighted, principally
for his work as Commissioner of the Medical Census in Ireland.

Though acclaimed for his medical and literary accomplishments—he
was the author of some twenty books, including one on Swift and the
standard textbook on aural surgery—Sir William was often satirized in
the Irish press for his imperious manner and for his seemingly dwarfish
appearance, particularly when compared to Lady Wilde's impressive
height and weight. His cleanliness—or lack of it—became the subject of
a query that reportedly circulated at the time: "Why are Dr. Wilde's nails
black?" The answer: "Because he scratches himself." Most significant for
an understanding of both Oscar and Willie was their father's sexual promiscuity, which in time became a national scandal. Before he married, he
had had at least three illegitimate children, but in 1864, the year of his
knighthood, at the age of forty-nine, he became the subject of a libel suit
that the Irish press capitalized upon when Oscar was ten and Willie
twelve.

Lady Wilde had brought a suit against a Mary Travers, whose father
was a professor of medical jurisprudence at Trinity College, Dublin. Ten
years before, Mary, then aged nineteen, had begun as Sir William's
patient and subsequently became his mistress. They were often seen
together around Dublin; indeed, Sir William even invited her to the
Wildes' home in Merrion Square. For ten years Lady Wilde tolerated
these indiscretions, though it may be assumed she harbored a smoldering
hostility toward them both. When Lady Wilde could no longer tolerate
the unstable, insolent girl, she wrote to Prof. Travers objecting to what
appeared to be an "intrigue" on his daughter's part. Mary then brought
suit against Lady Wilde for libel.

Lady Wilde, or "Speranza," as she had referred to herself earlier when
she published poems and essays, had a prominent place in the Young
Ireland revolutionary movement of the 1840s. An agitator for Irish independence, she was a major voice though a minor poet. When she
married, she settled into domestic life and later maintained a salon, to
which she invited writers and artists. Visitors to Merrion Square were
often struck by the strange ambience and her even stranger costumes
covered with jewelry copied from ancient Celtic relics.

Her lofty manner and huge physical stature—perhaps the original of
Oscar's domineering Lady Bracknell in *The Importance of Being Earnest*—impressed all who saw her. One referred to her as "the gigantic
lady . . . of the warlike songs" (White, 1967, p. 87). Oscar and Willie

were also physically huge, and may later have felt a closer identification with their mother than with Sir William. Lady Wilde may also have had a profound influence on the development of Oscar's personal myth—that of the outcast homosexual artist—for as one of the saviors of Ireland she saw herself doomed and martyred. When Oscar was born in 1854, she wrote to a friend: "A Joan of Arc was never meant for marriage, and so here I am bound heart and soul to the home hearth" (Wyndham, 1951, p. 50).

At the trial, Mary Travers protested that Sir William had committed an "outrage" against her in his office, but she admitted to seeing him thereafter and to obtaining money and gifts from him. The jury, convinced she was not a victim, awarded her a farthing's damages, its estimate, presumably, of the value of her lost virginity. In all of this, Oscar and Willie could not have been shielded from the scandal that filled newspapers and was the talk of Dublin.[1]

Sir William, who had not appeared in court, spent most of his last years at his country house at Moytura, in the West of Ireland, where he drank excessively and undertook archeological expeditions. During school holidays, the three Wilde children—Willie, Oscar, and their sister, Isola, who died in 1867 at the age of nine—assisted him in his explorations. He died in 1876, aged sixty, his final years marked by severe depression. Lady Wilde was left with a small income derived from rents.

Sir William's disgrace and exile were undoubtedly a source of family shame and guilt. Later, the images of the promiscuous father and the crucified figure became for Oscar pervasive self-images that were also embodied in his art. Willie, it may be conjectured, was also deeply affected by the event and by his parents' mutual hostility. Schafer (1967) has written that "in the instance of 'borrowed guilt,' which refers explicitly to identifying with the guilt of a parent, not only a superego position is taken over, but also fantasies concerning id and ego tendencies and properties that warrent such guilt" (p. 142).

Of Oscar and Willie's early relationship, little is known other than the facts of their schooling. When he was ten, Oscar was sent to the Portora Royal School (founded by King Charles II) in Enniskillen, Ulster, where Willie was already a student. Oscar preferred his private reading of English novels and poetry to the required curriculum, but in his final year

---

[1] Wyndham (1951) cites a ballad reportedly chanted by Trinity College Students at the time of the trial:

> There's an oculist living in Merrion Square,
> Who has skill that's unrivaled and talent that's rare;
> And if you will listen, I'll try to reveal
> The matter that caused poor Miss Travers to squeal! [p. 100]

there (1871) he distinguished himself by winning prizes for Greek Testament and a Gold Medal in Classics. Willie, however, made his presence known by his conviviality, as a former classmate later wrote in an unpublished letter (Louis Purser to A.J.A. Symons, January 28, 1932):

> My personal recollections of Willie Wilde are nothing but delightful. . . . He was clever, erratic and full of vitality. He was no systematic student. He never shone at examinations and took very little part in games. He was something of a "character" in the school, was a bit given to boastfulness, and used to be considerably ridiculed on that score. But he was very kind to and friendly with younger boys. . . . He was a tolerable pianist, and I remember with gratitude many a time he played for his juniors. . . . [Clark Library]

In 1871 Oscar won a scholarship to Trinity College and followed Willie there as he had followed him to Portora; indeed, he shared rooms with him in his second and third years. Willie obtained his degree in December 1873; in the following year Oscar received a scholarship to attend Magdalen College, Oxford. While at Trinity, Willie, a member of the University Philosophical Society, delivered an impassioned speech defending prostitutes—an interesting point, in view of the notorious sexual promiscuity of his father, who presided at the meeting.

In 1876 Willie contributed some poems to *Kottabos*, the college magazine. Among them is one titled "Salome," the subject of which was commonplace in nineteenth-century French literature; however, Willie's depiction of this destructive femme fatale may well have aroused in Oscar an early interest:

> The sight of me was as devouring flame
>   Burning their hearts with fire, so wantonly
>   That night I danced for all his men to see!
> Fearless and reckless; for all maiden shame
> Strange passion-poisons throbbing overcame
>   As every eye was riveted on me,
>   And every soul was mine, mine utterly—
> And thrice each throat cried out aloud my name!
>
> "Ask what thou wilt," black-headed Herod said,
> "God wot a weird thing do I crave for prize:
> Give me, I pray thee, presently the head
>   Of John the Baptist." 'Twixt my hands it lies.
>   "Ah, mother! see! the lips, the half-closed eyes—

> Dost think he hates us still now he is dead?"
>
> [Tyrrell and Sullivan, 1906, p. 172]

The poem lacks the hypnotic Symbolist rhythms, the suggestiveness and shocking perversity of Oscar's later one-act "Salome," a fresh dramatic rendering of the ancient story.

Another poem by Willie, titled "Faustine," combines the eroticism of much late nineteenth-century verse with the paganism that Swinburne had made fashionable (indeed, Swinburne had written a poem of the same title in 1862):

> Because bright jewels my fair bosom deck,
> And Love's hot lips—close press'd—cling fast to mine,
> Because rose-garlands crown the cups of wine,
> And all Love's ministers are at my beck,
> Think you I mourn—repent—or ought I reck
> How tongues wag? Think you I weep and pine,
> Shedding salt tears as bitter salt sea-brine,
> Because his arms lie warm around my neck?
>
> Look you! we live but once—this life I know;
> No other wot I of beyond the tomb—
> I laugh to scorn your devils down below—
> Your torture-fires—your everlasting gloom!
> I seek no heaven, I dream no God above,
> I fear no hell, save living without Love!
>
> [Tyrrell and Sullivan, 1906, p. 128]

Willie's poetic gifts may be slender, but his capacity for imitative verse is spectacular. Despite the mediocrity of expression, one cannot overlook the concern with guilt, disguised here as pagan insouciance. Oscar, meanwhile, was also publishing in *Kottabos* in the 1870s and 1880s, as well as in other magazines such as the *Irish Monthly*. No doubt Oscar and Willie saw each other as rival poets. To be sure, Oscar had the greater gift, though many of his early attempts, reprinted in *Poems* (1881), were no less imitative than his brother's. Indeed, one critic commented: "The author possesses cleverness, astonishing fluency, a rich and full vocabulary, and nothing to say. Mr. Wilde has read Messrs. Tennyson, Swinburne, Arnold, and Rossetti with great pleasure, and he has paid them the compliment of copying their mannerisms very naively" (Beckson, 1970, p. 37).

Following his graduation from Trinity College, Willie studied law and was called to the bar, though he apparently never practiced. He preferred the skating rink, which had captured Dublin—a "craze" in the 1870s but a cause of distress to Lady Wilde, who complained that Willie gave her "no rest about the £5 for the rink, and I hate the rink" (White, 1967, p. 239). Still, she doted on him, hoping he would marry into wealth but worrying whether he would ever find the "right" woman. Her concern over Willie and his seeming irresponsibility, especially in money matters, became for Oscar an increasing irritation, finally deep distress. In the late 1870s Willie was still without direction, as Lady Wilde implies in one of her letters: "Willie has spent *all his money* and is now in debt to the bank and all his personal debts are unpaid . . . meanwhile he is joking and enjoying life" (p. 240).

In the early 1880s, Lady Wilde and Willie decided to leave Dublin for London. To a friend in Sweden she wrote: "We have arranged to leave Ireland, and this is my last note from the old family mansion in Merrion Square. Both my sons prefer residing in London, the focus of light, progress and intellect, and we have taken a house there, and disposed of this on very good terms" (p. 241). But to Oscar, who had been living in London since his graduation from Oxford in 1878, she wrote of the difficulty involved in making the change: "Willie in London, looking after rooms as lodgings, but all are so dear! I think a house would be quite beyond us involving two servants. . . . But it is certain we quit Dublin even if we go into furnished lodgings in London. . . . Willie has good openings with the press. . . . I think after all Willie is more suited for it than anything else" (p. 241).

As Holroyd (1979) has pointed out, Willie's journalistic career was quite extensive: drama critic for *Punch* and *Vanity Fair* in the 1880s; leader writer for the *Daily Telegraph*; editor of Christmas numbers for a variety of magazines. Lady Wilde's remark that he was "more suited" to journalism than anything else reveals her acceptance of his limitations, while she continued to believe that Oscar's brilliance would lead to literary acclaim. Binstead (1927), who knew him at the time, wrote that Willie did not view the "journalistic life" as "irksome." Arriving at the newspaper office at noon, he would arrange with the editor to write a "leader," say on the anniversary of the penny postage stamp; he would then spend the rest of the day at restaurants and taverns, with a bit of time at the British Museum to "grub up a lot of musty facts," and would then retire to his club to write "three great, meaty, solid paragraphs" (pp. 231–232).

Oscar's view of journalists as the modern vulgarians was initially formed by his exposure to widespread ridicule at the hands of reporters during his lecture tour of America in 1882. He invariably referred to journalists satirically or scornfully despite the fact that he had himself edited *The Woman's World* in the mid-1880s and had done extensive reviewing for various publications. Perhaps with Willie in mind, he was later to write (1889): "Lying for the sake of a monthly salary is of course well known in Fleet Street, and the profession of a professional leader-writer is not without its advantages. But it is said to be a somewhat dull occupation, and it certainly does not lead to much beyond a kind of ostentatious obscurity" (p. 318). Indeed, Willie's journalism was for the most part anonymous, hence impossible to identify. For this reason, Oscar was able, in the summer of 1884, to substitute for Willie as a drama critic for *Vanity Fair* (it is not known how many other journalists were contributing drama criticism to the same periodical).

At this time in their lives there was apparent harmony. When Oscar married in May of that year, Willie looked for rooms for the couple while they honeymooned in Paris. Before the engagement, Lady Wilde had written to Oscar urging him to establish "a settled life at once. Literature and lectures and Parliament, receptions, etc., for the world and small dinners for genius and culture—at 8 o'clock. Charming this life, begin it at once. Take warning by Willie" (White, 1967, p. 257)—an indication, perhaps, that she was no longer satisfied with Willie's life as a journalist and that she now associated that life with Willie's fatal attraction to alcohol.

By 1888, Lady Wilde and Willie were living in Chelsea, at 146 Oakley Street, where she again established her salon for obscure and indigent artists and writers. As one visitor (Maxwell, 1937) later described the setting: "Lady Wilde lived in Chelsea in a very small house which she kept darkened with heavy curtains over the windows and as she, unlike the house, was very large, ungainly too, one wondered how she got about and up and down stairs in the obscurity without an accident. Artificial light was turned on for parties and one saw Lady Wilde as really a vast terrifying person, with a strangely toned voice and a lace-clad head that nodded portentously" (p. 95). Oscar and Willie often attended her soirées: the "vast terrifying person" maintained her fascination and, to some extent, her control over her two sons.

On October 4, 1891, Willie, aged thirty-nine, married Mrs. Frank Leslie, aged fifty-five, the proprietor of the Frank Leslie Publishing Company in New York. There had been no engagement, nor had any preparations been made for the ceremony. Willie had arrived by steamship from Le Havre just four days before. During that time, they dined together regularly, Mrs. Leslie captivated by bearded Willie's joviality and wit,[2] but unaware, apparently, of his drinking habits. Urged by Lady Wilde, in all probability, to effect a marriage of wealth and status, Willie provided Mrs. Leslie with an image of old-world charm and sophistication. He was the brother, after all, of the famous Oscar Wilde whose novel, *The Picture of Dorian Gray*, having appeared in *Lippincott's Monthly Magazine* the previous year, had caused a sensation. Within two days of his arrival, Willie proposed.

After a brief private ceremony at the appropriately named Church of the Strangers on Mercer Street, they drove to Delmonico's to receive some friends, then left for a week's honeymoon in Niagara Falls. One recalls Oscar's prophetic remark after he visited the falls on his lecture tour in 1882: "Every American bride is taken there and the sight of the stupendous waterfall must be one of the earliest, if not the keenest, disappointments in American married life" (Lewis and Smith, 1936, p. 163). To Oscar, Lady Wilde wrote: "I hope you wrote to Willie. He seems in radiant health, hope and happiness. God keep them happy and wise and living in truth and trust. I think it is an altogether fine and good thing for Willie. Her influence must work great good in him and give him the strength he wants" (White, 1967, p. 261). In another letter, she wrote to Oscar: "you are the leading man of England as Willie is of New York" (p. 260).

Lady Wilde's dream of a healthy and happy Willie—indeed, like most of her dreams—was to be shattered in less than a year, for Mrs. Leslie (an extraordinary woman, born illegitimately in New Orleans, an actress when young, later a journalist and finally owner of her husband's company) suffered immediate disillusionment. She later said of Willie: "A more scholarly and accomplished man never came to America. I had hoped he would be of great assistance to me in my business. . . . He couldn't lead a London club life here in New York, and his attempt to do so was his chief fault" (*New York Herald*, June 9, 1893, p. 12).

Mrs. Leslie had known the Wildes since the early 1880s. In 1881 she had suggested that Oscar undertake his celebrated tour of America, and in April 1883 she visited London with a letter of introduction to Willie, then living with Lady Wilde in Park Street; indeed, she hoped upon her return to establish a salon similar to Lady Wilde's. The precise course of Mrs. Leslie's early relationship with Willie is unknown, but, according to Madeleine B. Stern (1953), he "professed to adore her" (p. 156).

---

[2] Though the painter Jacomb-Hood (1925) recalls that Willie was "quite as brilliant as a writer and talker as his better-known brother" (p. 117), Lillie Langtry (1925) wrote: "Some said his [i.e., Oscar's] elder brother, Willie, was as clever in his way, but I found him quite uninteresting" (p. 85).

Willie settled into Mrs. Leslie's luxurious apartment upon their return from Niagara Falls and rapidly became a celebrity, known not only for his jovial wit but also for his idleness. The critic James Gibbons Huneker (1923) later recalled Willie as a "companionable pagan. Every ten minutes he would light a fresh cigarette, every fifteen ask for another drink. He invariably preluded with 'I have a zoological feeling that I may be thirsty.' Getting up at five in the afternoon finally got on the nerves of his wife . . ." (p. 157).

The marriage had begun disastrously, for Willie, drunk on his wedding night, continued drinking for a week. Later, Mrs. Leslie complained: "He was of no use to me either by day or by night" (Stern, p. 160). And, in tears, she revealed to a friend that Willie was impotent. He spent his time at the Lotus Club at Fifth Avenue and Twenty-first Street running up liquor bills of fifty to seventy dollars weekly (which Mrs. Leslie paid), gossiping about London society, or reciting parodies of Oscar's poetry—an instance of open hostility toward his brother.

Apparently regretting his behavior and wishing a reconciliation, Willie wrote a sonnet to Mrs. Leslie, who published it in one of her magazines in an attempt, perhaps, to announce not only her husband's remorse but also her control over his dissipation:

AD AMICAM MEAM

If through excess of love for you, my sweet,
  My passion did my temperate reason blind,
  If fretful fancy made my lips unkind,
And words rang harsh, and thoughts were all unmeet
To make the conquest of yourself complete,
  Forgive me, sweetheart! Trust me, you will find
  My love one day deep in your life entwined,
And tendrilled round your innermost heart-beat.

Into Love's water have I cast a stone,
  Where gently mirrored lay your face so fair;
But now the rippling circles, wider grown,
  Have blurred the clear gray eyes and golden hair.
Love! Can no love for all my faults atone?
  Should the waves quiet, will you still be there?
                                    [Stern, 1953, p. 157]

The waves, however, did not grow quiet, for Willie's extravagance and idleness continued. Accordingly, Mrs. Leslie progressively began to reduce his allowance. In order to raise some cash, Willie contributed four signed articles—headlined "Willie Wilde's Letter"—to the *New York Recorder*. The first of these, published on March 20, 1892, with the subheading "The Celebrated London Journalist's First Writing in This Country," begins with the ironically self-conscious allusion to his reputation: "At the very serious risk of permanently imperiling that hard-earned reputation for cultivated indolence bestowed on me so lavishly by certain candid critics, I must perforce acknowledge that The Recorder has with a falconer's voice lured this tasseled gentle back to the old familiar paths that he fears may ultimately lead to honest toil" (p. 12). An informal essay of little literary distinction or wit, it contrasts the style and practice of English and American journalists.

On March 27 another "letter" appeared, consisting of observations about America, such as the habit of numbering streets instead of naming them after illustrious figures or events, a practice that Willie found "inartistic" and "unpoetical" but "very wise and very simple." In his "letter" of April 10 he speaks of oratory and the use of the English language; and in his final "letter," on May 1—mostly on baseball—he labors the point that hissing the umpire is "uncivilized." Willie's indolent pen is much in evidence in these "letters."

At the end of his final "letter," he told his readers that by the time they read it, he would be at sea on the S.S. *Alaska*. Before he and Mrs. Leslie embarked for England, she confided to her friends: "I'm taking Willie over, but I'll not bring Willie back" (Stern, 1953, p. 161), and she informed Lady Wilde that she could not continue to support the idle Willie any longer. In London, she instructed her solicitors of her intent; they, in turn, hired a private investigator to keep Willie under surveillance. Divorce proceedings, meanwhile, were undertaken against him. Interestingly, Lady Wilde was amused by the newspaper stories of the divorce. One might have expected resentment at the exploitation. To Oscar she wrote (undated letter, Clark Library): "About Willie most [of the newspapers] are very amusing—one is headlined in large capitals 'Tired of Willie!' & then a synopsis of the divorce case is given. All because 'Willie *won't get up*—& won't work.' Mrs. Leslie has stopped all his *allowance*—so he has nothing now but what he earns." It can only be conjectured why she wrote to Oscar in this manner: possibly, she had long since resigned herself to the inevitability of the divorce, but, more significantly, there is apparent narcissistic pleasure in her account of the stories.

Willie's New York experience suggests a period of depression, perhaps brought on by his parasitic experience with Mrs. Leslie, a maternal surrogate. If Lady Wilde had found it difficult to provide money for Willie, Mrs. Leslie had provided luxury; but as the proprietor of a major publishing firm she was a formidable figure, as "vast and terrifying" as Lady Wilde. Willie's apparent resentment over this arrangement, it may be thought, resulted in flagrant self-indulgence calculated to infuriate Mrs. Leslie and to punish himself for having yielded all control.

In an unpublished paper titled "The Masochistic-Narcissistic Character," Arnold Cooper asserts that so interwoven are masochism and narcissism that they are, in fact, "one and the same": "Being disappointed or refused becomes the preferred mode of narcissistic assertion to the extent that narcissistic and masochistic distortions dominate the character. . . . To the extent that masochistic-narcissistic defenses are used, the aim is not a reunion with and fantasied control over a cruel and damaging mother. Original sources of gratification have been degraded, and gratification is secondarily derived from the special sense of suffering." To be sure, Willie acted out a complex masochistic fantasy, which, indeed, also dominated his more successful brother but in a different mode and with more disastrous results.

Oscar, meanwhile, was enjoying a phenomenal success in the theater. *Lady Windermere's Fan*, his first society comedy, had premiered in February 1892, and drama critics generally praised its striking wit. Hyde (1975) states that upon returning to London, Willie saw the play and published an unfavorable review (unsigned), but Oscar reportedly remarked: "After a good dinner, one can forgive anybody, even one's own relations" (p. 137). As notices began appearing, Lady Wilde wrote to Oscar: "You have had a splendid success, and I am very happy and very proud of you" (p. 137). She also informed Oscar that she was sending all the good notices to Willie in New York. This presumably was intended to assure Oscar of her admiration and to remind Willie of his less exalted position in life; no doubt it was also an expression of anger toward Willie for destroying his promising marriage. On Willie's side, there was undoubtedly resentment toward his mother for her constant mailing of good reviews, a reminder to him of his own failure in life.

Oscar was still maintaining a cordial relationship with Willie, if only on the surface, for in a letter dated July 1893, Oscar wrote that he could not invite him and a friend to The Cottage at Goring-on-Thames (where he was at work on his next play, *A Woman of No Importance*), but enclosed a check with the facetious remark: "a small piece of paper, for which reckless bankers may give you gold, as I don't want you to die;" he closed "With best love" (Wilde, 1962, p. 343). The tone is characteristically playful, but the letter reveals Willie's continuing propensity for borrowing, a dependency that was likely to arouse resentment. Oscar's remark about not wanting Willie "to die" suggests, perhaps, its opposite.

In early September, Max Beerbohm, on holiday at Broadstairs, Kent, and longing for London, saw a good deal of Willie, who was also staying there. In a letter to his friend Reggie Turner, Beerbohm—in his maliciously comic manner—informed him that Willie has been "his only consolation" but adds:

> He is very vulgar and unwashed and inferior, but if I shut my eyes I can imagine his voice to be the voice of Oscar. Who was it that said 'Scratch Oscar and you will find Willie'? It is a very pregnant saying: if Oscar had not been such a success in life as he has been he would be the image of Willie. It was Willie, by the way, who was found by his host in the smoking-room filling his pockets with handfuls of cigars—wasn't it dreadful? [Beerbohm, 1964, p. 63]

After returning from Broadstairs, Beerbohm wrote to the painter Will Rothenstein, as he had written to Turner, that he had seen "a good deal" of Willie, but he writes of him in darker tones: "Quel monstre! Dark, oily, suspecte [sic] yet awfully like Oscar: he has Oscar's coy, carnal smile & fatuous giggle & not a little of Oscar's esprit. But he is awful—a veritable tragedy of family-likeness" (Lago and Beckson, 1975, p. 21).

In later years, Beerbohm recalled dining with Willie, who had asked him for ten shillings. When granted the sum, Willie, in high spirits, whistled for the waiter, who responded angrily. "Don't you whistle for me," he said; "I am not a dog." Max concludes:

> You know, I will never forget it. Everything went out of Willie. He began to stammer out apologies to the waiter. 'But, my dear fellow,' he kept mumbling, 'my dear fellow . . . I didn't mean . . . I meant nothing. . . .' It was awful, you know—that sudden capitulation. In that moment, I believe, he really saw, and perhaps for the first time, the dingy failure of his life; even behind the bulwark of that ten shillings, he saw himself facing tragedy and defeat, he saw that there was nothing ahead for him, that he would never recover, that he would never find a clearing in the shambles he had made for himself. He saw the end, and I saw it, too. [Behrman, 1960, p. 239]

What was Willie doing in Broadstairs in 1893? An unpublished letter dated September 30 (Clark Library), from a correspondent named A. Mynoos to Oscar's wife, Constance, reveals that Lily Lees, a young lady whom Willie later married, has "confessed that she & Mr. W. Wilde have been living together as man & wife" at Malvern and Broadstairs and that the "wretched woman" had tried to obtain "a powder to prevent the birth of a baby, & she says he has treated her with great brutality." The correspondent continued: "Mr. W. is always asking his mother for money & stamps his foot & swears at her if she hesitates." She concludes that Lady Wilde is in "bed and suffering": "Cannot anything be done? You & Mr. Oscar are so good to her, but she conceals the state of affairs. The house is not safe or wholesome, Lady Wilde is always being asked for money & *worried to death*." The last phrase is underlined twice. The letter-writer is "afraid Lady Wilde will utterly break down & die if something is not done to prevent the tormenting worry."

Oscar was furious with Willie over the Lily Lees episode. In a letter (October 8, Clark Library), to Oscar, Lady Wilde tried to calm him down. The depth of her sons' mutual antagonism is also manifest: "the dissonance[?] between you & Willie is very distressing to me. . . . Do try & be more kind & conciliatory with Willie, & help him with your advice. This wd. do him good, but coldness & hostility do no good to anyone." As for Lily, Lady Wilde adds: "I believe Miss L. got up the whole story [concerning her pregnancy] just to try & force on the marriage, which will *never be* now—Willie was very angry with her—& she will not come to this house again."

On February 4, 1894, Lady Wilde revealed to Oscar that "Willie is *married* to Miss Lees—tho' not yet publicly announced" (Clark Library). Lady Wilde felt the burden of her elder son more than ever before. In her letter she complained that "Willie is utterly useless—& now, just when my income has fallen so low, he announces the marriage & the whole burden of the household to fall upon me. . . . Miss Lees has but £50 a year . . . and Willie is always in a state of utter poverty." Lily Lees's stepmother had apparently objected to her intention of marrying Willie; she had £2,000 to leave but was determined to alter her will if Lily married him. After their marriage, they consequently had little to live on; hence, they had to live with Lady Wilde, who complained to Oscar of her "immense dislike of sharing a house with Miss Lees, with whom I have nothing in common. The idea of having her here is quite distasteful to me" (White, 1967, p. 264). However, she soon overcame her aversion to Lily: "Willie and his wife get on very well here. Mrs. Willie is sensible and assists me in arranging the house and is very good-tempered" (p. 264).

By this time relations between Oscar and Willie had reached the breaking point. One can only speculate on the numerous causes of Willie's chaotic anger toward Oscar and toward their mother, who had always lavished praise on Oscar and had always reminded Willie of his drifting life. On September 18, 1893, at the time of Willie's liaison with Lily, Lady Wilde had written to Oscar: "You have always been my *best & dearest help in every misery*" (Clark Library). Her dependence on Oscar for financial and emotional support could only have further alienated the irresponsible Willie. By March 1894, after Willie's marriage, Lady Wilde had received a letter from Oscar, which is not extant, on the subject of his relationship with Willie. She responded (March 29, Clark Library): "I am truly sorry to find that you & Willie meet as enemies. Is this to go on to my death? Not a cheering prospect for me to have my two sons at enmity, & unable to meet at my deathbed." Oscar replied in a letter, also not extant, to which Lady Wilde refers in a lengthy letter (undated, Clark Library) that in its obsessive repetitions and desperate pleading reveals deep-seated guilt for her inability to maintain harmony between her sons:

> My dear Oscar
>
> I have read your letter carefully, & now make reply. You are, I know, anxious to aid the happiness of my life—but it will *not* make me happy to know that my two sons meet in society & do not speak & are hostile to each other, which all the world will look on and sneer, & make sarcastic remarks on you both. Already several have done so, & it is commonly said that *you hate* yr. brother. Now this does *not* make me happy; nor to find that you will not come here for fear of meeting him. On the contrary, I would suggest quite a different line of conduct on yr. part. Try & *do Willie good.* Be a friend to him. Speak truly & wisely, *but kindly.*
>
> He is very susceptible to kindness, & he would greatly appreciate your taking interest in him. He feels your coldness most bitterly. Now do try another plan if you want to help *me* & make my life happier. *Come* here, hold out yr. hand to Willie, & say—Let us be friends as brothers should. Give him good advice. It s[houl]d be of use. He is sickly and extravagant. *Preach to him*, but do it *kindly.* Willie has some good points, & do try & help him to be better. I am *miserable* at the present position of my two sons—& at the general belief that you *hate your brother.* Give up all bitter thoughts, & simply hold out your hand, & say, "Let us be friends, & help our Mother as we can best." I pity Willie in this that he does not get a sixpence from Moytura & so I am content to give him what I can. At my death he will at least have something—but till then I try & help him a little & I really think that if you treated Willie *kindly* he wd. get on better. He has a high opinion of you but feels bitterly your open & profound hatred[?]—while the condition of affairs between my two sons makes me *wretched.* So if you

want to make me happy do as I ask you. *Come here* at once—& offer your hand to Willie cordially & sincerely—& forget & forgive all past enmities—& above all, try & do him good by *kindly advice* & live as brothers; it is a sacred relation—& I feel so desolate when you say you will not come here, & that you hate Willie.

He has never injured you. Why should you hate him? If he has taken help from me in money, why, that *does not injure you*, & I don't want you to hate Willie on my account. That does not make me happier. So, do try & make me happy, by a friendly feeling towards Willie. You may do him good by *kindness*, you never can do him good by insolent behaviour[?]. Do as I ask—come to the house here, & be *friendly*, & let the past bitterness die. Otherwise, *I shall die* [of] despair. I cannot live & see you & Willie hostile to each other—& I know that you could if you chose greatly influence Willie for good by simple friendly kindness. You will both have to meet by my coffin, & I want you to meet before that in friendly feeling.

Come then & offer him yr. hand in good faith—& begin a new course of action. Not insulting him by coldness before yr. friends, & so causing the horrid remark that *you hate yr. brother*—I shall hope to see you soon—if not I'll die of grief. I have not [the letter ends here, incomplete].

Lady Wilde's narcissism, probably a major factor in the disturbed relationship between her sons, is evident in her initial remark that her sons' hostility would be sneered at by "all the world." In her attempt to unite her sons, it may be that she was intensifying, unconsciously, their mutual hostility at the expense of her elder son, for clearly she believed that the bad Willie needed the aid of the good Oscar.

In August and September of 1894, Oscar took rooms at The Haven in Worthing, where he wrote most of his theatrical masterpiece, *The Importance of Being Earnest*. Coming at a time when he was alienated from Willie and when his mother was pleading for reconciliation, the play takes on far greater significance than Oscar was willing to admit when he wrote facetiously to a publisher that it was a " 'trivial' play . . . written by a butterfly for butterflies" (Wilde, 1962, p. 382). *The Importance* is, after all, principally concerned with two brothers who are unaware that they are related; ironically, they discover that they are, in fact, what they have pretended to be.

The initial denial of brotherhood by the playwright is revealing; by the end of the play, however, discovery will occur and harmony ensue, a fulfillment of Lady Wilde's wish. Could such harmony be Oscar's defense against intolerable anxiety and deep-seated antagonism toward Willie and perhaps toward his mother for her attempt to control their anger? The misplaced Jack—from carriage to handbag—will discover who his parents are (knowledge initially denied him by the playwright) so that when the discovery is finally made, he announces: "Algy's elder brother! Then I have a brother after all. I knew I had a brother! I always said I had a brother! Cecily—how could you have ever doubted that I had a brother?" (Wilde, 1899, p. 504). Jack then introduces his "unfortunate brother" to the others, after which he admonishes Algy: "Algy, you young scoundrel, you will have to treat me with more respect in the future. You have never behaved to me like a brother in all your life" (p. 505). The relationship between Oscar and Willie is much in evidence, despite the defensive displacement of elder and younger brothers. The elder brother, Jack, discovers that he was christened with the name of his father, perhaps an unconscious allusion by Oscar to the fact that Willie was named after his father, Sir William. Indeed, for that reason Willie's indiscretions may have seemed to Lady Wilde—and perhaps to Oscar as well—an unfortunate repetition of her husband's dissolute life.

Indiscretion and deception are central to *The Importance*. The good, devoted Jack, who cares for his ward, Cecily, has invented a wicked, extravagant brother named "Ernest," who lives in town and whom Jack must, on occasion, assist out of the "most dreadful scrapes," a now more readily understood analogy between the good Oscar and the wicked Willie. Likewise, Algy has a device of his own, as he explains to Jack: "You have invented a very useful younger brother called Ernest, in order that you may be able to come up to town as often as you like. I have invented an invaluable permanent invalid called Bunbury, in order that I may be able to go down into the country whenever I choose" (p. 438). Algy's invalid is symbolically equivalent to the wicked Ernest; they function as doubles in the analogy: good/healthy//wicked/ill.

When Jack appears in Act II to announce his imaginary brother's death—a further instance of denial—the Rev. Chausable says to him: "You have at least the consolation of knowing that you were always the most generous and forgiving of brothers" (Wilde, 1899, p. 465). To be sure, Oscar was far from being such a brother, but perhaps he thought of himself as such or expressed the ideal that should govern such relationships. After Jack's announcement of the "death" of Ernest, Algy appears, pretending to be the wicked brother. The attempt at denial fails. Cecily remarks to Jack: "However badly he may have behaved to you in the past he is still your brother. You couldn't be so heartless as to disown him." Cecily, the instrument of reconciliation, concludes: "I'll tell him to come out. And you will shake hands with him, won't you, Uncle Jack?" The reconciling image of handshaking is precisely what dominates Lady

Wilde's lengthy letter, quoted earlier. When Algy appears with Cecily, she again makes use of the device: "Uncle Jack, you are not going to refuse your own brother's hand?" Jack: "Nothing will induce me to take his hand" (p. 469).

The original four-act version was reduced to three at the urging of George Alexander, the actor-manager who played the role of Jack. In it, Oscar had included a speech by the Rev. Chausable: "Mr. Worthing, your brother has been unexpectedly restored to you, by the mysterious dispensation of Providence, who seems to desire your reconciliation. And indeed it is good for brothers to dwell together in amity" (Wilde, 1956, p. 73). Was this removed by Oscar as part of the pattern of denial that dominates the play? Algy's response to the Rev. Chausable, however, was retained, in slightly altered form, in the three-act version: "Of course I admit that the faults were all on my side. But I must say that I think that Brother John's coldness is to me peculiarly painful" (p. 73). Indeed, "coldness" is the very charge made by Lady Wilde against Oscar in his relationship with Willie, as expressed in two letters previously quoted. When Jack finally submits and shakes Algy's hand, has Oscar also submitted, presumably unconsciously, to the urgent request by Lady Wilde that he take Willie's hand? To be sure, the reconciliation at this point in the play occurs between two "brothers" who are unaware of their true relationship—a gesture, so to speak, without substance.

In the four-act version, a scene entirely removed from the final stage version, involving the arrest of Algy for debt by the solicitor Gribsby, suggests further that the play may be read, in part, as an acting out of a seemingly unresolvable problem involving Oscar and Willie. The following exchange occurs when Gribsby flourishes a bill charged to "Ernest Worthing" and Jack continues the pretense that Algy is Ernest:

> JACK: You mean now to say that you are not Ernest Worthing, residing at B.4, The Albany? I wonder, as you are at it, that you don't deny being my brother at all. Why don't you?
> ALGY: Oh! I am not going to do that, my dear fellow; it would be absurd. Of course, I'm your brother. And that is why you should pay this bill for me. What is the use of having a brother, if he doesn't pay one's bills for one?
> JACK: Personally, if you ask me, I don't see any use in having a brother. As for paying your bill, I have not the smallest intention of doing anything of the kind. [Wilde, 1956, pp. 78–79]

He concludes that incarceration would do Algy "a great deal of good." But Jack again submits and agrees to pay the bill.

At that point, Gribsby, of the firm of Gribsby and Parker, reveals that he is also Parker—another double. He explains: "Gribsby when I am on unpleasant business, Parker on occasions of a less serious kind"—an equivalent to Algy's Bunbury and Jack's Ernest. Double lives, however, must be eliminated before the final harmony may occur. (In *The Picture of Dorian Gray*, a novel of the double life, Dorian's attempt to destroy his other self in the portrait in order to free himself of haunting conscience fails; indeed, the novel may be read as Oscar's unconscious attempt to destroy the external manifestation of his own inner division.) In the three-act version of *The Importance*, Algy says that he "killed Bunbury this afternoon. I mean poor Bunbury died this afternoon" (Wilde, 1899, p. 493). Jack disposes of Ernest, as has been seen, by announcing his death of apoplexy in Paris. However, in the four-act version, when Algy asks about the "profligate brother" Ernest, Jack informs him: "I have made up my mind to kill that brother of mine" (Wilde, 1956, p. 39). And on two subsequent pages, Jack repeats that he intends to "kill" his "brother." These allusions to metaphoric killing were deleted in the three-act version. Is it possible that the sentiment voiced by Jack—even as fantasy—was entirely too close to a desire felt by Oscar?

Later in the four-act version, Miss Prism urges Cecily not to speak with Algy-Ernest, for Jack would not approve: "For the past three years he has suffered much through the conduct of his brother. We have already today had a sad but vivid object-lesson of the inevitable results of profligacy and extravagance" (Wilde, 1956, p. 97). Saying goodbye to Algy, Miss Prism urges: "If you would only take your brother as your example, all would be well" (p. 99). To be sure, the play may be read as psycho-biography—certainly the relationship between brothers is central—but as a theatrical vehicle, "a highly original fusion of Wilde's idiosyncratic redemptive comedy and his basically anarchic assumptions" (Shewan, 1977), it transcends its autobiographical sources and remains one of the wittiest in the language.

With the extraordinary success of *The Importance* in February 1895, Oscar had two plays in West End theaters (*An Ideal Husband* had opened in January). Meanwhile, Oscar's own double life with renters had become, among his friends, one of deep concern. His relationship with Lord Alfred Douglas, moreover, had become increasingly distressing to the Marquess of Queensberry, Lord Alfred's father, who repeatedly warned Wilde about his liaison with "Bosie." On the opening night of *The Importance of Being Earnest*, Queensberry appeared with a bouquet of vegetables (believed to be carrots and turnips, symbolizing Wilde's sexual preference), which he planned to throw at the playwright when he made his appearance on stage at the end of the play. Prevented from entering the theater, Queensberry proceeded to Oscar's club, where he left his calling card with the words "For Oscar Wilde, posing Somdomite," misspelling the epithet.

At the urging of Lord Alfred, who hated his father, Oscar pressed a libel suit against Queensberry. The latter, with the help of private investigators, gathered incriminating evidence. Faced with the possibility of exposure, Oscar dropped the suit, but Queensberry's attorneys provided the public prosecutor with sufficient evidence to seek an arrest warrant. In his first trial in late April, 1895, Oscar was brilliant in his responses on the witness stand, but the jury could not reach a decision. A new trial was consequently ordered.

Released on bail, Oscar was refused rooms at various hotels, the work of Queensberry's hired thugs, who followed him about town and even into two suburban localities to inform hotel managers who he was. Robert Sherard, who was one of Oscar's friends in the final years and whose *Life of Oscar Wilde* (1906) is the earliest biography, tells what happened long past midnight when Oscar made his way to his mother's house in Oakley Street, Chelsea, where Willie and his wife were living. Oscar, said Willie, "came tapping with his beak against the window-pane" and knocked on the door. When Willie opened it, Oscar entered disheveled and exhausted, and—in Willie's reported words—"fell down on my threshold like a wounded stag." He staggered into the narrow hall and sank into a chair, crying out: "Willie, give me a shelter or I shall die in the streets" (p. 358). The story may be factually true, but—if we can believe Sherard—is clearly dramatized by Willie to suggest his moment of triumph: Oscar falling, in more than one sense of the word, at the feet of the scorned Willie.

When William Butler Yeats went to Oakley Street to visit Oscar, as he reports in his autobiography (1922), he was met by an Irish servant, "her face drawn and tragic as in the presence of death" (p. 191). Oscar was not there, but Willie received him with "Who are you; what do you want?" After Yeats informed him that he had brought letters of sympathy for Oscar, Willie, now friendlier, said: "Do these letters urge him to run away? Every friend he has is urging him to, but we have made up our minds that he must stay and take his chance." Yeats assured him that the letters were expressions of sympathy, nothing more, but Willie "threw himself into a chair and began to talk with incoherent emotion, and in phrases that echoed now and again his brother's style at its worst; there were tears in his eyes, and he was, I think, slightly intoxicated." Willie assured Yeats that Oscar could escape from England—there was a yacht ready to take him to the Continent, but, said Willie, Oscar was determined to remain. He then turned to his relationship with Oscar: "You must have heard—it isn't necessary to go into detail—that he and I have not been friends; but he came to me like a wounded stag, and I took him in" (p. 191). Here again is the "wounded stag" image that Sherard first recorded, and in Yeats's account a reinforcement of Willie's view of himself as Oscar's savior.

To Yeats, Willie also said that it was Oscar's "vanity that has brought all this disgrace upon him; they swung incense before him." During this conversation, Willie's wife, Lily, entered and "threw herself into a chair," saying in an exhausted voice, "It is all right now, he has made up his mind to go to prison if necessary." Yeats recalls what Oscar had said when he was arrested: "My poor brother writes to me that he is defending me all over London; my poor, dear brother, he could compromise a steam engine."[3] Rumor had it, says Yeats, that the "wounded stag" had not at all been "graciously received," that Willie, refusing to sit at the same table with Oscar, had dined at a nearby hotel at Oscar's expense. "Thank God my vices were decent," Willie reportedly said (p. 193). The idle drunkard had finally found grounds for asserting his moral superiority. One suspects that Willie's urging that Oscar remain in England to face the trial reveals a submerged wish to witness his destruction.

Convicted and sentenced to two years at hard labor, Oscar spent most of that time at Reading Gaol. At the end of 1895, a group of friends attempted to circulate a petition for an early release. The document had been written, in the main, by Bernard Shaw, who was convinced that Oscar had suffered enough already and that further confinement might render him incapable of continuing a literary career upon his release. Shaw was convinced that his signature on the petition would reduce it to "absurdity and do Oscar more harm than good" because of his own reputation as a "crank" (Hyde, 1975, p. 308). Willie was convinced that signatures would never be obtained, a prediction that proved correct.

With Oscar still at Reading Gaol, Lady Wilde died on February 3, 1896. Constance traveled from Genoa to inform him of her death—their final meeting.[4] To Willie she wrote that Oscar was an "absolute wreck compared with what he was" (Wilde, 1962, p. 399). In his lengthy letter to Bosie in March (later published as De Profundis), Oscar wrote of his mother: "You knew, none better, how deeply I loved and honoured her. Her death was so terrible to me that I, once a lord of language, have no

---

[3] On April 23, 1895, Oscar wrote to Ada Leverson: "Willie has been writing me the most monstrous letters. I have had to beg him to stop" (Wilde, 1962, p. 392).

[4] When Constance died in April 1898, Arthur Clifton, a friend of the Wildes, wrote to Robert Ross: "Willie had of course been to see if anything was left to him or his wife" (Clark Library).

words in which to express my anguish and my shame" (p. 458). According to Sherard (1906), Willie circulated a memorial card but provided no headstone for Lady Wilde's grave; after seven years, in default of payment, her remains were moved to an unknown site.

When Oscar was released from prison on May 19, 1897, some friends were there to meet him. Willie was not among them. Oscar went directly to the Continent to live out the remainder of his life and died there in November 1900. Little is known of Willie's last years, though Hyde (1975) states that continued alcoholism was a major cause of death. Katherine Tynan (1913) recalls that Lily, who nursed him in poverty and illness, made his last years happy, or "as happy as they could be." When Willie died on March 13, 1899, at the age of forty-six, Robert Ross, Oscar's close friend and later his literary executor, wired to inform him. Oscar responded: "I suppose it had been expected for some time. I am very sorry for his wife, who, I suppose, has little to live on. Between him and me there had been, as you know, wide chasms for many years." Beyond anger, perhaps in a moment of forgiveness, Oscar expressed his final words on Willie in his letter to Ross: "*Requiescat in Pace*" (Wilde, 1962). Anger had defined their relationship, had paradoxically and fatally united them with Lady Wilde, and had created the divisions and deceptions that found their way, through the alchemy of the imagination, into one of the great plays in the English language.

REFERENCES

Beckson, K., ed. (1970), *Oscar Wilde: The Critical Heritage*. London: Routledge & Kegan Paul.

Beerbohm, M. (1964), *Letters to Reggie Turner*, ed. R. Hart-Davis. Philadelphia: Lippincott.

Behrman, S.N. (1960), *Conversation with Max*. London: Hamish Hamilton.

Binstead, A. (1927), *Works*, vol. 1. London: T. Werner Laurie.

Cooper, A. (unpub.), The Masochistic-Narcissistic Character.

Holroyd, J.E. (1979), Brother to Oscar. *Blackwood's Magazine*, 325:230–240.

Huneker, J.G. (1923), *Steeplejack*, vol. 2. New York: Scribner.

Hyde, H.M. (1975), *Oscar Wilde: A Biography*. New York: Farrar, Straus & Giroux.

Jacomb-Hood, G.P. (1925), *With Brush and Pencil*. London: John Murray.

Lago, M., & Beckson, K., eds. (1975), *Max and Will: Max Beerbohm and William Rothenstein, Their Friendship and Letters, 1893–1945*. Cambridge: Harvard University Press.

Langtry, L. (1925), *The Days I Knew*. New York: Doran.

Lewis, L., & Smith, H.J. (1936), *Oscar Wilde Discovers America*. New York: Benjamin Blom, 1967.

Maxwell, W.B. (1937), *Time Gathered: Autobiography*. London: Hutchinson & Co.

Schafer, R. (1967), Ideals, the ego ideal, and the ideal self. *Psychological Issues: Motives and Thought*, 5 (2–3): 131–176.
Sherard, R.H. (1906), *The Life of Oscar Wilde*. New York: Mitchell Kennerly.
Shewan, R. (1977), *Oscar Wilde: Art and Egotism*. New York: Barnes & Noble.
Stern, M.B. (1953), *Purple Passage: The Life of Mrs. Frank Leslie*. Norman: University of Oklahoma Press.
Tynan, K. (1913), *Twenty-Five Years: Reminiscences*. London: John Murray.
Tyrrell, R.Y., & Sullivan, E., eds. (1906), *Echoes from Kottabos*. London: E. Grant Richards.
White, T. de V. (1967), *The Parents of Oscar Wilde: Sir William and Lady Wilde*. London: Hodder & Stoughton.
Wilde, O. (1881), *Poems*. London: David Bogue; Boston: Roberts Brothers.
——— (1889), The decay of lying. In: *The Artist as Critic: Critical Writings of Oscar Wilde*, ed. R. Ellmann. New York: Random House, 1969.
——— (1899), *The Importance of Being Earnest*. In: *The Portable Oscar Wilde*, ed. R. Aldington & S. Weintraub. New York: Penguin, 1981. (The revised three-act stage version.)
——— (1956), *The Importance of Being Earnest: A Trivial Comedy for Serious People, in Four Acts as Originally Written by Oscar Wilde*. Intro. by S.A. Dickson. New York: New York Public Library. (Vol. I: the printed text; Vol. II, the manuscript facsimile; references in text are to Vol. I.)
——— (1962), *The Letters of Oscar Wilde*, ed. R. Hart-Davis. New York: Harcourt, Brace & World.
Wyndham, H. (1951), *Speranza: A Biography of Lady Wilde*. London: T.V. Boardman.
Yeats, W.B. (1922), *The Trembling of the Veil*. In: *The Autogiography of William Butler Yeats*. New York: Collier, 1965.

I am grateful to the William Andrews Clark Memorial Library, University of California, Los Angeles, for permission to publish previously unpublished material; and to the Estate of Oscar Wilde © 1982, for permission to publish excerpts and letters written by Lady Wilde.

The inconstancy of fame is the solace of youth. It was, at least, to Sir Max Beerbohm (1872–1956, knighted 1939), who successfully lodged his name in memory as a consummate dandy, parodist, essayist, caricaturist, and prose fantasist. The persistent excellence of his work is a marvel that found its spur in the apparently insuperable luster of his half-brother, Sir Herbert Beerbohm Tree (1853–1917, knighted 1909). Tree, whose last name is merely the *bohm* in *Beerbohm* Englished with an eye to advertising, is not so well known as he once was, but in his time he was the leading actor-manager in London. His day was a long one to Max, covering most of the younger brother's best years, so it will perhaps come as no surprise that the youth made of his elder a surrogate father, one to imitate and supplant, and that the elder tried to forestall this eventuality. As a consequence, we have in their twin careers a curiously mingled pair: on the one hand, Beerbohm was a writer who postured like an actor and got as much mileage from his dandyish costumes and bon mots as he did from his books; Tree, on the other, was an actor who loved to give speeches, who expatiated in prose, publishing essays on the theater and even, as his career began to give way to Max's, a collection of prose fantasies. Indeed, the power of the pen and the mastery of spectacle became confused, even iden-

4

The Radiance of a Family Fire: Max Beerbohm and Herbert Tree

ROBERT VISCUSI

tical, to the protagonists in this struggle: it was Herbert who first taught ten-year-old Max to draw caricatures, and it was Max who in such works as *The Second Childhood of John Bull* (1901) and *Rossetti and His Circle* (1922) made caricature and writing into forms of one another, the visual and the verbal so joining forces in these works that they possess the semiological variety of theater and the staying power of hieroglyphics carved in stone. Max won.

Knowing the outcome in advance merely prepares us to appreciate better the brilliance of the struggle. And "brilliance" is the appropriate word, because this is a play, as it happens, of lights.

Radiance

Summer morning, 1872, the Kensington Road. Rolling toward the City, passing the great bee-shaped Albert Hall to the right and the incomplete spire of the Albert Memorial to the left—and possibly peering out of the windows of their hansom with a persistent curiosity that their evident high urbanity often failed to mask, looking very proper and thriving, rode Julius Ewald Beerbohm, then sixty-two years old, with his three grown sons, Ernest, twenty-two, Herbert, nineteen, and Julius, Jr., eighteen. *Père* Beerbohm had come far and done well. Leaving his native Me-mel—then a Prussian, now a Lithuanian port on the Baltic—in 1830 at age twenty, he had enjoyed ten years as a Parisian dandy, then ten years as a settling businessman in London. In 1850, he had married as such a man should, not a minute too soon, and produced these sons and a daughter, Constance. Now his blooming boys were at work in the corn-factoring concern he had founded, while at home his second wife (sister of his deceased first) was about to give birth to his fourth son, his eighth and last child, Henry Maximilian. He had every reason to rejoice, but his pleasure was not to last long.

His three elder sons wished to avoid his path. He had set them early in it, sending them to his own Alma Mater, a German boarding school they had all hated and fled (Cecil, 1964, pp. 4–7). Soon they would flee his firm in the City as well. Julius, Jr., would become an impecunious *flâneur* and speculator. Ernest was to take up sheep-farming in Cape Colony, where he would marry a Zulu and drop out of family conversation altogether. And Herbert was dreaming of the stage.

Father warned, but Herbert persisted. His success had the unlikely glamour of the dreams that had inspired it. We get a glimpse of its quality by looking at him on another occasion, thirty-six years later, this time through the eyes of little Max, now grown up and a personage in his own right; though not yet married, Max had been by this time ten years dramatic critic of the *Saturday Review* and had a name as a dandy-about-town, as a parodist of genius, as an essayist of the first water. Still, as we can see, Herbert was ahead in the game:

> On a wintry and damp afternoon, in the year 1908, I was standing on the doorstep of my mother's house in Upper Berkeley Street, seeing off a man who had been lunching with us. A taxi stopped at the curb, and my brother Herbert stepped out of it in that dreamy yet ample and energetic way he had of stepping out of taxis. 'Oh, how are you, Mr. Tree?' my friend greeted him. 'I?' said Herbert, shaking the proffered hand and gazing round him. 'I? Oh, I'm radiant.'
> My friend, when I went to see him a few days later, said to me that this epithet, if any ordinary man applied it to himself, would doubtless seem rather absurd, but that Herbert's use of it was perfectly right and proper: he looked radiant, it was obvious that he felt radiant, and he told the simple truth in saying that he *was* radiant. My friend having spoken thus, looked in the mirror and, I remember, sighed.
> Herbert was for many reasons an enviable man, but I think that what most of us envied in him was that incessant zest of his. [Beerbohm, 1920a, p. 187]

Enviable zest belonged to this brother who Zeus-like had defied his father and prospered. Max was by comparison stifled: he was sent to ordinary upper-class English schools, Charterhouse and Oxford, by a grandfatherly parent who no longer provoked the outright defiance his first three sons had displayed. Max's rebellion sent him in the train of Wilde and Beardsley, where the flush of the cheek usually signaled some other cause than zest. Absinthe and furtive passions covered themselves in roses. Very fine, but not *radiance*, which Tree possessed and Beerbohm sought. It was, in practice, the essence of family power.

No wonder Max admired and envied. "Difficulties that would have crushed any man of no more than ordinary power to cope with them," Beerbohm (1920a) writes, "were for Herbert a mere pleasant incentive . . ." (p. 187). Max, who imitated his father in not marrying till near the age of forty, was after Oxford living at home a little impecunious while the household was running mostly on Herbert's bounty. And his whole youth was passed in watching the florid *bildungsroman* of this hero unfold.

Tree had begun acting as an amateur, rising quickly in the profession during the eighties, dealing easily with difficulty upon difficulty. He had followed a string of successes in leading roles by taking the next logical step, for those days, of leasing a theater, The Haymarket, and assuming the mantle of actor-manager, mounting his first production in 1887. Success led to greater success, and greater success led, in 1895, to Tree's decision to build himself a theater.[1] He obtained the leasehold on the site of the old Her Majesty's Theatre and built there a new house under the former name, this one a monument no less to the extravagant pretensions of actor-managership than to those of the Hanoverian Queen. From the extravagant Renaissance facade and towering mansard roof to the Fontainebleau chandelier looming over the gilt-and-plush auditorium, Her Majesty's Theatre justified in triumph both its namesake and its proprietor. George Bernard Shaw (1897), no complaisant flatterer, called it "quite the handsomest theatre in London," praising Tree's magnificence equally with his taste. Shaw made the most of Tree's open exploitation of the splendid name he had bought for the place:

> The first night was exceedingly glorious. Our unique English loyalty—consisting in a cool, resolute determination to get the last inch of advertisement out of the Royal Family—has seldom been better pushed. Not a man in the house but felt that the Jubilee was good for trade. Mr. Tree told us that he would never disgrace the name the theatre bore; and his air as he spoke was that of a man who, on the brink of forgery, arson, and bigamy, was saved by the feeling that the owner of Her Majesty's Theatre must not do such things. [Shaw, 1897, pp. 119–120]

Shaw aimed with his customary accuracy, for the figure in the carpet of Tree's career was a royal silhouette.

Partly it was a matter of business: theatrical dominance meant Shakespearean roles, so one had to be a convincing king. But there was will in it too. Tree (1913) made that plain enough:

> The actor, even though he be peasant born, will be able by the power of his imagination to acquire the rare gift of distinction. He will be able, by its aid to become a king—not the accidental king, who in actual life may lack dignity, but the king of our imagination.
>
> It is on record that Napoleon once administered a rebuke to Talma, with whom he had a dramatic affinity. The actor, it seems, in playing a Roman emperor, made violent gestures. Napoleon, criticising this exuberance, said, "Why use these unnecessary flourishes? When I give an order I require nothing to enforce it—my word is enough. This is no way to behave as an emperor." The first

[1] For full accounts of Tree's career, see Pearson, 1956; Bingham, 1979.

Napoleon was a great actor, and his dramatic instinct was not the least formidable among those qualities which made him such a power in the world's history.

As on the stage, so it is in real life; we are not what we are—we become what we imagine ourselves to be. [pp. 112–113]

Tree imagined to good purpose. His stage management came to be an eternal byword for meticulously and literally realized fantasy. He had in his production of A *Midsummer Night's Dream*, for example, real rabbits to scurry under the real leaves of real trees. An excess of his virtue, no doubt, but he employed it to better effect when he stepped onto the stage as Svengali or Richard II so utterly transfigured that his many followers would at first fail to recognize him.

And in private he might have been taken for some Prince. He by policy avoided the impression, as Napoleon had, that he needed to strive for effects. No grinding professional he. "Genius," he liked to say, "is an infinite capacity for not having to take pains" (Pearson, 1956, p. 17). This Byronic attitude represented, as it were, only the lordly approach to Tree's real pretensions. Between the glittering ceiling and the huge dome of his theater, he caused to be built for himself an apartment where, suitably off the ground, he entertained *en prince* and philandered *en pasha*:

> It consisted of two rooms, a large one which he fitted up as a banqueting-hall, and a smaller one which he used as a sitting-and-living-room, in the wall of which was a concealed bed. All round the rooms were painted murals depicting scenes from his productions. . . . He was happier in his theatre than elsewhere, and though a naturally timid man he would pass many nights when himself in the roof and the watchman in the basement were the only occupants of the building. In the large outer room he gave innumerable supper-parties after first nights and on occasions that could be described as special if they had been less frequent. [Pearson, 1956, p. 142]

Fortune favored this fantasy monarch. It happened that the decade of his greatest triumphs coincided with the reign of the sovereign he most nearly resembled, Edward VII, who appropriately knighted Tree in 1909. Both Tree and Edward VII were, as Beerbohm noted, Germans who lived most fully in the warm glow of public fantasy. And Tree himself underscored the parallels, going in summers to Marienbad, a favorite resort of the King, and, finally, imitating that royal prize bull most sincerely by siring a bumper crop of bastards. "Poor Herbert!" his wife said, "all his affairs start with a compliment and end with a confinement" (Pearson, 1956, p. 150). But in the light of the image of him sitting alone at night under the roof of his theater, the truth poignantly stands out that his royalty was a matter of art.

It was, nonetheless, a triumphant art, one that his little brother dearly wished to master. And Tree's single companion in that lonely theater, the watchman down below, may stand for us as Max's viceroy. There was much of the attentive sentry in Beerbohm. In that role we best consider him as dramatic critic: for twelve years, though he disliked the work, he sat in the dark watching Tree. He never attacked and sometimes even praised the family concern in print (Beerbohm, 1900, pp. 230–233). But mostly his was the fascination of the aspiring rival. "I have not," he remarked (1903) in the course of a review, "lately been impersonating an English king" (p. 535). If not lately, then when?

It was natural enough for Beerbohm to aim at being "the king of our imagination," considering that Herbert Tree had been for him from the earliest days a hero, a rival, a god, and even a father. In all of these guises, Tree was precisely *radiant*. It is a striking fact that he recurred to Beerbohm's imagination in the form of a red flame. The image had its source in the color of Herbert's hair. This is Beerbohm's first recollection of him, at a time when Herbert was twenty-two and Max three:

> Herbert seemed very tall, . . . and his hair was of a very bright red, at which I used to look up, with interest. It would seem that his hair had touched the imagination of other children before me. In the early 'seventies, young laymen were apt to be less wholly lay than they are now; and Herbert, at the age of eighteen, had felt it his duty to preach in the Sunday-school of a neighboring church, and had ceased to do so only when the children, presuming on his lack of sternness, began to call him 'Ha'porth o' Carrots. [Beerbohm, 1920a, p. 188]

This towering carrot had started, by the time Beerbohm's memory began to register his height and hue, to pursue heroic destiny; in 1878, Tree made his professional debut at the Globe, and of this occasion Beerbohm (1920a) wrote, "what I remember is scanty—just that memory of a bright redness high up . . ." (p. 189).

Bright redness became something more definite when, nine years later, while Beerbohm was at Charterhouse suffering the usual sensitive boy's griefs among the muscular Christians, Tree was summoning up the clouds of champagnes and celebrities for his opening at the Haymarket in his first production, a play by W. Outram Tristram entitled *The Red Lamp*. Max was overwhelmed by this glory:

Ripened judgement has not inclined me to think *The Red Lamp* the greatest play ever written. But I thought so on its first night—the first night of Herbert's management. And I saw it seventeen times, without changing my opinion. Herbert always let me sit in his dressing-room during the entr'actes, and there I met many of the most interesting men of the period—none of whom, however, interested me so much as Herbert. . . . and it seems to me, as I look back, that even during term-time, when my body was at Charterhouse, my soul was at the Haymarket Theatre. [Beerbohm, 1920a, p. 194]

The image of a red lamp became for Beerbohm both the form that male brilliance should assume and even the standard by which it would be judged.

He writes that Tree, as star of *The Red Lamp*, "interested" him more than "many of the most interesting men of the period"—whom he visualized, in any case, standing in a kind of cigar-smoke aureole around the great light. He would, two years after the essay just cited, transfer the same image to Dante Gabriel Rossetti, the man who pleased Beerbohm's ripened judgment as Herbert had his greener tastes:

Byron, Disraeli, and Rossetti—these seem to me the three most interesting men that England had in the nineteenth century. England had plenty of greater men. Shelley, for example, was a far finer poet than Byron. But he was not in himself interesting: he was just a crystal-clear crank. To be interesting, a man must be complex and elusive. And I rather fancy it must be a great advantage for him to have been born outside his proper time and place. Disraeli, as Grand Vizir to some Sultan, in a bygone age, mightn't have seemed so very remarkable after all. Nor might Rossetti in the Quattrocento and by the Arno. But in London, in the great days of a deep, smug, thick, rich, drab industrial complacency, Rossetti shone, for the men and women who knew him, with the ambiguous light of a red torch somewhere in a dense fog. And so he still shines for me. [Beerbohm, 1922, p. vi]

Rossetti and His Circle, which Beerbohm is here prefacing, uses caricature and caption to portray the Anglo-Italian poet-painter as the central radiance of a vast and influential circle that began with the Pre-Raphaelite Brotherhood and extended to include not only disciples like Burne-Jones and William Morris but even such remote luminaries as Tennyson and John Stuart Mill. The last disciple in the book is Oscar Wilde: Wilde, who for a crucial period in Beerbohm's youth occupied a central place in the young man's imagination, was a friend of Tree's. Most of Max's heroes were connected with his brother somehow in his mind. Indeed, "interest" and "radiance" and centrality for him all had sources in his images of Tree. Thus the whole enterprise of caricature—the impaling of heroes upon his pen—took place by the light of that red fraternal lamp.

A Family Fire

Max Beerbohm liked to watch fires. One of his more purposefully outrageous early essays bore the title "An Infamous Brigade" (Beerbohm, 1896, pp. 57–62). The brigade in question was a company of firemen who, he complained, ruined his pleasure by putting out a grand blaze he was enjoying one night. He called them vandals who destroyed beauty, and he proposed to counter them with a band of artists who would bring to fires their own hoses, filled with oil. Eleven years later, after a decade of theatrical reviewing, he returned to the theme:

> If I were 'seeing over' a house, and found in every room an iron cage let into the wall, and were told by the caretaker that these cages were for me to keep lions in, I think I should open my eyes rather wide. Yet nothing seems to me more natural than a fire in a grate.
>
> Doubtless, when I began to walk, one of my first excursions was to the fender, that I might gaze more nearly at the live things roaring and raging behind it; and I dare say I dimly wondered by what blessed dispensation this creature was allowed in a domain so peaceful as my nursery. I do not think I ever needed to be warned against scaling the fender. I knew by instinct that the creature within it was dangerous—fiercer still than the cat which had once strayed into the room and scratched me for my advances. [Beerbohm, 1907, p. 3]

"Sexualised fire," Gaston Bachelard (1938) has written, "is preeminently the connecting link for all symbols. It unites matter and spirit, vice and virtue" (p. 55). Fire, at the level Beerbohm is writing about here, has the force of utterly untamed libido, the transformation of desire that engulfs Don Juan or that Sodom and Gomorrah draw down from the sky. When he saw Tree and Rossetti as red torches, he paid tribute to the fetterless vitality and sexuality these men displayed. He desired to feed those flames even as he feared them. Like fire itself, his heroes brought together all categories and struck him with awe. And he watched the blaze in his grate with the same sense of his own lesser glory that he felt when he contemplated his big brother's radiance:

I look around the room I am writing in—a pleasant room, and my own, yet how irresponsive, how smug and lifeless! The pattern of the wallpaper blamelessly repeats itself from wainscot to cornice; and the pictures are immobile and changeless within their glazed frames—faint, flat mimicries of life. The chairs and tables are just as their carpenter fashioned them, and stand with stiff obedience just where they have been posted. On one side of the room, encased in coverings of cloth and leather, are myriads of words, which to some people, but not to me, are a fair substitute for human company. All around me, in fact, are the products of modern civilisation. But in the whole room there are but three things living: myself, my dog, and the fire in my grate. And of these lives the third is very much the most intensely vivid. My dog is descended, doubtless, from prehistoric wolves; but you could hardly decipher his pedigree on his mild, domesticated face. My dog is as tame as his master (in whose veins flows the blood of the old cavemen). But time has not tamed fire. Fire is as wild a thing as when Prometheus snatched it from the empyrean. [Beerbohm, 1907, pp. 4–5]

Bachelard (1938) suggests that there is such a thing as a Prometheus complex, and that this is the source of the intellectual's fascination with fire. It arises from "all those tendencies which impel us to *know* as much as our fathers, more than our fathers, as much as our teachers, more than our teachers. . . . The Prometheus complex is the Oedipus complex of the intellect" (p. 12). This aptly describes Beerbohm's feelings toward his big brother and toward the fire in the proscenium arch of his bedroom wall.

He knew that a fire, however papered-over and hidden out of reach, lurked in his own breast and could be made to burn as bright in him as in another man:

Fire is savage, and so, even after all these centuries, are we, at heart. Our civilisation is but as the . . . crust that encloses the old planetary flames. To destroy is still the strongest instinct of our nature. Nature is still 'red in tooth and claw,' though she has begun to make fine flourishes with tooth-brush and nail-scissors. Even the mild dog on the hearth-rug has been known to behave like a wolf to his own species. Scratch his master and you will find the caveman. But the scratch must be a sharp one: I am thickly veneered. Outwardly, I am as gentle as you, gentle reader. And one reason for our delight in fire is that there is no humbug about flames: they are frankly, primevally savage. [Beerbohm, 1907, p. 7]

No reader of Beerbohm's prose, no viewer of his caricatures, certainly no member of his family who knew his "sudden scathing careless remarks" (Grizel, 1975) could fail to recognize the frank, primeval savage beneath the thick veneer of Max Beerbohm.

He had three sisters as well as three brothers. Two of his sisters were writers as well, Constance and Dora. He was not fond of the idea that women should wield the pen, and when he found a woman novelist whose work was particularly "vital," he confesses, he threw it into the fire (Beerbohm, 1920b, pp. 239–246). While he could recognize that "a fire is a thing sacred to the members of the household in which it burns," Beerbohm (1907) held to the image of fire as something that was both privately and criminally his: "Personally, though I appreciate the radiance of a family fire, I give preference to a fire that burns for myself alone. And dearest of all to me is a fire that burns thus in the house of another" (pp. 10, 11–12). Here was the permanent Prometheus *in flagrante delicto*: free of the constraints of familial fellowship and, particularly, of his blazing brother, who was the radiance of *that* family's fire, he places himself here, like the watchman in Tree's theater, in the house of another, the cuckoo at the grate.

Even as he sat entranced in the Haymarket watching *The Red Lamp*, Max was cherishing his own flame, and Herbert had some sense of the danger. In that play, Tree had the role of Demetrius, head of the Russian Secret Police, arch-foe of the anarchist Terrorists. He glossed the situation thus in the opening-night program: "Where does Terrorism exist except in Society? One thing is clear as the sun at noon-day. Where do the Terrorists live, if not in the ranks of Society? With whom are they in daily communication, if not with its members?" (Tree, 1887). Max, who called himself a "Tory anarchist" (1920c, p. 181), was always there, the terror in society, watching, and Herbert knew it. Many years later, he made the point more explicit, comparing Renaissance and modern methods of assassination: "To-day we grind our axe with a difference. A more subtle process of dealing with our rivals obtains. To-day the pen is mightier than the sword, the stylograph is more deadly than the stiletto. The bravo still plies his trade. He no longer takes life, but character" (Tree, 1913, p. 235). Little Max, wide-eyed in his seat at the Globe or Haymarket, had grown into one of those pen-brandishing bravos who were the paid foes of such men as the monarch at His Majesty's.

Such were the imaginative terms in which the battle was waged. We can turn now to chronicling the engagements themselves.

"The Brothers of Great Men"

Max Beerbohm made his debut in the first number of *The Yellow Book*, with "A Defense of Cosmetics" (1894), a flamboyantly decadent essay that made him notorious. In a prose so riddled with paradox, oxymoron, hyperbole, and extravagant diction that it made Oscar Wilde's manner seem by comparison pale and chaste, Max defended the thesis that "Artifice must queen it once more in the town . . ." (p. 85). This proposition, supported by a varied and detailed knowledge of the catalogue of powders and rouges ancient and modern, offered him the chance, which he enthusiastically embraced, to represent the epicene career of a young dandy, himself, who had just left Oxford without a degree, in terms of the whole elaborate technique of masquerade for which his brother was already very famous. He left no doubt that this was his intention. Shortly after the essay had made his name a well-known term of opprobrium, Max had this exchange with an interviewer:

> "I am doing some work for the new *Saturday Review,* and I am in treaty with a publisher to produce a little book of studies and essays. At this moment I am writing a treatise upon 'The Brothers of Great Men,' including a series of psychological sketches of Mr Willie Wilde, Mr Austen Chamberlain, and others."
> "You are a brother of Mr Beerbohm Tree, I believe?"
> "Yes; he is coming into the series." [Leverson, 1895, p. 439]

Here he deployed his most cherished ambition as a strategem: exaggerated megalomania. Like Wilde and other dandies going as far back as Beau Brummell, Beerbohm was a virtuoso of the delusion of grandeur, always ready to imply that both his soul and his haircut had more to offer the nation than anything the Prince of Wales could claim; indeed, his two favorite subjects for caricature were himself, generally seeming to have carved and polished his own figure of ebony and ivory, and Queen Victoria's heir (afterward the namesake of Tree's theater), the always-very-belated-looking Edward VII, who flowers in Beerbohm's drawings like the rose of some ultimate decadence that appears once brandy and pheasant and fine ladies have all begun to fail to please. In his struggle with the magnificent Herbert, Max had ever ready the hyperbole of his own imaginings.

But this was not weapon enough. It was the stylo-stiletto that would do the work. And Beerbohm gives us much evidence to reconstruct the history of how he came to adopt this weapon. It is a history of masks, of hypocrisy. Like other licensed lunatics, Max hid his grandeur as virtue:

> I was a timid child, always on the side of law and order, a predilection which perhaps accounts for my having chosen to imagine myself a policeman, usually. But even this prosaic office I filled only

in the day-time. Night-beats, as tending to the possibility of conflict with ferocious burglars, I eschewed. After dark I was simply a man of the world. I was a very tall man of the world, with a large blond moustache and a pair of those small side-whiskers which lingered as a relic of the so very hirsute 'sixties. [Beerbohm, Taylor ms., pp. 2–3]

This retrospective conservatism opposed him to Tree, who, far from being on the side of law and order, "wanted to go on the stage. That, in those days, was a wild, an awful inclination, and somewhat horrified even my father" (Beerbohm, 1920a, p. 189). Though the father's horror subsided in the face of Tree's success, little Max continued on the side of right-eousness, choosing out from his brother's powers those which he could harmonize with his own filial rectitude and raising his hands in holy horror at the others:

In 1879, or thereabouts, I had acquired a habit of drawing pictures; and what I liked about Herbert, whenever he came to see us, was that *he* could draw pictures, too. I think I liked him all the better for that our styles did not clash. I drew *and* painted—especially painted. Herbert used pencil only. The subjects I chose were sol-diers, policemen, cottages, and knights in armour. These subjects he would sometimes essay, but only to please *me*: they did not really interest him, and his handling of them was (I still think) inferior to mine. What he excelled me in was Mr. Gladstone and Lord Bea-consfield. He could draw either of them equally well in profile or in full face, and as the features of both of them were both very familiar to me in *Punch*, whose cartoons I was fond of colouring week by week, I was in a position to appreciate his skill. I was a Conservative, and Herbert (to my wonder and grief) a Liberal. Yet his Lord Beaconsfield amused me not less than his Mr. Gladstone. My mother, too, was very fond of watching him draw, and for her he used to draw all sorts of people—people whom he had recently met. 'This is Whistler, the painter,' he would say, 'This is E.W. Godwin,' or 'Here's Oscar Wilde, the poet.' Henry Irving, however, was his favourite theme. And I remember him saying, one day, with some importance: 'The Routledges have asked me to dine on Sunday night, and Irving is to be there.' Whereat I communed with myself: 'Dinner? On *Sunday* night?' Mr. Edmund Routledge had the house opposite to my father's, and on the following Sunday, at my bed-time, I looked out at those lit windows, looked long at them. I was fascinated, in spite of myself, and, much as I pitied Herbert for being so unlikely now to go to Heaven, I was also envying him not a little, too. [Beerbohm, 1920a, pp. 189–190]

Henry Irving, very much the leading light of the theater in those days, had the fire Tree wished to steal. That he succeeded in taking Irving's place was one of the crowning proofs of Tree's success. Beerbohm had ample reason to set out after Tree in the same manner, for he was in a position to appreciate acutely the skill of the pencil that so enthralled his mother.

Indeed, he concentrated upon this skill. It was a way to wear one's flamboyance as respectably as possible. He employed caricature to shore up a position of absolute Tory orthodoxy according to the childhood terms outlined above.[2] And he held fast to his double childhood mask of policeman/man-about-town, keeping the policeman's moral superiority and the man-about-town's social superiority, both carefully wrapped into the pen of the dramatic critic, who was thus admirably armed to deal with the actor-manager's radiance. It did not matter, indeed it helped, that policeman or watchman or man-about-town is less glorious than the actor-manager. The critic is a moral hero, a hero without any embarrassing license to detract from his heroism.

Beerbohm made the most of this in sharpening his ironic quill. When, for example, he began his career as a dramatic critic, in his maiden essay he gave a long series of reasons "Why I Ought Not to Have Become a Dramatic Critic," including among them his brother's considerable fame and receipts, and concluding thus: "I daresay that there are many callings more uncomfortable and dispiriting than that of dramatic critic. To be a porter on the Underground Railway must, I have often thought, be very terrible. Whenever I feel myself sinking under the stress of my labours, I shall say to myself, 'I am not a porter on the Underground Railway' " (Beerbohm, 1898, p. 6). This kind of irony has been nicely named by Potter (1959) "The Petrifaction of the Implied Opposite" (p. 38), and it here represents family warfare of a kind that is equally vivid and sophisticated. Of course the theater is an Underground Railway—dark, unpredictable, and tiresome in its wantonness, the palace of madness.

And how clearly Beerbohm scored by announcing his place there as porter! This, he seemed to say, is where my family has brought me. I need the money (he actually did say this), and my brother's entrée could only open me this door. I shall do it, but do not expect me to pretend along with these fools on the stage. And so he sat there, stiffly enough, wearing his impeccable toilette as the appanage of authority, no less faithful to his duties and no less unalterably classified by cloak and hat

---

[2] See, for example, the series "Mr Gladstone Goes to Heaven," Hart-Davis, 1972, pp. 584–596, done in 1898, showing the old Liberal very uncomfortable in Paradise and finally giving it up as a bad job when he comes across a thoroughfare called Disraeli Avenue.

than the most steadfast porter. Week by week, for twelve years he attended theaters and wrote his reviews. He never abandoned his posture
of protest, however. In 1908, after a decade of this, he wrote an essay
called "Dulcedo Judiciorum," wherein he claimed

> I frequent the courts whenever I have nothing better to do. And
> it is rarely, as one who cares to study his fellow creatures, I have
> anything better to do. . . .
>
> I can understand the glamour of the theatre. You find yourself
> in a queerly-shaped place, cut off from the world, with plenty of
> gilding and red velvet or blue satin. An orchestra plays tunes cal-
> culated to promote suppressed excitement. Presently up goes a
> curtain, revealing to you a mimic world, with ladies and gentlemen
> painted and padded to appear quite different from what they are.
> It is precisely the people most susceptible to the glamour of the
> theatre that are the greatest hindrance to dramatic art. They will
> stand anything, no matter how silly, in a theatre.
>
> . . . . In the courts I find satisfied in me just those senses which
> in the theatre, nearly always, are starved. Nay, I find them satisfied
> more fully than they ever could be, at best, in any theatre. I do not
> merely fall back on the courts in disgust of the theatre as it is. I
> love the courts better than the theatre as it ideally might be. [Beer-
> bohm, 1908, pp. 263–265]

This was the logical development of his strategy of protest and his posture
as critic: he had in his mind turned the theater into a courtroom where
he might pass judgment on the glamorous Lothario who lived in the
dome. Naturally, an actual courtroom, without all the things that made
the theater the theater, pleased him more, gave him more of what had
become his essential pleasure in watching.

Thus it is that his clearest description of his delight in Herbert arises
from a courtroom spectacle. What he likes best there, he tells us,

> is a disingenuous witness who is quick-minded, resourceful, thor-
> oughly master of himself and his story, pitted against a counsel as
> well endowed as himself. The most vivid and precious of my mem-
> ories is of a case in which a gentleman, now dead, was sued for
> breach of promise, and was cross-examined throughout a whole hot
> day in midsummer by the late Mr. Candy. The lady had averred
> that she had known him for many years. She called various wit-
> nesses, who testified to having seen him repeatedly in her company.
> She produced stacks of letters in a handwriting which no expert
> could distinguish from his. The defense was that these letters were

written by the defendant's secretary, a man who was able to imitate exactly his employer's handwriting, and who was, moreover, physically a replica of his employer. He was dead now; and the defendant, though he was a very well-known man, with many friends, was unable to adduce any one who had seen that secretary dead or alive. Not a soul in court believed the story. As it was a complicated story, extending over many years, to demolish it seemed child's play. Mr. Candy was no child. His performance was masterly. But it was not so masterly as the defendant's; and the suit was dismissed. In the light of common sense, the defendant hadn't a leg to stand on. Technically, his case was unshaken. I doubt whether I shall ever have a day of such acute mental enjoyment as was the day of that cross-examination. [Beerbohm, 1908, pp. 273–274]

Why was Beerbohm's pleasure so "acute"? Strong feelings were engaged. First, Beerbohm had himself been Tree's secretary, during the spring of 1895, on a tour to America; Beerbohm did the work so painstakingly that it never got done, so he was relieved of the job but still paid his wage; on that same tour, he became engaged to Grace Conover, an ingenue in Tree's company. Second, he would caricature himself, in "Genus Beerbohmiense" (see plate), as "physically a replica" of his brother. Then, he had seen at close quarters the daring in Tree's philandering: in addition to the usual casting-couch opportunities that routinely fell to him, Tree had a second family in Putney, where he fathered six children over a period of twenty years.[3] And though his wife, Maud Holt Tree, was a leading member of his company, Tree carried on blithely under her nose, going so far as to cast himself in the title role of Stephen Phillips's *Nero*, while casting Maud as Aggrippina and his current mistress Constance Collier as Poppaea. That was in 1903. Shortly afterward, Max repeated his earlier exploit, this time affiancing himself not to an ingenue but to a star, indeed to Miss Collier herself.

It was a daring move, but Tree won this battle without even trying. Constance Collier was a great beauty, accustomed to warmer passions and fatter purses than Max could command. In a very short time, she fell in love with another actor, Julian L'Estrange, and dropped Max; she continued, too, to be seen with Herbert. The lesson was not lost on Beerbohm. He wrote (April 12, 1904) to his best friend:

> she felt it would never do, after all, for us to marry—neither of us being the sort of people for the serious responsibilities of life. . . .

---

[3] See Bingham, 1979, for the details of this "complicated story, extending over many years."

It *is* a pity I was not born either rich or the sort of solid man who
could be trusted and would trust himself to make his way solidly
in the world.

Of course I am a success in a way, and may continue to be so for
some time; but that is in virtue of certain qualities in my defects:
it is in virtue of a sort of humble fantastic irresponsibility; for solid
worldly success this is no good at all. And I now, for the first time
clearly, see myself as on the whole a failure—I have never coveted
the *solid* quality until now, when I find that without it I cannot get,
and don't deserve, Constance. [Beerbohm, 1964, pp. 158–159]

Of course the galling thing about Herbert was that he managed to combine
a "fantastic irresponsibility" with that enviable "solid" ability to rake in
the silver. There was always a good deal of pessimism and skepticism
around Herbert, but he himself made a point of never yielding to it and
was in consequence as masterly in his evasions of trouble as the philan-
derer under cross-examination. "The gigantic risks of His Majesty's Theatre never, so far as I could see, caused him to turn a hair. He was glad
if things were going well; if they weren't, he had a plan for making them
do so within a few weeks. He could look Ruin in the face and say, 'Oh,
I'm radiant'; whereat Ruin always slunk away, drawing her hood over her
face—foiled again" (Beerbohm, 1920a, pp. 187–188). Judges, like Ruin,
wear hoods; and Beerbohm in the courtroom had acute delight in watching
the drama of his brother's life played out with fresh and "authentic" actors.
But he played not only judge in that scenario. He was the secretary, too,
who posthumously became the great man's "author."

"He Could Have Done So"

Bernard Shaw once summed up the missed chance of Tree's career:

Tree should have written his own plays. He could have done so.
He had actually begun to do it as Shakespear and Molière had, by
tinkering other men's plays. The conflict that raged between him
and me at the rehearsals [of *Pygmalion* in 1914, where Tree as
Higgins constantly tried to revise the play in a direction that *My
Fair Lady* afterward made very familiar] in his theatre would then
have taken place in his own bosom. He would have taken a parental
pride in other parts beside his own. He would have come to care
for a play as a play, and to understand that it has powers over the
audience even when it is read by people sitting around a table or
performed by wooden marionettes. It would have developed that
talent of his that wasted itself in *jeux d'esprit* and epigrams. And it

would have given him what he was always craving from authors, and in the nature of the case could never get from them: a perfect projection of the great Tree personality. What did he care for Higgins or Hamlet? His real objective was his amazing self. That also was Shakespear's objective in Hamlet; but Shakespear was not Tree, and therefore Hamlet could never be to Tree what Hamlet was to Shakespear. For with all his cleverness in the disguises of the actor's dressing-room, Tree was no mere character actor. The character actor never dares to appear frankly in his own person: he is the victim of a mortal shyness that agonizes and paralyzes him when his mask is stripped off and his cothurnus snatched from beneath his feet. Tree, on the contrary, broke through all his stage disguises: they were his robes of state; and he was never happier than when he stepped in front of the curtain and spoke in his own immensity to the audience, if not as deep calling unto deep (for the audience could not play up to him as splendidly as that), at least as a monarch to his courtiers. [Shaw, 1920, pp. 251–252]

"Parental pride" clearly played a dominant part in the life of this man who fathered at least ten children. (On record are three by his legitimate wife, six by his wife in Putney, and one by an American actress, though there are rumors of others, particularly in America.) Authorial ambitions surfaced in many ways, too: Tree always kept a diary, wrote thousands of letters, notes for many of his productions, speeches for dramatic societies, interpolated scenes for many plays.

Tree founded not only a family and a theater, but the Royal Academy of Dramatic Arts as well. But none of this fathering had quite the permanent effect of the written word. Tree came to acknowledge this position, as shall be seen, but too late. Beerbohm, on the other hand, had recognized it from the start. Even before taking up his post at the *Saturday*, he wrote an essay entitled "Actors" (1897, pp. 27–32) where he gave the picture of actor-and-audience as monarch-and-courtiers and asked whether actors ought not to be envied all the applause they receive. Clearly, this question was always alive to him. His answer was a "formula": *"The actor's medium is himself."* "Ponder my formula!" he exclaimed. "The actor's art is evanescent, and he must needs, therefore, be rather hectic in his desire for fame" (p. 30). Writers and painters could afford to wait. Lest the point be missed, he repeated it in his conclusion, using as instances two of his own favored exemplars:

'Into the night go one and all.' But the gods are not ruthless. They have been kind to these players. We need not weep. In their days, these players have been blest supremely. What other artists, save singers, can match their laurels? Their art dies with them, but I think that in the immediateness, the directness of their fame, they are supremely recompensed. Great writers, great painters, must needs suffer many years of insult or of neglect. Most often, when the tardy paean is sung in their honour, they are too old or too bitter to be gratified by its sound. Nor is the paean, even if they still care to hear it, so loud and so near as to the actor. Mr. Meredith does not receive one 'call' at the end of any chapter, howsoever noble. When Mr. Whistler puts the finishing touches to a paper-lithograph, how exquisite soever, even Mr. Joseph Pennell does not clamber upon the window-sill and throw in a bouquet. Yet may both Mr. Meredith and Mr. Whistler be accounted lucky. Artists, not less great than they, have died without honour, consoled only by the sure knowledge that their work will survive gloriously. [Beerbohm, 1897, pp. 30–31]

Those bouquets at the windowsill remained, nonetheless, desirable, and Herbert continued to receive them by the ton: the ever growing fame of the great man made the little brother ever more determined.

There is, for example, in his work the very strong theme of the writer who would never be remembered at all had Max Beerbohm never written about him. This is central in *Seven Men* (1919), particularly in the story of "Enoch Soames," a poet so minor that when he sells his soul to the devil for the chance to visit the British Museum a hundred years later and learn of his posthumous fame, the only reference to himself he can find is as an imaginary character in a story by Max Beerbohm. There are echoes of the same notion in the story of "A.V. Laider," a gifted and compulsive liar (like Tree) whose fabrications exist nowhere but in Beerbohm's prose, and in Hilary Maltby of "Hilary Maltby and Stephen Braxton": Maltby is a writer who might have turned out like Beerbohm himself had not his social climbing led him to marry a woman who was "a lineal descendant of the Emperor Hadrian" (1919, p. 104). Beerbohm, under his own name, is narrator in all these tales, and the characters all resemble him to a degree (as indeed Tree did as well) but are not so successful as he at writing. The one most like Tree is "Savonarola" Brown, who figures as Beerbohm's steady companion at "second nights" during Beerbohm's years as a critic. Brown, like Tree, secretly is rivaling Shakespeare, in his case by composing a blank-verse tragedy that bears more than a passing resemblance to the tragedies that Stephen Phillips composed for the proprietor of His Majesty's Theatre. Brown's "Savonarola" is given in full, four of its five acts having been completed before the long arm of coincidence, which is much in evidence in the play, took the form of a "motor-omnibus" and ran Brown over, killing him in the middle of a conversation with Beerbohm on the theme of coincidence. Brown's play, written shortly after Tree's death, resembles not only Phillips's ersatz Shakespeare but Tree's notorious extravaganzas—his *Julius Caesar*, which featured all of Rome at the famous funeral speech of Mark Antony, or his *Antony and Cleopatra*, which had interpolated a vast spectacle showing Constance Collier as Queen Cleopatra in an apotheosis as the Goddess Isis, a scene that marks Tree as the true precursor of DeMille. "Savonarola" has a parody of the crowd scene in *Julius Caesar*. It also features such grandiose stage-directions as this:

> *Re-enter Guelfs and Ghibellines fighting.* SAV[ONAROLA] *and* LUC[REZIA BORGIA] *are arrested by Papal officers. Enter* MICHAEL ANGELO. ANDREA DEL SARTO *appears for a moment at a window.* PIPPA *passes. Brothers of the Misericordia go by, singing a Requiem for Francesca da Rimini. Enter* BOCCACCIO, BENVENUTO CELLINI, *and many others, making remarks highly characteristic of themselves but scarcely audible through the terrific thunderstorm which now bursts over Florence and is at its loudest and darkest crisis as the Curtain falls.* [1919, p. 207]

This comes as close as Tree ever could to writing the plays that, according to Shaw, he should have written. It is not very close. Not only is the hand Beerbohm's, but the pen it holds is poisoned, making of the things Tree actually did the satirical capital of what is surely the classic parody in its kind. For Beerbohm takes on not only Tree and Phillips but even their god Shakespeare.

"The Total Body of That Spirit"

What Tree could, should, have done, Beerbohm did. Not only did he install himself as chronicler of that extravagant Edwardian theatrical world which Tree ruled, so that it remains more alive in Beerbohm's bejeweled prose than in any quire of dull photographs of its lost glories; and not only did Beerbohm in tale and parody and essay carve into the printer's stone his own signature across all that Herbert had done and failed to do; but Beerbohm also took the positive step of writing, as perfectly as it has ever been done, "the projection of the great [Beerbohm] personality." Self-portraiture is the evident theme of all his work—from his caricatures, where he is his own favorite subject, to his essays, where his own imaginings and failings and desires and triumphs fill out the fullest full-length psychological presentation of a writer's own mask since Montaigne.

But self-projection was only a part of the issue. For Beerbohm as for

Tree, the center of the struggle was not some "self" but the ability to occupy the place of the father. Beerbohm wrote that Tree had always been a hero to him, but that his brother Julius, on the strength of a mustache (and let it be added, the paternal cognomen) had been a "god." "In the early months of '84 my classification of the two brothers underwent a sudden change. Herbert became a god, Julius sank to the level of a hero. For Herbert was engaged to be married; and being married had always seemed to me an even finer thing, a thing more essential to the full glory of the adult state, than having a moustache" (Beerbohm, 1920a, p. 192). Beerbohm was alive to the sexual symbolism, that is, not just of the hirsute face but of the event as well; and he found it overwhelming. The floral arches that the gardener erected for the wedding inspired awe: "I remember the surprise I felt when the gardener's brother said to me: 'They're not what you might call awful grand, but they're what you might call rustic.' To me they appeared awful grand" (Beerbohm, 1920a, p. 193). The dynastic implications in the event loomed large in Herbert's own mind and lodged themselves in Max's recollection: "And at the wedding-breakfast there were sillabubs, my favorite dish. I remember Herbert saying that they sounded Biblical—'And Sillabub, the son of Sillabub, reigned in his stead,' a remark which shocked but amused me" (Beerbohm, 1920a, p. 193). The recollection seems a startling confirmation of Jane Austen's dictum that everything happens at parties, for Herbert's remark had the ring, in retrospect, of clear-eyed prophecy: when, nine years later, old Julius Beerbohm died, Tree came into the family kingdom in every way: his name gave them all a measure of reflected glory, and his income kept all of them, from impecunious Julius to impractical Max and his doting mother, afloat.

Max tried countering this in all the ways reviewed: his power as a critic; his sharp tongue which kept him and Herbert in a state when they were together of, as Beerbohm (1920a) wrote, "terrified love" (p. 200); his caricatures and the ability they had to keep his mother fascinated; his actress fiancées, the first two of whom he recruited from Herbert's troupe. But none of this, finally, would do. Max needed two things: first to marry, and he finally did marry, in 1910, to an actress of course, but one prudently chosen, with an independent income and no ties to Tree; second, to establish in writing his own claims upon the dynastic mantle. This he did with his one novel and intended masterpiece *Zuleika Dobson, Or an Oxford Love Story*, which he published in 1911, in the second year of his marriage. With this novel, he established himself as a man in his own right.[4] It is dedicated *Illi Almae Matri*, and has at its heart the documentation of the son's claims over the mother's body.

[4] For a fuller account of its place in his plans and family position, see Viscusi, 1979a.

Closer to the epidermis, as it were, of the novel are other familial themes. There is Zuleika herself, described as "a lithe and radiant creature" (Beerbohm, 1911, p. 2), who carries much of Dora, Max's sister and Herbert's half-sister, a woman whose favor both of them valued.[5] There is the river Isis, with whom Zuleika in a moment of apotheosis becomes identified, like Constance Collier as Cleopatra. There is the hero of the book, the Duke of Dorset, a nonpareil undergraduate who represents Max dreaming of being as overpowering as Herbert; and there is Noaks, the Duke's pathetic double and rival, who represents the realities that Max's dreams of himself brought out. There is the Warden of Judas, Zuleika's grandfather, who figures in this novel as the totem of tradition, a kind of walking Dead Father. At one point he is described as a "mummy" (p. 134). Most important of all, there is Max himself, who appears in the novel under his own name; and with him, in a moment of divine apotheosis, there is the Great Nourishing Mother Herself, in the form of Oxford.

It is a fantasy, and never a more thoroughly realized one filled the arch at His Majesty's. As Julius and Herbert had been gods, so now Max, married and independent, portrayed himself ascending to that rank. Zeus, he tells us, in 1863 fell in love with Clio, Muse of History. He wooed her in the form of various historiographical monographs, but his suit did not prosper until Hermes whispered to him that Clio had a secret addiction to novel-reading. As a special favor to his new mistress, Zeus allowed that for once an historian might be given the novelist's powers of "invisibility, inevitability, and psychic penetration, with a flawless memory thrown in" (p. 174). The favored person was Max Beerbohm. And he was given to report Zuleika's fateful visit to Oxford, in which all the undergraduates would perish for love of her. Beerbohm gives this account in the central chapters of the novel. Zuleika has at this point humilated the Duke in a particularly degrading way, and Beerbohm in protest has decided to use his divine gifts to please himself.

Herein he plays the incestuous god. He floats out over the meadows that border the Colleges:

> The scent of these meadows' moisture is the scent of Oxford. Even in the hottest noon, one feels that the sun has not dried *them*. Always there is moisture drifting across them, drifting into the Colleges. It, one suspects, must have had much to do with the evocation of what is called the Oxford spirit—that gentlest spirit, so lingering and searching, so dear to them who as youths were brought into ken of it, so exasperating to them who were not. Yes, certainly, it

---

[5] For a full account of the family themes in *Zuleika Dobson*, see Viscusi, 1979b.

is this mild, miasmal air, not less than the grey beauty and gravity
of the buildings that has helped Oxford to produce, and foster eternally, her peculiar race of artist-scholars, scholar-artists. [Beerbohm,
1911, p. 180]

Thus he establishes that Oxford is a woman—moist and scented, and so
sexually desirable—and accounts for his own ability to exasperate Herbert,
who could not number among his advantages the Oxford education that
their father had procured for Max. The passage creates as well a noble
category—"artist-scholars, scholar-artists"—into which Max, however
peculiar and marginal he might have seemed at the moment, could slip,
there to keep company with Lewis Carroll and Cardinal Newman and
A.C. Swinburne—lingering gently, it might be, and forever searching in
the murk the dim frescoes that Rossetti and Burne-Jones and Morris had
made to sanctify eternally the walls of the Oxford Union. Once all this
was established, Beerbohm could set in his musical prose the full grandeur
of his claims:

> And on that moonlit night when I floated among the vapours of
> these meadows, myself less than a vapour, I knew and loved Oxford
> as never before, as never since. . . .
> I floated up into the higher, drier air, that I might, for once, see
> the total body of that spirit.
> There lay Oxford far beneath me, like a map in grey and black
> and silver. All that I had known only as great single things I saw
> now outspread in apposition, and tiny; tiny symbols, as it were, of
> themselves, greatly symbolising their oneness. There they lay, these
> multitudinous and disparate quadrangles, all their rivalries merged
> in the making of a great catholic pattern. [Beerbohm, 1911, pp.
> 181–182]

Oxford in that passage becomes not just Alma Mater but Mother Church,
Mother England; and to Max is given to see "the total body of that spirit."
At the end of his contemplation of her, Love moves him to weep:

> My equanimity was gone; and a tear fell on Oxford.
> And then, as though Oxford herself were speaking up to me, the
> air vibrated with a sweet noise of music. It was the hour of one. . . .
> [Beerbohm, 1911, p. 183]

Consummation follows this midnight rendezvous, where the radiance has
been a dandy's sexually ambiguous moonlight,[6] showing the body of Ox-

---

[6] For the debt of this moonlight to Oscar Wilde, see Riewald, 1953, p. 139.

ford "in grey and black and silver," a map in the monotone that belongs both to dandies and to writers. Beerbohm here has *written*, as fully as it can be done, his own kingdom, has made Oxford into Mother and made Mother his own in the form of a text, the substantial stone and mortar of the Colleges dissolving into "tiny symbols, as it were, of themselves, greatly symbolising their oneness"—greatly symbolizing, that is, their resolution into the body that Beerbohm claims for himself.

This, Beerbohm's moment of greatest achievement, did not stand alone in his career. Others responded to his grandiosity. G.K. Chesterton had cast him as Auberon Quin, the middle-class king of England, in *The Napoleon of Notting Hill* in 1904 and been a little taken aback to see how literally Beerbohm accepted the notion (Beerbohm, 1964, p. 160). Virginia Woolf (1925) dubbed him "prince of his profession" (p. 46). But no one so intimately felt the paradoxical radiance of Max's moonlight as did Herbert.

The Seed of Abraham

A struggle between brothers so far removed in age much resembles the struggle of father and son, for it is not merely a battle, it is a contention of love. The two are rivals and mutual dependents in many spheres. They help one another through the long dance of waxing and waning, each taking pride in the other's achievements, each understanding the other better than he can find words to say. Beerbohm and Tree, trapped in their "terrified love," kept at a mutually respectful distance. But Herbert helped Max for a long time, and Max expressed a certain sympathy for Herbert, and never so deeply as in his assertion (1920a) that the two were more alike than would appear to be the case:

> For twenty years after its completion [His Majesty's] was a source of immense happiness to him; it enabled him to realize his dreams; it fulfilled him. He achieved there things that he could not have attempted elsewhere; and these were the things nearest his heart and most agreeable to his ambition. I shall always be thankful for His Majesty's. For my own pleasure in play-going, let me admit, I prefer small theatres. And for my own delight in the genius of Herbert as an actor I liked His Majesty's less than the Haymarket. Robust though he was in mind and body, it was not in sweeping effects that his acting was pre-eminent. The full strength of his art was in its amazing delicacy. His humour and imagination, and his beautiful power for pathos, found their best expression in ways that were subtlest. Subtleties have a hard time on a large stage, in front

of a large auditorium. Herbert had to adapt his method to his surroundings. He did this with great skill and success; but I often
wished he had not to do it at all. Apart from his acting—and his
acting was but one of the many parts of him—I am entirely glad for
him that he had His Majesty's. [p. 201]

This amounts to an assertion—not unusual from one brother to another,
perhaps—that he understood Tree better than Tree understood himself.
It implies as well that Max himself had remained truer to the essential
"Genus Beerbohmiense"—that quality in the common seed that made
them sons of their father—than Herbert had done.

Such assertion and implication, here surfacing in eulogy, must have
formed a steady theme of Max's conversation *en famille*, and their efficacy
in reaching Herbert would not have depended much upon whether Max
said them to him in person, or by way of Dora or Constance or Maud or
Mama: Max, a gifted talker, had everyone's ear when he wanted it. And
the persistent theme that Herbert had somehow gone wrong, not merely
in bed where it was evident but in his art where he seemed to have
conquered the world, joined with Beerbohm's reminders of the immortality of writing and his ever increasing hegemony in the world of letters
(his "A Christmas Garland Woven by Max Beerbohm" [1912] gave him
acknowledged parodic mastery over every consequential writer then living in England)—all this penetrated to Tree. In the last few years of his
life, he began to think of writing. He published his essays in 1913. In
1916, a year before his sudden death, he was in California making a film
of *Macbeth*, snatching, as it turned out, at his one chance at the actor's
hope of a writer's immortality. The film, when it was finished, put him
to sleep at the first screening: a suitable result, for he had not enjoyed
Hollywood weather (it rained endlessly) or the process of making films.
To while away the hours in California, Tree made what, had he lived,
might have been the start of a new career. He wrote a book of stories.

They are not very good. But for beginner's work they are masterful.
Tree clearly had learned a good deal from his brother's work, for the
stories are written in a vein about halfway between Max Beerbohm and
Robert Louis Stevenson: prose fantasies echoing with conscious and unconscious self-portrayal. Had Tree continued as he began, given his remarkable determination and very extraordinary powers of concentration,
he might have done something very fine indeed. As it stands, however,
the most noteworthy thing in *Nothing Matters* (Tree, 1917) is "The Lament of a Lilliputian Twin," a story in which Tree confesses that his
brother has usurped him:

I am a freak of Nature. I am one of two, or two of one. I am, in

short, a semi-detached twin. We (how hateful to me is our plurality!)
are known to fame as "The Royal Lilliputian Twins." By all civilisation we are recognized as the champions of the twin world, while
from the Crowned Heads of Europe we have received the homage
due to the phenomenal condition by which Nature has singled—or
rather has doubled—us out for distinction among our fellow-men.
It is in no spirit of idle boast that I claim at least an equal share of
that Divine Right which is conferred by kings upon themselves; for
it is, after all, more difficult to be a twin with four legs and two
heads than it is to be a king with one head and two legs. Indeed,
it is my opinion that there would be lacking in my dual state no
element of superiority over the rest of mankind, were it not for the
fact that my other half is an utterly contemptible, not to say loath-
some, being. While I am sympathetic, high-minded, proud, but of
delicate physique, my brother is unintelligent, coarse, cunning, and
self-indulgent, but robust. We have two brains, but one stomach.
Imagine the horror of sharing a stomach with a man one despises!
I am called Ham; my brother is known as Abra. We were christened
Abraham; but, characteristically, my brother has usurped the first
two syllables, leaving to me the Ham, the smaller share of our joint
name. [pp. 125–126]

This might have been an ordinary Doppelgänger tale, of the kind that
writers from Poe to Conrad regularly turned out, were it not for the last
two sentences.

Tree's purpose had been to be a glorious son who would take his father's
place. "And Sillabub, the son of Sillabub, reigned in his stead." But now
he saw his rival brother had overtaken him. The last sentences of the
paragraph will not resist this translation: "I am called Tree; my brother
is known as Beerbohm. We were christened (and I meant forever to be
known as) Beerbohm Tree; but, characteristically, my brother has usurped
the first two syllables (Sillabubs), leaving to me the smaller share of our
joint name." *Abra* means *father*, even as *Beerbohm* was the family pat-
ronym; *Ham* here is bitter sarcasm for *actor*. By the end of Tree's life,
when this was written, his little brother, who had stood to him in the
relation of son to father or at least of vassal to lord, was well on his way
to reversing the situation. Beerbohm it was, childless though he was to
remain, who was going to carry the name forward into time. Tree's efforts
at immortality did not prosper: his film-making was forgotten, and among
his children was no legitimate son to bear his name. (One of his illegitimate
sons, Carol Reed, became a film director and was even knighted, as his
father and uncle had been, but always hid the truth of his parentage.)
Tree's name, glorious in its day, would survive only in the shady modesty

of theatrical history. But Beerbohm had already achieved the permanent little niche in literature that was to be his. A book is always there, and every new reader can give it new life. *Beerbohm* was going to mean *Max* Beerbohm.

Max was King in the family Lilliput after Herbert died. But victory has its price. Though Max Beerbohm lived thirty-nine years after Tree's death, and though he went from honor to honor, becoming in the fullness of time a knight and an honorary doctor of Oxford University and a Rede Lecturer at Cambridge and a Grand Old Man of the BBC, Max had lost in Herbert his real inspiration. Only one of his books, *The Dreadful Dragon of Hay Hill* (1928), was begun any appreciable time after Tree's death: it is, among Beerbohm's books, the one real failure. Everything else that he published between hard covers during those four decades was the completion of a project he had started while the other Royal Lilliputian Twin still contested the throne with him.

The contest had been, as suggested in the opening of this chapter, a play of lights. And these were, finally, to Beerbohm, Tree as the sun and himself as the moon. At the close of "Savonarola" (1919) the eponymous hero who so resembled Tree has died, as has Lucrezia Borgia, his mistress in the fantasy. The Pope offers for them a funeral oration which concludes, "In deference to this our double sorrow/Sun shall not shine to-day nor shine to-morrow," while the sun obligingly falls below the eastern horizon *"leaving a great darkness on which the Curtain slowly falls"* (p. 218). Beerbohm surely felt that darkness as he lingered in damp gloomy London for the better part of three years after Herbert's death, seated regally next to Tree's relict Lady Maud, going through the great man's innumerable papers, long diaries, mounds of letters, slicing out the thousands of references to matters that the dowager did not wish posterity to learn soon or easily or ever at all. At the same time he was cajoling Bernard Shaw and Desmond MacCarthy and others to write something to put into the memorial volume alongside his own memoir and the lucubrations of Tree's wife and daughters, which Max of course had to edit into presentability.

For most of this time Beerbohm's own wife Florence waited dutifully for him in Rapallo. There, in a small villa perched on a cliff overlooking the Ligurian Sea, the Beerbohms had set up house after their marriage. There, when the funeral games were over, Max would return to live out his interminable retirement, sitting, most days, on the tessellated pavement of his terrace, avid of the powerful Italian sun.

Brilliant and warm and progenitive of cataracts of flowers, that sun still could never do for Max what Herbert had. "I shall always miss him,"

Beerbohm (1920a) wrote. "He was a great feature in my life, and I am always wishing him back again" (p. 202). But there were only the fruits, a little dry as it turned out, of victory. Max, as the years went by, sometimes liked to talk to Florence of Miss Dustworth and Miss Libman, two pathetic spinsters who lived dreary lives before the War, lives brightened only by their visits, in cheap or complimentary seats, to the theater. Dreary ladies, one with a small settlement, both failed actresses, they cannot get along without one another. Not very interesting people, whose whole lives revolve around a glamour they have never done more than watch, they preoccupy aging Max. His own withered career and Florence's, for she was once an actress of promise and is now rather a tiresome hostess who always interrupts her husband's stories when his admirers come to luncheon, must be in his mind. He is not sure he should make so much of Miss Dustworth and Miss Libman: "Perhaps I have written . . . at too great length about them. I admit they are not remarkable women; not ladies exactly; narrow, uncultivated, without any fairness of vision. But am I mistaken in thinking there is a sort of awful cosiness about them? Florence thinks I am utterly mistaken in this opinion. Which of us is right? I will abide by your decision" (Beerbohm, 1972, p. 108). Of course, Miss Dustworth and Miss Libman are Florence and Max. It would appear that, secure in his fantastic imperial Italian retreat, the Royal Lilliputian turned upon himself the ironic eye and pen that Herbert had so long and beautifully withstood.

"Be It Cosiness" was the title of one of Beerbohm's earliest essays (1895). There, with the mock-stageyness he put on so well, he announced, at age twenty-four, his "retirement." He did not retire then, or even at age thirty-seven, when he bid farewell to his readers in the *Saturday* and left with Florence for Italy. But with Herbert's death came to Max a genuine retirement, a kind of perpetual veteran ease and boredom and "awful cosiness" that must at times have worn the color of an appropriate purgatory. Nothing again struck him so vividly as the memory of Herbert, suddenly stricken in the act of paring a peach for dessert, and perhaps the victor after all: "When I saw him early next morning, he lay surrounded already with the flowers he had been fondest of. His face was both familiar and strange. Death, that preserves only what is essential, had taken away whatever it is that is peculiar to the face of an actor. Extreme strength of character and purpose was all that remained and outstood now. But at the corners of the lips there was the hint of an almost whimsical, an entirely happy smile. And I felt that Herbert, though he was no longer breathing, was somehow still 'radiant' " (Beerbohm, 1920a, p. 202).

To picture Herbert immobilized forever and sealed in a box and carried at a stately pace behind the plumed horses down the Kensington Road—and yet, somehow, still radiant for Max—this is to consider once again the formidable paradox of fire, in which the images of fatherhood and rebellion, order and disorder, civilization and savagery change places perpetually like dancers. Freud (1932) speaks of Prometheus as the great civilizer, punished by the "gods" of libido for denying the deep homosexual pleasure that lies in extinguishing a fire with a stream of urine, the contest of a man's phallus with the furious insubstantial licking points of flame, a contest that ends with a satisfaction of hisses and smoke. Watching Max watch Herbert leads to a further reflection: that civilized—or overcivilized or "decadent"—man will seek to keep the fire burning, as indeed Prometheus did, but will take in the prospect a doubled pleasure that even Freud seems to share, mixing with his delight in its comfort a vicarious sharing of its joy. Max, it will be remembered, liked to imagine bringing artists to a conflagration dressed as firemen, carrying hoses filled with oil. If to sustain fire is to sustain civilization and to yield to the order of father and elder brother, there still may be some subtle revelry to be found in doing so with exuberance, as if obedience were rebellion and a man in tails could be a god. But that pleasure passes, and in its place arrives the duty of keeping the fire alight. Max fondly liked to think that Herbert dead was still radiant. But he wasn't. Max had won. It was he now who wore the mask of the family fire. And like Prometheus he was left at last with its burden, living out his long years on a cliff over the Mediterranean, rather fretful at times, and somewhat careful of his health.

REFERENCES

Bachelard, G. (1938), *The Psychoanalysis of Fire*. Boston: Beacon Press, 1964.
Beerbohm, M. (Berg ms.), *Notebook*. Unpublished manuscript. The Berg Collection. New York Public Library.
———— (Taylor ms.), *The Mirror of the Past*. Unpublished manuscript. Robert H. Taylor Collection, Princeton, New Jersey.
———— (1894), A defense of cosmetics. *Collected Edition*, 1:85–106, retitled The pervasion of rouge. London: William Heinemann, 1922.[7]
———— (1895), Be it cosiness. *Collected Edition*, 1:129–138, retitled Diminuendo. London: William Heinemann, 1922.
———— (1896), An infamous brigade. *Collected Edition*, 2:57–62. London: William Heinemann, 1922.
———— (1897), Actors. *Collected Edition*, 2:27–32. London: William Heinemann, 1922.

[7] I have followed Riewald (1953) in accepting *The Collected Edition of the Works of Max Beerbohm*, London: William Heinemann, 1922–1928, as standard; wherever possible, I have referred the reader to this edition.

———— (1898), Why I ought not to have become a dramatic critic. *Collected Edition*, 8:1–6. London: William Heinemann, 1924.

———— (1900), At Her Majesty's. *More Theatres: 1898–1903*, ed. R. Hart-Davis. New York: Taplinger, 1969, pp. 230–233.

———— (1901), *The Second Childhood of John Bull*. London: Stephen Swift, 1911 (first exhibited 1901).

———— (1903), Ibsen's 'Epilogue.' *More Theatres: 1898–1903*, ed. R. Hart-Davis. New York: Taplinger, 1969, pp. 532–535.

———— (1907), The fire. *Collected Edition*, 3:3–14. London: William Heinemann, 1922.

———— (1908), Dulcedo judiciorum. *Collected Edition*, 3:263–277. London: William Heinemann, 1922.

———— (1911), Zuleika Dobson, or an Oxford love story. *Collected Edition*, 6. London: William Heinemann, 1922.

———— (1912), A Christmas garland woven by Max Beerbohm. *Collected Edition*, 5. London: William Heinemann, 1922.

———— (1919), Seven men. *Collected Edition*, 7. London: William Heinemann, 1922.

———— (1920a), From a brother's standpoint. In: *Herbert Beerbohm Tree: Some Memories of Him and His Art*, ed. M. Beerbohm. London: Hutchinson, pp. 187–202.

———— (1920b), The crime. *Collected Edition*, 4:239–246. London: William Heinemann, 1922.

———— (1920c), Servants. *Collected Edition*, 4:161–182. London: William Heinemann, 1922.

———— (1922), *Rossetti and His Circle*. London: William Heinemann, 1922.

———— (1928), The dreadful dragon of Hay Hill. *Collected Edition*, 10:3–86. London: William Heinemann, 1928.

———— (1964), *Letters to Reggie Turner*, ed. R. Hart-Davis. Philadelphia: Lippincott.

———— (1972), Miss Dustworth and Miss Libman. *A Peep into the Past and Other Prose Pieces*, ed. R. Hart-Davis. Brattleboro, Vt.: The Stephen Greene Press, pp. 105–108.

Bingham, M. (1979), *'The Great Lover': The Life and Art of Herbert Beerbohm Tree*. New York: Atheneum.

Cecil, D. (1964), *Max: A Biography*. London: Constable.

Felstiner, J. (1972), *The Lies of Art: Max Beerbohm's Parody and Caricature*. New York: Knopf.

Freud, S. (1932), The acquisition and control of fire. *Standard Edition*, 22:187–193. London: Hogarth Press, 1964.

Grizel, Sister Margaret, O.S.M. (1975), Letter to the author concerning Sister Dora Beerbohm, O.S.M.

Hart-Davis, R. (1972), *A Catalogue of the Caricatures of Max Beerbohm*. Cambridge: Harvard University Press. (References to Beerbohm's caricatures in this essay are by Hart-Davis's catalogue numbers.)

Leverson, A. (1895), A few words with Mr Max Beerbohm. *The Sketch* (London), 8:439 (January 2).

Pearson, H. (1956), *Beerbohm Tree: His Life and Laughter*. London: Methuen.

Potter, S. (1959), *Supermanship*. New York: Random House.

Riewald, J. (1953), *Sir Max Beerbohm, Man and Writer: A Critical Analysis with a Brief Life and Bibliography*. The Hague: Martinus Nijhoff.

Shaw, G.B. (1897), Her Majesty's. *Our Theatre in the Nineties*, 3:117–120. London: Constable, 1954.

—————— (1920), From the point of view of a playwright. In: *Herbert Beerbohm Tree: Some Memories of Him and of His Art*, ed. M. Beerbohm. London: Hutchinson, pp. 240–252.

Tree, H. (1887), Opening Night Program for *The Red Lamp*, play by W. Outram Tristram. Theater Collection, New York Public Library.

—————— (1913), *Thoughts and After-Thoughts*. London: Cassell.

—————— (1917), *Nothing Matters and Other Stories*. Boston: Houghton Mifflin.

Viscusi, R. (1979a), A dandy's diary: the manuscripts of Max Beerbohm's *Zuleika Dobson*. *Princeton University Library Chronicle*, 40:234–256.

—————— (1979b), *The Dandy Dante: Max Beerbohm's Epic Allegories*. Unpublished doctoral dissertation. New York University, New York, N.Y.

Woolf, V. (1925), The modern essay. *Collected Essays*, 2:41–50. New York: Harcourt, Brace & World, 1967.

The testimony is unanimous: both brothers, their survivors, and the scholars agree that their relationship was superb and mutually supportive. The written remains show reciprocal solicitude over and over: Aldous for Julian's sinusitis and nervous breakdowns; Julian for Aldous's flickering and fluctuating vision. They also commiserated over money and over their separation. When they were together, the air crackled: "I always returned to my work," Julian writes, "stimulated and refreshed, my mental and spiritual batteries recharged" (J. Huxley, 1973, p. 96). Lady Juliette Huxley, Julian's widow, adds,

> To see and hear them together were some of the best moments of my life, their minds the same Huxley brand of steel, their interests so much alike with the profound difference of their temperaments. They loved each other deeply and expressed it most intellectually. [Personal communication]

Under strong attack from D.H. Lawrence, infuriated by evolutionary and psychological ideas, Julian the scientist was reinforced by Aldous the novelist; they considered Lawrence anti-intellectual (J. Huxley, 1970, p. 160). Each supported the other in intellectual risk and in social reform. They overlapped like the logical circles of a Venn diagram, but each had his own preoc-

5

Brothers Under the Skin: Aldous and Julian Huxley

PHILIP WEST

cupations. The relationship was not fixed, however; each brother on occasion sallied across the borders into the concerns of the other.

However voluble the brothers in person and in print and however unanimous the second- and third-hand evidence, arriving at significant conclusions involves complex methodological problems. The principals are dead, not to be queried. I knew neither of them alive. Secondary sources must be considered as having filtered data through their own personalities. While these limits apply to most studies, in the case of Aldous and Julian, fire is even more telling. In 1961 a brushfire in the dry Los Angeles hills consumed all of Aldous's papers except the manuscript of *Island*. He lost everything he had accumulated toward his memoirs: books, manuscripts, letters from others, including those from Julian. Hence, in the absence of an autobiography, it was given Sybille Bedford (1974) to produce the authorized biography of Aldous. Julian, on the other hand, produced two volumes of memoirs (1970, 1973) but no one has undertaken a biography. The letters he received from Aldous are included in the standard edition, but his letters to Aldous are lost. To infer the relations of the brothers from one's memoirs and the other's letters is risky: like listening to a series of phone calls, the present speaker only, half from Julian's end, half from Aldous's.

Aldous, for example, asked Julian to visit the nineteen-year-old Maria Nys, later Aldous's first wife, and send him an opinion. It appears not to have been entirely positive; the response it provoked from Aldous was "chilly" (Bedford, 1974, p. 94). When Julian was on the verge of proposing to Juliette Balliol, he kept it entirely to himself. It is telling as to the closeness of the relationship of the brothers that Lady Ottoline Morrell wrote Aldous to ask whether a romance was afoot, and just as telling that Aldous wrote back that he knew nothing. The one-sidedness of the direct correspondence has the effect of making Aldous seem often to be admonishing Julian—gently, though, in the style of his "soft impeachment" of being in love with Juliette. Finally, one labors under the traditional misgivings about authorized biographies and selective publication of letters that plague studies of such great Victorian figures as the ancestors of Aldous and Julian, T.H. Huxley and Matthew Arnold among them. Julian (1973, p. 169), for example, complains mildly that Laura Archera, Aldous's second wife, included in *That Timeless Moment* things better left unsaid about Aldous's last years.

The brothers' interactions around money seem at once cooperative but distant. When Aldous's London agent, Pinker, went bankrupt frittering away such funds as authors' royalties, Aldous authorized Julian to act for him after his own lights; when Julian and Juliet needed furniture, Aldous passed on to them some used furniture. Julian sent Aldous a check unsolicited for it, but Aldous returned the check with an expression of embarrassment over the condition of the goods (Smith, 1969, p. 302). Julian seems to have felt financial pinches more than Aldous, and they may have made some contribution to the depressions to be discussed later. Though Julian felt disdain for H.G. Wells, the promise of big money kept him involved in the collaboration on *The Science of Life*.

It is interesting how many of Aldous's letters to Julian begin with a paragraph mixing money and health before moving on to ideas. Julian (1970) records a childhood story of his involvement—involuntary—in helping Aldous. The occasion was a 1901 unveiling of a statue of T.H. Huxley:

> my own family was there, together with Gran'moo and hordes of Huxley aunts, uncles and cousins. Aldous was not quite five years old, and found the lengthy ceremony very trying. Suddenly my mother whispered, 'Give me your top hat.' 'What for?' I muttered. 'For Aldous to be sick in—he's turning green.' 'I won't,' said I, unwilling that my sacred headgear [Julian had just entered Eton] should be so profaned. 'But you must,' she said, 'we can't have him making a mess on the floor before all these grand people.' 'No, No,' I hissed, clutching the precious object, carefully ironed for the occasion, behind my back. And then Aldous miraculously restrained himself, and my hat was saved. [p. 47]

Julian told this story in the late 1950s to the Duke of Edinburgh when, standing by the same statue, he was about to inaugurate a Huxley wing of the Natural History Museum: "By then I was able to see its comic side."

Julian's sinuses were a perpetual trial; Aldous uncovered in Los Angeles a musical treatment devised by a Dane, Dr. Christian Volf.

> One listens through ear-phones to a record of synthetic sounds in the lowest musical octave and the effect is to give an intense internal massage, vibrating the bones of the skull, stimulating nerve activity and circulation and resulting, in cases of congestion, in immediate discharge. I have heard of many people who keep sinusitis at bay simply by listening to the record every morning before breakfast. [Smith, 1969, p. 626]

Aldous also found for himself the Bates system of eye-training, a quasi-meditational form of muscle relaxation, and it did do him some good, though not enduring. Aldous was in general less sanguine about the medical establishment than Julian, but that was part of his solitary nature, a sharp contrast with Julian's preferences for organizations and their lower-paying but steady salaries; his mental compensation came from knowing his place in the structure. Aldous, by contrast, was not likely to accept an external definition of his own place.

Of the two nervous breakdowns Julian tells us much about, the second clearly had a financial aspect. The first, in 1912, was "due to unresolved conflicts about sex" (J. Huxley, 1970, p. 153); writing that it was "a real 'nervous breakdown'—in modern terminology a depression neurosis, a horrible experience, a hell of self-reproach, repressed guilt, a sense of my own uselessness and the futility of life in general" (p. 97), he compares it with the Dark Night of the Soul. He had written about that experience in the interval in *Religion Without Revelation* (1927):

> Most disorders of this type are apparently paralyses of action caused by the mental house being divided against itself, and squandering all its energy in civil war; this is combined, for most of the time at least, with extreme depression, worry, and self-reproach. To the sufferer they are the extremest blackness of the soul's night, a practical demonstration that not only heaven but hell is within us, and that neither the one nor the other need seem deserved. [p. 125]

The breakdown, Julian noted, rendered him "profoundly miserable, as well by paralysing my energies [as] by threatening to tear my mental being in half" (p. 120). Julian was aware of the difference between his self-assured exterior and the internal reality of "intense activity of work to make up for the assurance . . . of which a divided self is robbed" (p. 120). It became a treadmill of insecurity, overwork, exhaustion, illness, depression, and breakdown.

The 1912 breakdown was treated by long convalescence in a sanatorium in Surrey. "The one incident I remember," Julian (1970) writes, "from that depressing interlude is of a robin perching on my window-sill and, after some effort, disgorging a tiny black pellet" (p. 97). Julian adds that the pellet consisted of "wing cases and other hard parts of small insects, so I was able to add a mite to my ornithological knowledge." More interesting is the symbolic value of this incident toward his cure: the bird's effort, the vomiting, the blackness of the pellet. The description of his added knowledge as a "mite," a small insect, may well, by way of unconscious punning, identify his psyche with the robin's stomach.

The 1944 breakdown followed his forced resignation from the London Zoo and a resultant loss of income. He returned from an exhausting trip to Africa "yellow with jaundice and deeply depressed," suffering from hepatitis (J. Huxley, 1970, p. 279). He remembers treatment by electroshock without anesthesia, and Juliette's signing a release from liability for broken bones; convalescence in this instance took place at Colorado Springs.

In 1945 Aldous wrote Julian a long letter of consolation. The nearest he had been to a breakdown was only "a long spell of insomnia," but he found the threat in it, like that in a breakdown, more severe because "mind is so much closer to the essential Self than the body" (Smith, 1969, p. 525). In *Religion Without Revelation*, Julian had considered breakdowns a form of the Dark Night of the Soul; in the letter Aldous describes the mental disciplines that restore light. Both Aldous and Lady Ottoline Morrell had recommended the work of the Swiss psychiatrist Vittoz. Aldous writes,

> What Vittoz's methods do bring out very clearly is the great importance of doing physical actions consciously and voluntarily, not permitting them to be done hugger-mugger and automatically, in a blind, thoughtless process of 'end-gaining' that totally ignores the 'means-whereby'. [p. 526]

This openness, awareness, and self-discipline, Aldous argues, corresponds to the higher states described in non-Western sacred writings; error consists in "improper ways of attending to things and by using consciousness, not to let go and open up but to tighten the grasp upon personal prejudices and bad habits" (p. 527). He recommends one seek "the grace of aesthetic experience . . . and the grace of mystical experience, which can only come when alert passivity is carried . . . to the point of complete humility and selflessness . . . , where thinker, thinking and thought are one" (p. 527). In *Religion Without Revelation*, Julian had gone no further toward a solution than to cite such Romantic nature poets as Wordsworth; Aldous's letter is, in speech act if not in form, a small sermon. And it would seem that Maris saw Julian much as Aldous did:

> Julian came and went like a dream. . . . Every minute of his stay was perfect and I believe he enjoyed it as much as we did. Poor Julian, . . . whenever he is not talking about his own affairs—and I must say very interesting—he has such a sad look in his face, perhaps that is why he must keep his mind crammed and crammed with outside business. [Bedford, 1974, p. 531]

The inability to deal with outside business is apparently what drove Aldous to inside business. Had Aldous his sight, both he and Julian would have ended up biologists; Julian recalls that he and Aldous had the same biology teacher at the beginning, a man memorable for his expression "the key to the Absolute": for Julian it meant a particularly pure laboratory fluid, for Aldous the purest transcendental idea.

Aldous's vision appears to have been a lifelong problem. "Whether the disorder was organic or psychosomatic in origin," Woodcock (1972) writes, "it is impossible now to determine for lack of evidence dating from that period" (p. 43). His vision may have been weak before he entered school; by 1912, "for practical purposes he was totally blind" (Smith, 1969, p. 39). An infection of *staphylococcus aurens* had afflicted him with *keratitis punctata*; in 1912 he underwent surgery for scarring on the cornea; he retained faint light perception in the left eye: "at best he could tell night from day, sunlight from dark shadow" (Woodcock, 1972, p. 44). With the aid of a powerful magnifying glass, he could read with his left eye. He learned Braille, both letters and music, and touch-typing; his friend at school Lewis Gielgud also learned Braille in order to keep up their correspondence. At this time, 1914, Aldous published his first piece in, of all things, *The Climbers' Club Journal*, a mountain climbers' student publication at Balliol College; typical of Aldous's ability to "see eternity in a grain of sand," he wrote about climbing staircases. The most significant advance in his vision occurred when he discovered the Bates method in 1939: he experienced for the first time in his life stereoscopic vision. In 1942 he wrote and published a defense of Bates, *The Art of Seeing*. Bates assumed "that eye disease and defects of vision are not merely physical in origin, and that as far as they are physical they arise usually from failure to allow the eye to function properly" (Woodcock, 1972, p. 237). Aldous's responsiveness to this treatment seems the chief base for Woodcock's hypothesis that his eye problems may well have been psychosomatic. One might raise, further, the question of whether his blindness and Julian's depressions might be variant symptoms of some common etiology now not traceable. In any case, the benefits of the Bates treatment dissipated by 1951 and for the last decade of his life Aldous suffered cataracts. Nonetheless, it was Aldous who persuaded Julian to paint a still life with him during one visit (Bedford, 1974, p. 238).

The tactility of Braille keys an important characteristic of Aldous's experience of both nature and art. We will see below that much earlier than 1912 he was preoccupied with skin, the body's ultimate sensor of the external world. Thus, his friend Kenneth Clark remarked on his close-up scrutiny of paintings, his preoccupation with texture, and his taste for drapery in Renaissance and Baroque art (Woodcock, 1972, pp. 41–42).

During one drug experience described in *The Doors of Perception* (1954), he meditates on his own crossed legs, "those folds in the trousers—what a labyrinth of endlessly significant complexity! And the texture of the gray flannel—how rich, how deeply, mysteriously sumptuous!" (p. 30). The average representation of the Madonna or an Apostle, he states, comprises ten percent of a painting: "All the rest consists of many colored variations on the inexhaustible theme of crumpled wool or linen" (p. 31). In *Heaven and Hell* (1954), Aldous associates a negative visionary experience with "a body that seems to grow progressively more dense, more tightly packed, until he finds himself at last reduced to being the agonized consciousness of an inspissated lump of matter, no bigger than a stone that can be held between the hands" (p. 136). Or perhaps as small as a pellet disgorged by a robin. Aldous remarks, too, that many of the punishments in Dante's *Inferno* involve "pressure and constriction."

> Dante's sinners are buried in mud, shut up in the trunks of trees, frozen solid in blocks of ice, crushed beneath stones. The *Inferno* is psychologically true. Many of its pains are experienced by schizophrenics, and by those who have taken mescalin or lysergic acid under unfavorable conditions. [p. 136]

Under favorable conditions, however, these drugs provided Aldous inner sight and insight.

Although he concedes in *The Doors of Perception* (1954) that he was and for as long as he could remember had always been "a poor visualizer" (p. 15), and that "most visualizers are transformed by mescalin into visionaries" (p. 45), he makes exceedingly small claims on his own behalf: "What the rest of us see only under the influence of mescalin, the artist is congenitally equipped to see all the time. His perception is not limited to what is biologically or socially useful" (p. 33). Although he seems to identify with "the rest of us" and to distance himself from the "artist," whose experience is not drug-induced and intermittent, Aldous does link himself with the artist in a shared experience of drapery: "For the artist as for the mescalin taker draperies are living hieroglyphs that stand in some peculiarly expressive way for the unfathomable mystery of pure being" (p. 33). They stand for pure being in that they are structures or patterns rather than entities or ideas. Later we shall find Aldous describing the inadequate forms of conscious, verbal knowledge in the language of crystallography; his mescalin experience, though similarly geometrical, involves the shifting grids of topology.

The typical mescalin or lysergic-acid experience begins with per-

> ceptions of colored, moving, living geometrical forms. In time, pure
> geometry becomes concrete, and the visionary perceives, not pat-
> terns, but patterned things, such as carpets, carvings, mosaics.
> These give place to vast and complicated buildings, in the midst of
> landscapes, which change continuously, passing from richness to
> more intensely colored richness. [pp. 96–97]

The drugs also offered Aldous an experience of color long denied him.
The primary common feature of the experience of the visionary is of light;
everything is "brilliantly illuminated and seems to shine from within."
Colors "are intensified to a pitch far beyond anything seen in the normal
state, and at the same time the mind's capacity for recognizing fine distinctions of tone and hue is notably heightened" (p. 89). This is characteristic of all descriptions of otherworldly Paradises and earthly Golden
Ages. Reflective gemstones, translucent stained glass, precious metals:
all have value as intensifiers of light and color. Painting, dramatic spectacle, and the illumination of cities lift the mind—except when "it occurs
nightly and celebrates the virtues of gin, cigarettes and toothpaste" (p.
115).

Imagery of the experience of light against dark pervaded Aldous's work
even before he began his drug experiments. It keys the fairly standard
"dialectic of opposites—nihilism—mysticism, flesh-spirit, corruption-re-
generation—which dominates his thought and work. . . . [T]he search for
light in darkness . . . is the grand metaphor of his life . . ." (Woodcock,
1972, p. 41).

The deficiencies of Aldous's physical vision and his weakness as a mental
visualizer "combined to enhance his eventual desire for a visionary life
that would overleap the physical world, real or imagined" (Woodcock,
1972, p. 44). It is a most touching image, finally, of Aldous in the California
desert standing as close as he could get to a Yucca tree—they fascinated
him—and puzzled by the buzzing about him at the mass emergence of
indiscernible locusts.

Finally, Aldous's cancer. Everyone knew Aldous was not well in 1963,
but Aldous knew it better than any of them. Julian and Juliette saw him
off to California: "The last we saw of him was at the airport—he said
goodbye, and opened his brief-case to take out some papers . . ." (J.
Huxley, 1973, p. 223). A few days later he wrote them to say that he had
had a malignant tongue tumor since 1960; it was destroyed by radiation
treatment, but spread to the lymph glands of the neck. One was removed
but another mass appeared and was treated; one nerve controlling the
vocal cords was permanently damaged and Aldous left in a generally
weakened condition. His wife, Laura, wrote shortly after to say that

"Aldous really had terminal cancer and that there was no hope of his recovery . . ." (J. Huxley, 1973, p. 224). Aldous died in less than two months; Julian organized the British memorial service at Friends' House, the Quaker headquarters, and edited the collected addresses and the appreciations of friends who did not speak that day into *Aldous Huxley: A Memorial Volume* (1965). He and Laura also selected Sybille Bedford to produce a suitable biography. This reminds us of Lady Huxley's statement, "They loved each other deeply and expressed it most intellectually."

As one would expect, the brothers provided each other material. For example, Julian and H.G. Wells were collaborating on *The Science of Life*. Throughout, Wells badgered Julian to produce copy, to keep pace, to keep profit before his mind and even to slight his teaching. Julian (1970) describes Wells's letters as "blasts."

> *My dear Huxley,*
>   You will know that Brown [Curtis Brown, a literary agent] has turned down part of Book III as boring. He objects to the evolution of the Horse being done in such detail. I have now re-read Book III. He is wrong about that section, but he is right about objecting to Book III as it stands. The only interest of that horse stuff lies in its controversial value, and Book III begins so lazily, loosely and slackly that only the initiated will grasp the bearing of this horse material. [p. 163]

Wells concludes his long critique of Julian's 150,000-word manuscript, "Look at this letter! If it was an article I could get 1500 dollars for it. Look at the waste of time and attention, Oh my collaborator!" Some of the deleted material appears in "The Evolutionary Process," Julian's lead essay in a collection (J. Huxley, Hardy, and Ford, 1954) of which he was senior editor; the other contributors, in benevolent insubordination, seized the foreword to turn the volume into a festschrift in his honor. Here the "horse stuff" is more lighthearted.

> During its 50 million years of evolution, the horse stock reduced the number of its toes, and increased the complexity of the grinding pattern of its teeth. But any further complexity of tooth-pattern would be less efficient for grinding-up grass stems, and clearly a reduction of the number of toes below one per foot would not be advantageous. [pp. 8–9]

More economically and in more dignified context, Aldous had quoted the "horse stuff" in a form fit for *The Perennial Philosophy* (1944):

> There is no reason to suppose that, between the thirteenth century and the twentieth, the human mind underwent any kind of evolutionary change, comparable to the change let us say, in the physical structure of the horse's foot during an incomparably longer span of geological time. [p. 17]

This condensation of his idea had given Julian the hint for a less ponderous use of it later on. A similar instance of such cross-pollination occurred near the end of Aldous's career, when he derived a major essay from one of Julian's simple, concrete observations. In his remarks at the memorial service for Aldous, Julian (1965) recalled a recent conversation with his brother:

> Only this year, when I was talking about Rachel Carson's *Silent Spring*, and explaining how our butterflies and poppies and hedgerow flowers were disappearing and our song-birds and falcons were being poisoned by pesticides, he said, "It is dreadful: they are destroying half the basis of English poetry." [p. 24]

In *Literature and Science* (1963), his last book, Aldous develops Julian's observation into a seven-and-a-half-page essay on the differences between what scientists know about nightingales and what poets have made of them. The longest of the thirty-eight sections of the book, it is number thirty-seven, a comprehensive demonstration of one mind's encounter with the Two Cultures in a mood of healing and wholeness.

Literature, Aldous argues, links experience and discourse always in surprising ways; science does, too, sometimes, but whatever rifts occur are produced by science, which "de-poetized man's world and robbed it of meaning" (p. 111). Aldous asserts that the only way to restore meaning is to abandon the quest for "symbols standing for things outside the world" in order to embrace the world's intrinsic poetry: "Its significance is the enormous mystery of its existence and of our awareness of its existence" (p. 111). Such satisfaction is not merely perceptual but cognitive. The poet finds a new nightingale.

"There is," Aldous continues, "subject matter here for a richly ramifying essay, a poem, at once lyrical and reflective, a long chapter in a Proustian novel" (p. 112). Aldous had written Julian years before that the true man of reason combines the lyrical and the critical, Shelley and *The Edinburgh Review*. His Proustian exercise in memory surveys the nightingale in recent English poetry. From Ovid's *Metamorphoses*, VI, oddly overlooking Milton's *Il Penseroso*, through Keats's "Ode to a Nightingale," through Matthew Arnold's "Philomela," on to Eliot's "The Waste Land"

and "Sweeney Among the Nightingales," Aldous establishes a poetic continuity against which to gauge the losses brought on by science's discoveries: (1) not the female but the male nightingale sings; (2) his song is not for courtship but for territorial challenge; (3) he sings not from pangs of love or sorrow but because his digestive system wakes him every four or five hours; (4) his existence is threatened because he lives on caterpillars being decimated by insecticides; and (5) after the eggs are hatched, "glandular change within the cock nightingale's body puts a stop to all singing. . . ." and he is left only an "occasional hoarse croak" (p. 116). This new data is, nonetheless, potentially poetic: "To ignore it is an act of literary cowardice" (p. 117). Between Ovid and Keats, the Middle Ages and the Renaissance held radically different poetic views of the nightingale; if the view changed once, it can change again, and it must. What science tells us focuses the imagination on the significance inherent in the natural object, the meaning within the world. "Far more deeply interfused," writes Aldous, alluding to Keats, "than any scientific hypothesis or even any archetypal myth . . . is the Something whose dwelling is everywhere, the essential Suchness of the world, which is at once immanent and transcendent" (p. 117). The science-produced rift between the Two Cultures is healed only by a perennial philosophy.

The large questions the brothers had to resolve as individuals were also the ones they often discussed together. They involve a psychological approach to the philosophical problems raised by the Two Cultures, a philosophical dispute over the dissociation of twentieth-century sensibility. C.P. Snow's *The Two Cultures* defined the problem, the solution to which, he claimed, lay mainly in the hands of science. Opposing him was the literary critic F.R. Leavis, who claimed it lay in the hands of the humanities. This dispute had the dimensions of a family argument for Aldous and Julian insofar as it perpetuated a disagreement between the Huxley side of the family and the Arnold side. The amazing veneration they both had for T.H. Huxley was due to his unique ability to transcend the conflict, straddle the split, and achieve a wholeness despaired of since the death of the ideal of the Renaissance Man. Aldous and Julian's formulation of the problem centered on the Victorian doctrine of work: the question changed from "What is there to be done?" to "What shall we decide to do?" Aldous tries to temper Julian's sanguine expectations about what can be accomplished through formal organizations: the larger the less. "Two major obstacles," he tells Julian in a letter, "in the way of intellectuals doing anything in groups and as groups were (a) egotism, first personal and then national and professional and (b) the mind's infinite capacity for irrelevance" (Smith, 1969, p. 539). In an unusually long letter,

Aldous lists several reasons why he is "dubious about the whole idea of progress" (p. 551). His interest in the Orient emerges in a passage discussing his fourth reason; in it he describes the pith of a lecture he heard by "a Chinaman": "We understand more than we know; you know more than you understand" (p. 553). "Genuine improvements, I come to feel more and more strongly, can only be achieved on a small, a human scale—by decentralization of power, production and population, through self-governing co-operative groups working for themselves and not manipulated by government managers and experts" (p. 554). About six weeks later, Aldous concludes another long letter to Julian, recently named Director General of UNESCO: "I wonder," writes Aldous, "if there is any hope, through Unesco, of persuading the technologists" of anything having to do with "a human scale." After contrasting the attractions of uranium with those of wind-power as substitutes for the already troubled supply of oil in the Middle East, he concludes that uranium and aggressive atomic power provide the technologists an irresistible temptation: "I suppose there is not the faintest hope that such perfectly obvious considerations will be heeded" (p. 557).

These late statements firm up an early attitude. The frequency with which Aldous addresses in letters to Julian the questions "What is to be done?" and "What is not to be done?" appears motivated not only by Aldous's own processes of finding his own stance in relation to society but also by Julian's suggestions or example or invitations. For example, in 1928 Julian invited him to join the editorial board of the short-lived review *The Realist*. Aldous accepted, "so long as it doesn't entail any work beyond occasionally contributing; for I'm afraid I'm not sufficiently preoccupied about the future of the human race to be prepared to read manuscripts or do anything of that sort" (p. 303). This position, of course, was modified over the years, in part due to the influence of Julian. In 1948 Aldous writes him, just before a visit to Paris: "I will bring with me the article I did on population last year. ['The Double Crisis'] is rather long, but I think covers a lot of ground" (p. 582). His précis in the letter concludes, "The more we advance technologically, the dottier we become. And the dottier the parents, the super-dottier the children. So that the advance is by geometrical progression" (p. 583). Although Aldous writes about exceedingly large and complex social issues, his conclusions usually have to do with the individual psyche.

Such concern links directly with a lost letter from Julian. Aldous writes, "I was interested by the passage in your letter about the new Ideal Man. I have long been interested in the history of such ideal men" (p. 463). Aldous lists the Renaissance Man (an "all-round Greek-through-rose-coloured spectacles"), the *honnête homme* of the seventeenth century, the *philosophe* of the eighteenth, and the "respectable man" of the nineteenth, and accepts Julian's designation of Social Man for the present century. In accepting the ideal of a particular kind of man, one accepts "as its corollary the ideal of the divine state. I have now come to feel that all these ideals are disastrous, because incomplete" (p. 463). Aldous argues instead for a Brahmin class idealizing Theocentric Man, "not primarily concerned with human values at all, but merely with the business of knowing and making actual in themselves the ultimate reality of the world" (p. 463). It would have been enlightening to know whether Julian's description of Social Man was as analytical, evaluative, and autobiographical as was Aldous's of Theocentric Man.

Aldous describes his own activity another way: "doing one's best to prevent the oncoming of mental sclerosis in oneself, to keep the mind open to the world and to that which transcends the world and gives it sense and value" (p. 428). This, says Aldous, is "the only genuine contribution." And in 1959, recommending Jacques Ellul's *La Technique* to Julian—one of innumerable short reviews in the letters—Aldous finds technique developed "according to the laws of [its] own nature and not at all according to the laws of human nature . . . extremely depressing" (p. 859). The only hope Aldous sees involves "tempering technique, ever more perfect, and ever more all-embracing and totalitarian, with a kind of Zen training in spontaneity, in de-conditioning, in becoming open" (p. 859). The alternative Aldous poses to Julian, later printed as a series of articles and even later as *Brave New World Revisited*, enables technology to bypass the conscious and rational self in order to engage "the psycho-physical machine. . . . A dictator who systematically made use of existing methods and subsidized research in their refinement could, by the use of drugs, sleep-teaching hypnosis, subliminal projection and the latest advertising techniques based upon motivational research, establish a high degree of control over his subjects and make them positively enjoy their slavery" (p. 837).

Although Aldous distinguishes Theocentric Man from Social Man, when he comes to discuss "What is to be done?" he turns to the most subtle social instrument of all, language, and to religion:

> The techniques of applied semantics must be supplemented by the techniques of applied religion. . . . If I had the necessary equipment of knowledge, I might attempt the job myself; but I haven't and the best I can do is to attempt, as I intend to, a kind of fictional hint, adumbration and prolegomenon to the desired and necessary systematization and synthesis. I don't know whether there is any so-

lution to human problems; it seems doubtful. But if there is, it lies, I am convinced, in applied semantics and applied religion. [p. 453]

Thus, when Julian writes to ask his opinion of the title *Omnibus* for a one-volume collection of his work, Aldous counters by referring to the recent volume, *A Newman Synthesis*: "Why not a Julian Huxley Synthesis?" Even better, he suggests, "Take a hint from St. Thomas Aquinas and his *Summa contra Gentiles*. Why not a *Summa contra Credentes*?" (p. 884). Such a suggestion follows from Aldous's remarks in his 1940 letter on applied semantics and applied religion; in it he describes making notes "for a kind of novel, which I hope to make into a philosophical Summa, couched in fictional form" (p. 453). The measure of the brothers' openness to new theology in new language may be taken as well by their advocacy of the work of Teilhard de Chardin. New ideas need new words; in *Essays of a Humanist*, Julian (1954) writes,

> Comparative study makes it clear that higher animals have minds of a sort, and evolutionary fact and logic demand that minds should have evolved gradually as well as bodies and that accordingly mind-like (or "mentoid", to employ a barbarous word that I am driven to coin because of its usefulness) properties must be present throughout the universe. [p. 205]

Justly, the word appears not to have caught on. Julian was right, however, in expressing admiration for Teilhard de Chardin's new word, *noösphere*. In the process of praising and explaining it, he adopts a metaphor of Aldous's. *Noösphere* denotes "the special environment of man, the systems of organized thought and its products in which men move and have their being, as fish swim and reproduce in rivers and the sea" (J. Huxley, 1954, p. 203). The Biblical phraseology adds dignity to a metaphor from Aldous's principal letter on semantics, addressed to Julian. "We live," Aldous asserts, "in language as a fish in water; but all languages embody fossilized neolithic metaphysics" which tempt us to settle easily for "neolithic prejudgments implicit in the language we use" (Smith, 1969, p. 452). While Julian was preoccupied his life long with biological and cultural evolution, Aldous worked with the linguistic.

Aldous writes Julian that he believes society has imposed some sort of taboo on the study of language. By "study" he means no shallow rote memorization but "analysis." He does mean "taboo" as it is understood in the study of comparative religion. "This powerful taboo against the analysis of language makes one suspect (what every person of deep religious insight has always insisted to be true) that most people don't want to think correctly about the world because they get a lot of short-range fun (which outweighs for them the long-range miseries that follow) from thinking incorrectly and acting stupidly" (Smith, 1969, p. 443). Aldous specifies that the linguistic insight corresponds to religious insight.

That the brothers shared a deep interest in language is evident from Aldous's letter replying to another lost letter of Julian's: "Yes, I agree with you about the interestingness and importance of the Ogden-Richards work on language" (Smith, 1969, p. 491). He endorses it as an "excellent scholastic discipline" and recommends it as specific for the "muddle" of Carlyle, St. Paul, or Plato. Julian remarks in *Memories* and *Memories II* how often he and Aldous exchanged lists of recommended reading; while it would be helpful to know which books on language Julian thought worth recommending, we have only the little syllabus sent by Aldous: Korzybski's *Science and Sanity*, Irvine Lee's *Language Habits and Human Affairs*, Jespersen, and especially Leonard Bloomfield's *Language*. Aldous develops the argument begun in a letter to Julian five years earlier.

> The vast majority of people continue to think and act as though things were the signs of words, not words of things. Sometimes I think that the reason for this strange state of affairs must be a kind of instinctive self-protective instinct on the part of existing society. For of course the effects of broadcasting a knowledge of semantics, of teaching all men the habit of analysing the language they not only use, but actually swim in, like fishes in the sea, would be profoundly revolutionary. So much so that it may be doubted whether any of the most sacred institutions and ideas would remain unaffected by the educational reform. [Smith, 1969, p. 491]

Not only does Aldous bring together his ideas about the self-protective drive of society with language as its defense mechanism, he also connects language with the shields of organized religion. From the 1940 letter to Julian about "neolithic metaphysics," he nets again the metaphor of men swimming like fish in a sea of language, but the idea that lodged in his mind for further examination is "instinct." When he gets echoic, even repetitive, as in the phrase "a kind of instinctive self-protective instinct," it is sign that he knows so little about the idea he can't let go of it. A sign, too, of the mind's floundering about with the idea is the pseudospecific "a kind of." The same vagueness had characterized Aldous's getting under way in response to Julian's comments on the new Ideal Man: "I was interested by the passage in your letter about the new Ideal Man. I have long been interested in the history of such ideal men" (Smith, 1969, p. 463). Aldous began this later letter agreeing with Julian on the "interestingness" of the work of Ogden and Richards. With this word Aldous buys time in his letters. It is, like authentic personal letters between intimates, first-draft and informal. Theorists of the psychology of composition would term it pre-writing or, perhaps, field-exploration, but the pseudoscientific jargon covers only an old pre-psycholinguistic process of rhetorical invention, *in-venire*, to come upon what is already there to be found. Aldous's discussion of language in this letter concludes with a series of questions about the prospects for man "condemned to do his talking and non-mathematical thinking in terms of an instrument which cannot in the nature of things express the truth" (Smith, 1969, p. 492).

As Aldous's 1943 letter on language appears in part to have been stimulated by receipt of Julian's large book, *Evolution*, so was his 1953 letter by receipt of *Evolution in Action*. Of the first Aldous wrote, "I have not had time to do more than turn the pages and read occasional passages." He compliments Julian on its "enormous scope . . . and . . . masterly lucidity"; he admits he doesn't read the journals in which it might be reviewed. Of the second book Aldous wrote, "I have had time, so far, only to glance here and there . . .; I shall read the whole with pleasure and much profit" (Smith, 1969, p. 664). In both cases these brief opening paragraphs pass as quickly as possible in the language of workmanlike reviews so that Aldous can get down to what's on his own mind. If the brothers were not so mutually supportive, though, his praise might sound exceedingly faint.

In contrast, Aldous is excited by von Bertalanffy's *Problems of Life* to the extent that he wishes he knew more mathematics and chemistry.

> How paradoxical it is that, when life develops organizations complex enough to be capable of thought, the emergent mind should revert, in its always simplified abstractions and generalizations, to patterns of symbols comparable in their subtlety and complexity only to organizations in the inorganic world, not to those in the living universe. Our thought-patterns are on the level, more or less, of crystallography; whereas the patterns of our physiology, the patterns of the relations between our physiology, our thought-patterns and the living and inorganic world are of an immensely higher order of complexity. Hence, of course, the mess in which we find ourselves. Even with the best will in the world—and the will is generally rather bad—we *cannot* think completely realistically about ourselves and our situation. [Smith, 1969, pp. 664–665]

A hierarchical conception of the universe underlies this analysis: man is superior to the animals, which are superior to the plants, which are superior to the rocks. While both Julian and Aldous look to an improvement of the human species along the lines foreseen by Teilhard, the comparison of thought-patterns with crystallography bodes ill. The species is sinking to a common denominator lowest of all; the avoidance of complexity parallels man's avoidance of the truth that semantics puts at his disposal. To Aldous it is not a matter merely of apathy or defense but of lack of will. Mundane, negative, immediate decisions rule out options long-range, positive, and in some sense celestial. Julian agrees; in "The New Divinity" (1954, p. 221), he writes, "To say that God is ultimate reality is just semantic cheating, as well as being so vague as to become effectively meaningless. . . ." Julian himself allows such blurring in, for example, his essay on love in *New Bottles for New Wine* (1957). He asks, "What do we know about love?" Aldous would ask, "How do we know about love?" For Aldous, how we know is what we know: love is an activity, a process. For Julian it is an entity objectified, moved from inside the psyche to outside. Julian fails in this essay to answer his question.

> It is almost impossible to give a formal definition of anything so complex and general as love. All I can do is to indicate some of the range of meanings comprised in this one little word. There is mother-love and self-love, father-love and grandmother-love, and children's love for their parents; there is brotherly love (which gave Philadelphia its name) and the love of one's country; there is being in love, and making love; one can say that a man loves his food. . . .
> [p. 213]

And on for another paragraph. As soon as he focuses on the "one little word," he veers off into compounds of two words, away from the center of meaning. He does not discuss the nature of love but, instead, the conglomeration of lovers and love-objects colloquial speech allows. Here it is not a matter of penetrating what Aldous called "neolithic metaphysics"; and as the essay grows, Julian wanders even further from the point. Enlarging the scope, he changes the questions and finally the subject. Julian maps out the minefield but neither disarms nor detonates anything. His tendency is to accumulate individual items of data and generalize from their more extensive coordination; Aldous takes one item and penetrates it. Aldous takes chances, Julian the safer way. Julian's significances emerge from social support, common enterprise, institutional sponsorship. Hence Aldous writes alone, while Julian edits. Responsibility for ideas focuses in Aldous, defocuses outside Julian. Aldous is centripetal, Julian centrifugal. Typically, Julian writes the introductory essay to *The Humanist Frame* (1961) but leaves the concluding essay to Aldous: it is an act of deference both editorial and brotherly.

In some sense, Julian deferred to Aldous all his life. Julian (1957) reports that from the time he was twelve and Aldous five,

> I knew in some intuitive way that Aldous possessed some innate
> superiority and moved on a different level of being. . . . As a child,
> he spent a good deal of his time just sitting quietly contemplating
> the strangeness of things. His godmother once saw him gazing out
> of the window, and asked what he was thinking about. He looked
> round, said the one word *Skin*, and turned his gaze out the window
> again. [p. 21]

Here Julian is at his most exact. The word itself was probably the subject of Aldous's meditation, and monosyllables are best for everyman's home-spun exercises in what the psycholinguists call "satiation." One takes a monosyllable—the best, they say, have not more than five phonemes—and repeats it and repeats and repeats: it has meaning for a few moments, then it becomes ambiguous, then the primary meaning comes to have no more primacy than any of the other meanings, then all the meanings become equally contingent, then all equally arbitrary, and the mono-syllable—flush with meaning—is flushed of meaning. The empty sounds must be left alone for a few moments before they can be reinvoked, re-created by means of a word, everyman his own Adam. It's a linguistic experience of the Fall of Man: retroactive inhibition, as the behaviorists might say. "Don't touch that tree!" We can keep the commandment only after it has been over-broken. But man tastes no fruit; rather, his tongue slips into speech, into concepts, into forbidden knowledge, Milton's grand theme. No wonder Aldous (1963) holds that "poetically speaking, *Paradise Lost* is *Syntax Regained*—regained and completely remade" (p. 29).

It seemed strange to Adam, no doubt, and it seemed a vehicle for encountering "the strangeness of things" for Aldous. He was well aware of the phenomenon.

> When isolated from the other words in relation to which it makes
> the ordinary, accepted kind of sense, a word takes on a new prob-
> lematic, mysteriously magical significance. It becomes more than
> an idea; it becomes an *idée fixe*, a haunting enigma. It is possible . . . to
> talk oneself out of one's own familiar identity simply by repeating
> the syllables of one's own name. And something analogous happens
> when one isolates a word, pores over it, meditates upon it, treats
> it, not as an operational element in some familiar kind of sentence,
> but as a thing-in-itself, an autonomous pattern of sounds and mean-
> ings. [A. Huxley, 1963, p. 34]

In short, *Syntax Lost* is *Paradise Regained*: the fixed idea becomes obsessional not because it is inflexible but because, in constant flux, it becomes a "haunting enigma." With the removal of context, the sentence within which the word occurs, it becomes impossible to commit the mind to any one meaning. The diachronic experience of sentence making is reduced to a synchronic problem of a new type: not which word of many best fits a sentence but which meaning of many best fits a word. As if "Aldous" were name distinctive enough, he claims he can even "talk [him]self out of [his] own familiar identity." Like common nouns, the proper noun becomes isolated, individual, apart, private. As if by naming-magic, as the name of the seer, so the person. Numinous syllables serve the blind seer, while luminous sentences serve the sighted scientist: this distinction is Julian's. Satiation, for Aldous, amounts to a theory of crea-tivity. In the chapter on silence in *The Perennial Philosophy*, he begins (1944, p. 216) with a quotation from St. John of the Cross: "The Father uttered one Word; that Word is his Son, and He utters Him for ever in everlasting silence; and in silence the soul has to hear it." The second Person of the Trinity is the first Person's "Om"; this created universe is the second Person's sentence. John's Gospel opens, "In the beginning was the Word, and the Word was with God, and the Word was God. . . . By It were all things made, and without It was made nothing that was made." Against a background of eternal silence, a macrosilence, the Father satiates the name of his Son; against a background of temporal silence, a microsilence, the contemplative satiates over a numinous syl-lable.

It is significant that *The Perennial Philosophy*, too, focuses on numinous syllables. The doctrine is derived from the fourteenth-century mystical treatise *The Cloud of Unknowing*. "And if thou desirest to have this intent [of pure contemplation] lapped and folden in one word, so that thou mayest have better hold thereupon, take thee but a little word of one syllable, for so it is better than of two; for the shorter the word, the better it accordeth with the work of the spirit" (A. Huxley, 1944, p. 277). *The Cloud* recommends such positive words as "God" or "Love" and such negative words as "Sin"—that is to say, polar opposites. The mind has two principal cognitive strategies, one of condensation, the other of at-tenuation. In the condensation, the mind crams the monosyllable with as much significance and associational richness as possible; in attenuation, the mind unpacks the syllable to rederive by rote memory and associa-tional recollection all that had been condensed.

The Cloud of Unknowing also provides a *locus classicus* for the dis-cussion of "What is to be done?" Here the distinction hinges on the differences between Action and Contemplation; the vehicle for its discussion is the allegorical interpretation of the differences between Martha and Mary. Martha embodies the Active Life; hers is the lesser calling and her Old Testament male counterpart is the leader Moses, who never entered the Promised Land of contemplation. Mary embodies the Contemplative Life; hers is the better part and her Old Testament male counterpart is Aaron, who did lead the People into the Promised Land, a foreshadowing of Heaven. The Active attenuates a text into allegory, the Contemplative condenses it into a numinous syllable. *The Cloud* itself alternates these activities, which lend themselves to the Two Cultures as well as the two Huxley's: science and Julian lean toward the Active side, Aldous and the humanities to the Contemplative.

From applied semantics to applied religion: the transition is not tortuous. Theoretical religion—questions of Trinity or of angels and pinheads—interests the brothers very little. In *Religion Without Revelation*, Julian pays attention to the Trinity only to re-allegorize it to fit a radically different psychology from that of St. Augustine. Julian's book treats theology as a myth system understood through psychological euhemerism. Not to attribute the whole approach to the influence of Aldous, one notes nonetheless that as early as 1916 he is writing Julian with the first of many reading lists; this one recommends "Blake perpetually, with a foundation of Jacob Behmen; that will keep your religion all right, the importance of which I cannot overemphasize" (Smith, 1969, p. 96). The connection with semantics is even closer in a 1938 reading list: "Korzybski on the problems of semiosis; the Abbé Bremond on the history of religious psychology" (p. 438). Aldous characterizes religion as an "obstacle race":

> One covers the course with intellectual hedges, chevaux-de-frise, pitfalls, booby-traps; having done which one spends enormous ingenuity and subtlety in circumventing these obstacles. In the intervals the theologians make the most remarkable psychological discoveries, record astonishing insights. [p. 438]

With growing knowledge only of the *homme moyen sensuel*, he concludes, modern psychology is shallow and incomplete. Aldous sounds most a scientist in a much later letter to Julian, in which he decries Western religion's preoccupation with concepts and symbols; oriental religions, in contrast, "are all of them forms of transcendental pragmatism" (p. 438). "What matters is the experience, not the conceptual system in terms of which the experience is explained. . . . To my mind, the problem of religion is one which has to be approached operationally. If you do A, then B is likely to happen; if you do X, then you will probably get Y" (p. 827). It is more than a little tempting to consider Aldous's *The Perennial*

Philosophy, The Doors of Perception, and *Heaven and Hell* one work in polar companionship with Julian's *Religion Without Revelation*; we should have to retitle Aldous's *Revelation Without Religion*.

Julian (1970) writes often about experiences, beginning the time he was at Eton, of heart-filling joy and peace in the contemplation of Nature: the deeps of space on a starry night or—even while awaiting his turn at bat in cricket—the complex structures of a common plant. "I had a strange cosmic vision—as if I could *see* right down into the centre of the earth, and embrace the whole of its contents and its animal and plant inhabitants. For a moment I became, in some transcendental way, the universe" (p. 55). He adds that he has heard from Aldous of such effects being produced by LSD, but "I, subject as I am to occasional fits of depression, have never dared to take this or any other hallucinogenic drug." In the auto-biographical chapter of *Religion Without Revelation*, "Personalia," he had already described his nervous breakdowns in accord with traditional doctrines of, for example, the Dark Night of the Soul, a transitional phase of the mystical experience.

> Almost all religious mystics have passed through a period of conflict and discipline, in which the body and its desires are mortified. This process may eventually be accomplished and the discipline become perfect, but it involves in its earlier stages a great deal of repression; and I suspect that even in the end the "Mortification" of desires is not literal but that they are repressed from their normal outlet and harnessed in new ways. In any case, the possibility that conflict may be felt to contribute to the intensity of desired states of mind should, I think, be considered in discussing the psychology of mysticism. [1927, p. 55]

In describing the consolations he found, similar to those of the Romantic nature poets, he defines mysticism in a parenthesis: "Mystical (because irrational, given, and so transcending itself as to cause every highest and deepest fibre of the mental being to vibrate)" (1927, p. 122). From *De profundis* to *O altitudo*, the depressed psalm of David to the third heaven of St. Paul, the "given" euhemerizes the theological concept of grace. Julian asserts that the experiences of the nature poets are identical with those of the mystics; they differ only in the focus of attention. Mystics see the Dark Night as "an abandonment of the soul by God"; "with me," writes Julian, "there is no reference of the distress suffered to the action of any personal or supernatural being whatever" (1957, p. 124). The mystic enjoys the advantage of being able to understand his experience in the context of an "all-embracing intellectual framework," and his mind finds it "ready-made" (p. 124). For Julian, though, the Dark Night of nervous breakdown is "a practical demonstration that not only heaven but hell is within us, and that neither the one nor the other need seem deserved" (p. 125); that is to say, there can be a dis-graceful, negative "given," too.

Julian also describes in mystical terms an experience he had on army maneuvers of sudden problem solving after a long period of incubation; he mentions Poincaré's classic essay on mathematical discovery and compares his own experience with that of St. Theresa.

> But only once before had I had such a complete sense of outside givenness in an experience—the only occasion on which I had a vision (of a non-hallucinatory but amazingly real sort: such, of a religious case, abound in the records of mystics such as St. Theresa). This of mine had no connection with morals or religion; it was a seeing with the mind, a seeing of a great slice of this earth and its beauties, all compressed into an almost instantaneous experience. [1927, pp. 134–135]

The "slice of the earth" rings geological, again the influence of Teilhard. The structuralist shift from diachronic perception (digging a hole straight down and encountering the past in reverse order of its occurrence) to the synchronic dimension (exposing a bank so as to make visible many strata at the same time): here not the word is numinous but the image.

In his chapter on "Psychology and Religion," Julian addresses the mystical experience in less personal terms. He considers mystical phenomena to be lower-level mental activity than logic or moral effort because mere images are substituted for concepts. The Dark Night at this point in the argument requires the mystic to give up his "familiar and clear processes of thinking to an as yet unpractised, confused, and fitful faculty of . . . direct perception" (1927, p. 279). The pain resides not in any personal deprivation but in unfamiliarity, awkwardness, and fear, not in loss but in hesitancy to gain. An experience strictly understood in, say, the Middle Ages is given an even looser construction: "Art and literature help nowadays for many people to accomplish many of the functions of meditative prayer" (p. 283). However solicitous and nurturing of Julian Aldous was during and after the breakdowns, he nonetheless insisted, for example (and appropriately enough) near the end of *Heaven and Hell* (1954), that "visionary experience is not the same as mystical experience. Mystical experience is beyond the realm of opposites" (p. 138). His concluding paragraph is explicit: "There is . . . a heaven of blissful visionary experience; but there is also a hell of the same kind of appalling visionary experience as is suffered here by schizophrenics and some of those who take mescalin; and there is also an experience, beyond time, of union with the divine Ground" (p. 140). "Beyond time": Aldous's version of Julian's synchronic, numinous instant.

Aldous told Julian he had had only one bad experience with LSD. "All his other experiences with lysergic acid were of liberation and over-whelming beauty; this was doubtless due to his gentle and loving tem-perament" (J. Huxley, 1970, p. 55). Other friends of Julian's who tried it had experiences so awful that he never tried it himself. It must have appealed to Julian's sense of comparative religion that a chief provincial minister he met in India asked

> whether my brother Aldous's book, *The Doors of Perception*, in which he told of the transcendent and usually beautiful visions in-duced by mescalin and lysergic acid, was really serious, or was it intended as a parody of Indian yoga? I was able to assure him that it was indeed serious, a real contribution to our knowledge of the capacities of the human mind when suitably stimulated, whether by psychedelic chemicals, by fasting, or by meditation. I added my own private comment that the use of these methods *could* be dan-gerous. [1973, p. 156]

"Dangerous" refers only to the chemicals, not to fasting and meditation. In *The Perennial Philosophy*, Aldous discusses meditation at length, of course, but it is a little surprising to find digressions on scientific discov-eries that shed light on mental operations, like the newly formed schema of somatotypes or a discussion of diet and nutrition in the great ages of religion: periods of penance like Lent merely intensified year-round di-etary deficiencies which had effects on the chemistry of the brain; this material grew into Appendix II of *Heaven and Hell*. Julian (1973) quotes Aldous's opinion of Hinduism as "the primal curse of India and the cause of all her misfortunes" (p. 150). It has kept "millions upon millions of men and women content, through centuries, with a lot unworthy of human beings. A little less spirituality and the Indians would now be free—free from foreign dominion and from the tyranny of their own prejudices and traditions. There would be less dirt and more food." A diet that conduces to mysticism can be overdone with negative results to society. Even worse, a phenomenon viewed as a grace in Europe turns out to be in India a blight, the cause of a nation's starvation. Spirituality is not, then, an absolute value.

For both brothers, visionary or mystical experience is utterly individual and private. In *Religion Without Revelation*, Julian compared man in society to an atom in a chemical compound: politically he might contribute to forming one molecule, economically another. As visionary, though, a man-atom is as pure and contained as the symbol for his element in the box on a periodic table. Aldous (1944) puts it more vividly.

> We live together, we act on, and react to, one another; but always and in all circumstances we are by ourselves. The martyrs go hand in hand into the arena; they are crucified alone. Embraced, the lovers desperately try to fuse their insulated ecstasies into a single self-transcendence; in vain. By its very nature every embodied spirit is doomed to suffer and enjoy in solitude. [p. 12]

For Aldous this thought is especially poignant: his private experiences are much influenced by his deprivation. *Privatus*, the Latin ancestor of both words, keys the notions of loss, separateness, solitude connected with his blindness. The upshot of Aldous's study of semantics is an awareness of the multivalence of words: in ordinary discourse and in literature alike, the individual word, the element of a semantic compound, participates in one molecule politically, another economically, and so on. Correlative to this interest in private man and individual experience is his preoccupation with the individual word, the individual syllable, the numinous psychology of satiation.

For Aldous (1963) it doesn't much matter that, although "all our experiences are strictly private, . . . some experiences are less private than others" (p. 4). Generally, similar people facing the same general stimuli will react in similar ways. The use and understanding of language, for example, depends upon a semantic and structural commonality. Still, he maintains, "Every concrete particular, public or private, is a window opening onto the universal" (1963, p. 7). The metaphor modulates into the title *The Doors of Perception*, to say nothing of its source in Blake. Julian (1965) testifies, "His blindness was a help instead of a hindrance. It forced him to rely more on himself and less on books, to cultivate his memory and the art of quick and intense perception" (p. 22).

Aldous had implied in *The Perennial Philosophy* that when God—the Individual for Whom, paradoxically, Trinity is a crowd—created the world by agency of the Word, He was satiating. Adam unpacked the divinely numinous syllable in naming the animals; he reversed the process of satiation in discriminating among a wide variety of entities, by speaking a wide variety of words in recognition of the prior existence of these beings. This experience corresponds to that of Aldous under the influence of mescalin: "I was not now looking at an unusual flower arrangement. I was seeing what Adam had seen on the morning of his creation—the miracle, moment by moment, of naked existence" (A. Huxley, 1954, p. 17). Uncertain whether to describe it as "indefinite duration" or "perpetual present," Aldous means by the expression "moment to moment" a sequence of synchronous experiences. Heaven, more traditionally defined, consists of a Beatific Vision: one master synchronization of discrete synchronous experiences as one passes out of time into eternity. The diachronic dimension is necessarily to some extent the real arena of action; the synchronic dimension pertains to some extent to pure contemplation. Hence Aldous readdresses the problem he and Julian had often puzzled over, "What is worth doing?"

In *The Doors of Perception* (1954) he adverts yet again to the medieval allegories of the strife between Martha and Mary: "Mescalin opens up the way of Mary, but shuts the door on that of Martha. It gives access to contemplation—but to a contemplation that is incompatible with action and even with the will to action, the very thought of action" (p. 41). Abandoning action or the impulse to action, one comes to perceive the sources of perception as impersonal: "Our linguistic habits lead us into error. . . . We are apt to say, 'I imagine,' when what we should have said is, 'The curtain was lifted that I might see' " (p. 93). The language of medieval vision and dream is more precise in its syntactic form: *It thoughte me; It dremed me;* or *It semed me.* The question is not merely action against contemplation but activity against passivity: the agent seems outside the self. Strung up between Heaven and Hell, the mind seeks synthesis: "Significance here," Aldous writes of the drug trip, "is identical with being; for, at the mind's antipodes, objects do not stand for anything but themselves" (p. 95).

Finally, we recognize in the Martha-Mary polarity a kind of mitotic plate upon which the tendencies of the brothers separate in fruitful polarity. In *Literature and Science* (1963, pp. 40–41), Aldous asks, "Snow or Leavis?" The Two Cultures he perceives as each defined by a series of correspondences:

SNOW	LEAVIS
bland scientism	moralistic literalism
Nebuchadnessars	Levites of culture
public experience	private experience
objective reality	subjective reality
logic	intuition
social convention	idiosyncrasy
accumulated information	particles of information

Only the more mechanical figures in this controversy were forced to extreme positions; it would be inaccurate to add Julian to the Snow column or Aldous to the Leavis. The brothers both move to a more centrist position: they may be facing each other on the plate, but they are always connected and always in the same cell. The differences between the brothers are keyed in the restriction of fiction and drama to Aldous, editing to Julian. Both wrote essays and books of non-fiction. Although Aldous made his living at film scripts, Julian's documentary on gannets won an Oscar. Julian's strength was assimilating huge amounts of data into an established position; Aldous's strength was penetrating small amounts of data to intuit that position. They remember the figure best able to combine processes and synthesize positions, their grandfather, T.H. Huxley. It is not merely that they supported each other in separate enterprises; rather, they were also each other's best resource.

REFERENCES

Bedford, S. (1974), *Aldous Huxley: A Biography*. New York: Harper & Row.
Huxley, A. (1944), *The Perennial Philosophy*. New York: Harper & Row.
―――― (1954), *The Doors of Perception* and *Heaven and Hell*. New York: Harper & Row.
―――― (1963), *Literature and Science*. New York: Harper & Row.
Huxley, J. (1927), *Religion Without Revelation*. New York: Harper & Brothers.
―――― (1954), *Essays of a Humanist*. New York: Harper & Brothers.
―――― (1957), *New Bottles for New Wine*. New York: Harper & Brothers.
―――― (1961), *The Humanist Frame*. New York: Harper & Brothers.
―――― (1965), *Aldous Huxley, 1895–1963: A Memorial Volume*. New York: Harper & Row.
―――― (1970), *Memories*. New York: Harper & Row.
―――― (1973), *Memories II*. New York: Harper & Row.
―――― Hardy, A.C., & Ford, E.B. (1954), *Evolution as a Process*. London: George Allen & Unwin.
Smith, G. (1969), *The Letters of Aldous Huxley*. London: Chatto & Windus.
Woodcock, G. (1972), *Dawn at the Darkest Hour: A Study of Aldous Huxley*. New York: Viking Press.

"My brother Evelyn and myself," says Alec Waugh (1967) in his reminiscences, "were brought up in an atmosphere not only of books but of professional writing" (p. 17). Born five years apart, Alec on July 8, 1898, and Evelyn on October 28, 1903, the only children of Arthur and Catherine Raban Waugh were nurtured on the written and spoken word, for their father was both Director of Chapman and Hall, publishers of Dickens, and a critic and author himself. Frequent visitors to Underhill, their childhood home, included Edmund Gosse, E.V. Lucas, St. John Ervine, Ernest Rhys, and W.W. Jacobs, author of "The Monkey's Paw." Alec's first marriage was to Barbara Jacobs, daughter of the last-named dignitary, and Evelyn's first infatuation was with her younger sister, Luned.

The boys' father took immense pleasure in reading to his family in the evening, particularly from Dickens, a practice which, as Evelyn (1964) noted, emphasized "the cadences and rhythms of the language," so that he "never thought of the English language as a school subject, as matter for analysis and historical arrangement, but as a source of natural joy" (p. 72). This love for English, which the brothers shared, was reinforced during their formal education. At Oxford, Evelyn had many friends later to become prominent writers and critics, among them Graham Greene and Anthony Powell. Alec, who

6

"My Brother Evelyn and Myself ": Alec and Evelyn Waugh

ROBERT J. KLOSS

193

never went beyond public school, considered his seven-month impris-
onment in the Citadel of Mainz as his university education (1967, p. 74),
because when captured by the Germans in 1918 he was interned with
Gerald Hopkins, Hugh Kingsmill, and Milton Hayes. Daily these four
assembled in a common room, worked on novels, and read their manuscripts to each other, providing criticism and support. With such a rich
literary background, it seemed inevitable that the brothers would themselves become professional writers. Indeed, both had made significant
contributions before their mid-twenties.

Ironically, Alec seemed at first to have more promise. He wrote his
first novel, *The Loom of Youth*, in six and a half weeks and published it
in 1917 when he was only nineteen. An exposé of homosexuality in the
public schools, it was controversial by Edwardian standards, fictionally
recounting his own adventures at Sherborne, which was also his father's
school. The scandal resulting from publication prevented Evelyn from
attending Sherborne when his turn came.

Loom was dedicated to his father, whom Alec idolized: "For whatever
altars I may have raised by the wayside, whatever ephemeral loyalties
may have swayed me, my one real lodestar has always been your love,
and sympathy, and guidance." As Alec recounts in his *Early Years* (1962),
the two had always been close. "When I look back on my first years . . . I
find that every memory I have is connected with him. My nurses are
shadowy figures, my mother did not become distinct until a much later
day" (pp. 14–15). "I confided in him all my ambitions, all my problems.
I have never since been so completely myself with anyone" (p. 19). "I
never needed any company but his" (p. 77).

Evelyn resented this deep bond between the two, considering it a
conspiracy. When he was sixteen and wore to a party a tailcoat passed
down from Arthur through Alec to him, Evelyn announced, "It has come
down from generation to generation of them that hate me" (A. Waugh,
1967, p. 165). Alec himself confesses that "in a sense, Evelyn and I have
never been close. He is more than five years my junior and that gap was
made to seem greater when we were young by the war and by the
publication of *The Loom of Youth*. When he was a fag at Lancing, I was
in the public eye. He thought of me as an uncle rather than as a brother."
He further admits that Evelyn "was, inevitably, something of a nuisance
to me. Presumably I was to him. . . . It is probable that he realized that
I considered him a nuisance and that he resented it" (p. 163). He concedes,
as well, that "it is possible that I was not very kind to Evelyn. I can still
visualize the occasion when my mother lectured me on this point" (p.
164).

On his part, Evelyn tells in his autobiography (1964) the tale of the mother of one of his playmates remarking how sad it was for Evelyn to be an only child. " 'Oh, but he isn't,' one of them replied, 'he has a brother at school whom he hates.' This was a distortion of my regard for Alec, but it was true that he held himself aloof from, and greatly superior to, all our doings" (p. 66). Evelyn's biographer, Christopher Sykes (1975) tries to deny the brothers' estrangement, declaring that Alec exaggerated and that Evelyn's diaries and letters really reveal a hero-worship (p. 24), but the fact is that the brothers remained distant, both physically and emotionally, for most of their lives. Though they corresponded, they saw each other only about twenty times in the last twenty years of Evelyn's life (A. Waugh, 1967, p. 162).

The Loom of Youth began for Alec a career which has since seen the publication of more than forty books: essays, short stories, travel accounts, and novels. Much of the fiction is autobiographically based, like *Loom*, and contains recurrent themes or elements that appear in that novel, for instance, a passive victim, sexual flagellation, and homosexuality. Alec (1962), in speaking of the Sherborne incident, declares that every boy in public school practiced homosexuality as a consequence of conditions, but that "I had the bad luck to be found out" (p. 63). He was asked to leave school at the end of the term, soon took a commission in the Army, and was captured in 1918. "I was," he says of the expulsion, "the victim of a system which created a conspiracy of silence to conceal the reality of the public school boy's life" (p. 63). This sense of being a passive victim is what best characterizes the heroes and heroines of his novels.

Although, like Evelyn, Alec is essentially antipsychological, he is also astute enough to realize that the Sherborne incident was traumatic, that it "left scars of some kind," because for the rest of his life he had three recurrent dreams, and "the second is staged during my last term at school when I am involved in a scandal and threatened with expulsion" (1962, p. 66). Such scandals appear occasionally in the fiction itself. In *The Fatal Gift* (1973) and *Guy Renton* (1952), younger brothers are expelled from public school for the identical offense of homosexuality.

The Loom of Youth provoked further anguish in Alec later in life when Wyndham Lewis in 1932 published *The Doom of Youth*, a satire, and accused Alec of "homosexual tendencies," declaring that "all the feminine maternal elements were excessively developed in him" (A. Waugh, 1978, pp. 11–13). Alec sued for libel and eventually settled out of court. Ironically, though, he admits he was worried later that his son Peter would "turn out gay" (p. 280). Why he never makes clear. He does, however, through his characters, offer a number of curious theories on the origin of homosexuality, possibly in attempts to understand it himself. In *The Mule on the Minaret* (1965) and *A Spy in the Family* (1970), for example, he attributes it to a man's "being absorbed in his mother," and in *The Fatal Gift* (1973), observing that it is prominent among second sons of the aristocracy, he ascribes it to a "subconscious reaction against the occupancy of a second place" (p. 84). Repeated speculations like these demonstrate a fascination, if not preoccupation, with the condition. *A Spy in the Family* is itself a detailed exploration of lesbianism, homosexuality, and flagellation, woven through a thin plot line of intrigue and smuggling.

Much like his brother Evelyn, Alec began to travel soon after the failure of his first marriage, and in time became virtually an American by dividing his living between the United States and France, generally in favor of the former. For nearly half a century, when not writing in the Escurial Hotel in Nice, he was ensconced in the Algonquin in New York City or at the MacDowell Colony, where he met his third wife. During this time, he had, in addition to three wives, numerous affairs. Like most of his fictional characters, he had difficulty in his marriages, and, with his usual poor sense of psychology, proclaimed the difficulty to be genetic: in his autobiography (1978), he declared, "I was a born bachelor" (p. 249). With this rationalization, of course, he relieved himself of any responsibility to scrutinize his motivations in order to dispel the continual conflicts in his emotional relationships with women. His three wives were, in order, Barbara Jacobs, Joan Chirnside, and Virginia Sorensen, the writer.

The first marriage ended after a year—still unconsummated. "For this failure," he says, "my inexperience was entirely to blame. Young people today have no idea of the general ignorance at that time about the physiology of sex. Certain subjects were not discussed. . . . The failure to establish a physical relationship created a barrier between us. We could not be outspoken with one another" (1962, p. 155). Alec fails to note that thousands of other British marriages were succeeding around him, people of the same generation. He admits, though, that he rushed into the marriage out of what he calls "perpetual, persistent restlessness" and offers further rationalizations for its failure, suggesting that "monotony of atmosphere" and lack of their own home were significant causes (p. 160). He appears not to have suffered long in self-reproach, however, because by the time he was to meet Barbara to effect a rapprochement soon after their separation, he was "deeply committed to a sultry tempestuous romance" with a woman three years older than himself (p. 163). The hint of an oedipal choice here is reiterated in later emotional relationships with other women. He extols the virtues of a Tahitian maiden, Tamia, for instance, free and lovely and nubile, declaring that "this is

what I had come across the world to find" (p. 238), but three weeks later
he is bored and abandons her, lamely excusing himself by telling her his
mother is sick. Soon he is involved in another affair with the unavailable
"Ruth," herself married to a man twenty-five years her senior. The three
volumes of Alec's autobiography (1962, 1975, 1978) are full of statements
of fact regarding emotionally turbulent affairs like these, but they are
devoid of any self-analysis in regard to his motivation or the significance
of the events.

Given this, it is not surprising that his fictional characters engage in
little or no introspection and that the men and women in emotional
relationships find it impossible to confront each other at critical points.
Noel Reid of *The Mule on the Minaret*, for example, need only ask his
lover, Diana Benson, what has happened between them to discover why
she has been so cold to him recently; he does not. Myra Trail, the spy
in the family, need only ask her husband Victor what he was doing in the
Brompton Road when he should not have been there. Though urged by
a friend to do so, she does not, and, as a result, she is constrained, through
blackmail, into lesbianism, drug smuggling, and espionage. Eventually
she realizes that if she had asked, "None of this need have happened"
(1970, p. 238). Of course, but then, too, she could not have become a
passive victim.

Each of Waugh's characters lacks, as well, emotional commitment to
another human being. Guy Renton, in the novel of the same name (1952),
carries on a fifteen-year affair with a married woman, content to share
snippets of her life. Jill Somerset, in that eponymous novel (1936), declares
when eighteen that unless she can determine whether or not what she
feels is "really love, then I'll not commit myself" (p. 22). Myra Trail, even
after her belated discovery of the unnecessariness of it all, is not unhappy,
for she has learned the joys of lesbianism, and, though she continues in
her marriage, she looks forward at the end of her story to "delicious
bypaths" (p. 248).

Probably the epitome of these emotionally uncommitted victims is
Raymond Perrone, hero of *The Fatal Gift* (1973). The second son of a
peer, Perrone never had a homosexual phase in his development (says
Alec both as author and character in the novel) because he was introduced
to heterosexuality in his teens by a married aunt, who also taught him
the pleasures of flagellation and sadomasochism. A playboy, he drifts to
Dominica, in the Caribbean, and literally falls in love with the island,
which takes precedence over all else, including a wife and the peerage,
to which by a chain of events he eventually succeeds. But he fails in his
maiden speech in the House, returns to Dominica and, when offered an

important administrative post elsewhere, cannot leave the island because he has been hexed by a voodoo witch, the lesbian lover of his native mistress. All of this without an inkling of why the hero is incapable of healthy action, indeed, with the narrator himself wondering why. Like his brother's characters, Alec's seldom if ever indulge in analysis of themselves or others. They repeatedly offer the observation that it is not so important to discover the sources of one's "complexes" as to learn to live with them.

Island in the Sun (1955), doubtless Alec's best work, is an exception to this generalization. Here, in an amalgam of four plots previously unconnected and destined for separate tales (1967, p. 323), he has intertwined racial and class conflict in a British colony with both familial strife and, ultimately, murder. The plot sketches, as he originally conceived them, were these: (1) a woman kills a man by accident; (2) an American falls in love with the daughter of a West Indian planter; she discovers that she has "colored blood" on her father's side and believes she cannot marry because of it; her mother rescues her by revealing she is not her father's daughter; (3) a planter discredits a colored rabble-rouser by inciting a riot; and (4) a man returns home to discover the toilet seat up: what man has been there? These are the strands that Waugh weaves together in his eighteenth novel, and, as shall be seen, the changes he makes from inception to publication are pertinent.

The characters of this novel are well-defined, particularly those of the central figure, Maxwell Fleury, and his antagonist, David Boyeur, and their stated motivations work, at least superficially, to explain their actions. Despite this, the reader will discern that Fleury is still passive and afraid of emotional confrontation. The mainspring of the tale is Fleury's returning home to find the toilet seat up and the smell of an Egyptian cigaret in the house. Rather than ask what man has been there, he is instantly jealous of his wife, constructs a fantasy of her adultery, eventually kills his suspect, and, ultimately, foments a labor riot in which he himself dies. After he has murdered Colonel Hilary Carson, he feels uplifted because, he believes, of the discovery of his colored bloodline on the same day. That, he thinks, is "why he had felt himself rid of the burden that oppressed his boyhood" (p. 270), a burden that is never explained. He is wrong.

Indeed, he killed Carson partly because he became enraged when Carson taunted him about his ancestry, declaring that he had "a Tarbrush rubbed across his face" (p. 258). The burden that he feels lifted after the killing evaporates only momentarily. It is the burden of defending against the rage he felt toward his father in his competitive strivings with him. It is notable that Waugh has changed the sex of the murderer to a male, one who has slain an older man in jealous rage over a woman—not at a place where three roads meet, but still a fairly clear oedipal murder. Appropriately enough, Colonel Carson is directly linked to Fleury's father; he *was* the user of the toilet and the smoker of the cigaret. He was in the house, innocently, as chairman of a committee working secretly to honor Fleury's father, Julian, with a surprise gift for his years of service to the British community on the island. All of this Maxwell could have discovered merely by asking his wife. When he belatedly does learn of Carson's task that day, he says to himself, "[My] jealousy had invented the whole thing. None of this need have happened" (p. 247). These last, of course, are the identical words of Myra Trail, who, like Maxwell Fleury, failed to confront her spouse. And just as this failure led to the chain of events that led Myra to become lesbian while at the same time appearing to be a passive victim, so too Maxwell's failure leads him to kill a father figure while appearing to have been passively and accidentally brought to such action.

Further oedipal elements are evident in Fleury's hostile and rivalrous relationships with his father and late brother. The brother, long dead, once "was all his father cared about, how the elder son, the apple of his eye, was doing" (p. 33). In addition, Maxwell literally competes with his father for a seat on the new Legislative Council of Santa Marta and with a brother surrogate, David Boyeur, the colored union leader and rabble-rouser. In Council debates, he is constantly resentful and envious of both his father's and Boyeur's speaking abilities, which considerably over-shadow his.

Fleury's deliberate provocation of Boyeur and his peasants to kill him in the riot can thus be viewed as his passive way of punishing himself for his oedipal crime. That he needs to suffer is evident; at any point up to the murder he can still question his wife, and at any point afterward he can confess and receive a mitigated sentence, because the killing was, legally and technically, manslaughter, not premeditated murder. Further, he continuously reveals a compulsion to confess by making repeated slips in discussing the murder with the police inspector, Whittingham. Like Raskolnikov, he exemplifies Freud's famous criminal out of a sense of guilt. When he dies, he masochistically satisfies his need for punishment in a manner in keeping with his passive character.

Discussing this novel, Alec has called himself "a very minor writer" (1967, p. 321). This is probably an accurate assessment. Yet, *Island in the Sun* was to achieve a success—Book of the Month Club Selection, serialization, and filming—such as none of Evelyn's novels enjoyed during his lifetime. And there is some evidence that Evelyn was indeed envious.

In his diary (January 20, 1956), Evelyn calls the novel "highly enjoyable" (1976, p. 752) and says in a letter to his son Auberon, "It's very nice for him after so many years of disappointment and obscurity" (1980, p. 442). To Alec himself, he wrote (February 11, 1956) that he had read the book "with keen pleasure" but on the twenty-fifth of the same month commented to Anne Fleming that "it's rather good if you think of it as being by an American which he is really" (1980, p. 464). To appreciate this comment, one must know that Evelyn loathed Americans.

Soon after this, Evelyn instituted and won a libel suit for £5,000 against Nancy Spain, a *Daily Express* columnist. He wrote to Alec (April 24, 1956) that "the facts of the libel spring from a senile aberration of Lord Beaverbrook's [he was owner of the paper] who believes that you and I are consumed with mutual jealousy which he wishes to aggravate" (1980, p. 471). The facts, however, were otherwise. Frances Donaldson (1968) declared that the suit was precipitated when Miss Spain "made an unguarded statement comparing the sales of Evelyn's books inaccurately and unfavorably with the sales of his brother Alec's" (p. 87). The rivalry between the brothers, it would appear, was in continuous play.

They apparently never really saw eye to eye on matters important to each other, and Alec confesses never to have understood Evelyn. He recounts (1962) an interview Evelyn had with a psychiatrist during World War II to determine if he was fit for commando duty. When the psychiatrist had finished, Evelyn asked him a single question: "Why have you asked me nothing about the most important thing in a man's life, his religion?" "That is where," continues Alec, "I lack the key to Evelyn. I cannot enter imaginatively into the mind of a person for whom religion is the dominant force in his life, for whom religion is a crusade, as it is with Evelyn" (p. 218).

Alec lacked the key to Evelyn and would never have found it because he was searching in the wrong place. Religion is only one element in the complex pattern of Evelyn's life and works, and the more both are scrutinized the clearer it becomes that the key lies in Evelyn's emotional life. On at least half a dozen occasions in the latest biography, Sykes (1975) refers to Evelyn's "persecution mania" (p. 357), citing it to explain personal problems. Further, though he notes as well Evelyn's lifelong insomnia, unrelenting depression, hallucinations, tendencies toward cruelty, and homosexuality, he sees no relationship between them, nor does he discern them as part of a larger pattern that today would be recognized as paranoia. Symptoms of Waugh's condition appear very early in his childhood, and several open reactions occur during later crises. Since most of his life and work can be better understood in relation to this condition, a sketch of the classical theory of paranoia is in order.

The typical paranoid, as a child usually "the youngest member or the baby of a family" (Meissner, 1978, p. 21), finds it nearly impossible to establish a warm, loving relationship of trust with his mother. Feeling rejected, he cannot, as infants usually do, develop a sense of identity through an early symbiosis. He perceives his mother as rejecting and turns to the logical alternative, the father. This attempt to find a substitute leads, in the boy, to fears of passive homosexual desires. The child's lack of a relationship with the mother—who is often overcontrolling and se- ductive—results only in his rejection and humiliation. Feeling worthless, he attempts to compensate with feelings of grandiosity. These contradic- tory feelings alternate throughout his life.

As a consequence of the mother's rejection, the boy fears intimacy with women and avoids it. Further, he assumes that all close relationships must be purchased at the price of his independence and can only be had by adopting a passive, submissive attitude. He expects this because he learns early that his mother and father are not primarily motivated by love for him. Because their actions do not tally with their words, he tries to read the hidden messages in whatever they say. Thus begins the para- noid attitude of suspiciousness.

The boy's father, if not completely absent, is often rigid and distant, and the boy submits to authority only to escape what he interprets as sadistic attacks upon him. These are often seen as forms of rape and appear later in the symptomatology as fears of penetration, usually anal. This fear, as well, defends against the passive homosexual wish for the father and against the rage which the boy feels toward him.

During puberty, when sexual impulses become intensified, the future paranoid finds it difficult to transfer his emotional interest from members of the same sex to those of the opposite sex. He avoids women because he fears his sexual impulses and because he expects domination and rejection from them. He remains distant, as well, because of his deeply felt sense of inadequacy. He relates much better to men, but this ne- cessitates either strengthening his defenses against his homosexual wishes or yielding to them.

In the Schreber case, Freud (1911) showed that the fundamental conflict of the paranoid concerns these unconscious homosexual tendencies and that he defends against them by denial, reaction-formation, and projec- tion. Thus, the feeling "I love him" is converted by reaction-formation into its opposite: "I hate him." Because the affect remains, however, this is then projected and becomes "He hates me." This chain of defenses results in the delusions of persecution the paranoid typically suffers. Now, if the feeling of hate surfaces, as it will when the repressed returns, the paranoid rationalizes it away: "I hate him, but I am justified because he persecutes me." Comparable sets of defensive transformations create symptomatic delusions of erotomania and of grandeur.

In the former, "I love him" is converted by displacement into "I love her"; this is then projected, becoming "She loves me." In the case of the delusion of grandeur, the homosexual feeling "I love him" is absolutely denied and becomes "I do not love him. I do not love anyone. I love only myself." Clearly this delusion aids the ego in warding off the deep feelings of inadequacy, of being totally unlovable, that underlie the paranoid's exterior.

Evidence of these symptoms is plentiful throughout Waugh's life and works. In the latter, says Stopp (1958), "The passive, rather melancholy and isolated central figure will lose his first love, his Beata Beatrix, to the coarse-grained knight-robber of worldly success" (p. 76). Here, though unknowingly, Stopp has encapsulated the paranoid's basic situation as it appears in derivative form: the mother, preferring the father or another male figure, abandons the child, leaving him alone, depressed, and passive. This passive male strives to overcome obstacles, eventually emerging triumphant. Critics (Carens, 1966, p. 47; Sykes, 1975, p. 139) have noted this pattern of "the victim as hero," and instances spring readily to mind. Among those betrayed by women are Charles Ryder of *Brideshead Revisited*, Guy Crouchback of *The Sword of Honor* trilogy, Adam Fenwick-Symes of *Vile Bodies*, Cedric Lyne of *Put Out More Flags*, and, of course, Tony Last of *A Handful of Dust*.

Such preoccupation with betrayal begins early. Evelyn's first short story, published when he was twenty, appeared in the Oxford *Broom* (No. 3, June 1923), edited by his friend Harold Acton. Entitled "Antony Who Sought Things That Were Lost," it too dealt with betrayal and had a hero who "seemed always to be seeking in the future what had gone before" (p. 15). His obsession, then, evidently began earlier, very likely in the family home at Hampstead. He himself described his life there as one of "blissful happiness" (Sykes, 1975, p. 7), and Lane (1981) says that Evelyn had a "happy childhood in the afterglow of the Victorian era" (p. 17). It becomes impossible to maintain this claim, however, in the face of the evidence. Sykes observes, for instance, that this happiness was marred by "familiar psychological factors" (p. 7), and Alec focuses on their nature: "He adored his mother and his nurse. He resented his father's intrusion on their life together" (1967, p. 165). He was so strongly fixed on his mother that he was able to obtain "sanctuary" from any punishment by climbing into her chair. Sykes confirms this fixation and the antagonism toward the father: "He resented his father's prior claims over his mother, and Arthur Waugh's evening return was a moment of sorrowful wrath on the part of the young Evelyn" (p. 7).

Despite the apparently happy relationship with the mother, Evelyn did not feel secure, because of the presence of his older brother. On one occasion he remarked to his biographer, "I was not rejected or misprized, but Alec was their firstling and their darling lamb" (Sykes, 1975, p. 7). Alec acknowledges this and relates how Evelyn attempted to bind his mother to him by openly seeking an oath from her: he said to his mother, " 'Daddy loves Alec more than me. But you love me more than you love Alec.' That was indeed true, but my mother felt that she should not show favoritism. 'No,' she said, 'I love you both the same.' Then I am lacking in love,' he said" (1967, p. 174).

His mother's attempt to be fair is experienced by Evelyn as rejection, rejection so absolute as to make him feel unloved and unlovable. While his logic may not seem clear to us, it is the logic of narcissism, as Meissner (1978) calls it, that states "originally that if the subject is without a certain good, then everyone else must be in possession of it. . . ; if the [subject] is deprived to any degree, the deprivation is seen as absolute" (p. 640). This absoluteness causes the depression and rage found in the paranoid, as well as the lack of self-esteem and the delusions of grandeur which counteract it.

References to Evelyn's lifelong severe depression abound. Donaldson (1968) sees it as "a melancholia of Johnsonian proportions" (p. xiii) which he could almost not endure. He, of course, refused to recognize the condition, preferring to label it "boredom." Meissner (1978) summarizes the dynamics: "The psychology of depression is the psychology of disappointment and unfulfilled expectations. Disappointment evokes fury at those who frustrate the child's wishes and expectations, but when the frustrating object is also highly valued the frustrations come to represent abandonment. The wishes to destroy the object can be avoided only by turning the aggression against the self" (p. 141). As an alternative, the child can also project it, placing it in an external object where it can be disavowed. Paranoia can thus be seen as an important defense against depression (MacKinnon and Michels, 1971, p. 263; Meissner, 1978, p. 127).

An unfortunate event when he was eight further complicated Evelyn's childhood relationship with his parents. He fell ill and needed an appendectomy, then still a dangerous operation. As he recounts it (1964, pp. 55–57), his "parents were anxious" and he "was kept in ignorance of [his] condition." The doctor, "a strange man," came to his room and asked him to "smell this delicious scent," proceeding to chloroform the boy. The surgery was performed on the kitchen table, and when Evelyn awoke later, he found himself in his own bed with his legs strapped down, a precaution to keep him from moving and thereby opening the stitches. The strapping, which lasted "a week or ten days," apparently had harmed his legs, and he could not walk when recovered. A doctor prescribed electrical treatment, and the boy was sent, alone, to a girls' school on the Thames estuary, the mud flats of which purportedly had curative properties. Over fifty years later, in speaking of this, Evelyn would say, "For the first time in my life . . . I felt abandoned" (Sykes, 1975, p. 8). Though the mud and electricity ostensibly worked, it is more likely that the boy's inability to walk was an hysterical paralysis. It is not improbable that it lifted because Evelyn's physical therapist discovered how miserable the child was at the school and, after obtaining his parents' permission, took him in to live with her family. He became happy and was "cured" when he found himself loved once more and no longer a victim.

We have come full circle in trying to find the roots of Waugh's "victim as hero." It is as if he is impelled to reenact in his fiction the significant ordeals of his childhood in an attempt to undo their traumata. We see that this theme contains aspects of both the depressive and the paranoid position. When depressed, the individual is simultaneously victim and victimizer: victim because he has suffered an inconsolable loss; victimizer because the rage felt over this loss is terrifying and needs to be vented on someone. In the paranoid state, however, one can project the rage, not see oneself as a victimizer, and regard oneself as a pure, innocent victim. By this logic, then, it is better to be a victim than an aggressor, a potential murderer.

The fiction reflects, additionally, the family dynamics displayed in these incidents from Evelyn's childhood. "It has been observed," notes Stopp (1958) "that there is little of what may be termed family life in the novels . . ." (p. 12). Hinchcliffe (1966) concurs, observing "the almost inevitable lack of sympathy and understanding between the generations" (p. 294) and concluding that Basil Seal's efforts to find homes for displaced children represent the "broken family on a national scale" (p. 301). Hinchcliffe's summary delineates the fundamental situation in Waugh's fiction: "All of Waugh's major characters are the children of incomplete families. . . . [They] grow up spiritually maimed and unable to find the love that they crave so desperately" (p. 295).

One of the results of this desperate craving for love is the rage expressed when it is not forthcoming. This is evident in Evelyn's life. Whatever else he was, he was also a cruel and malicious man, to both friends and family. Sykes (1975) concedes that "the evidence of his early life shows that he always had a tendency to cruelty; his every book, indeed almost every writing from his hand, shows a deep underlying bitterness . . ." (p. 96). Evelyn himself (1964) reflected on his diaries, which he kept diligently from the age of seven onward, and enters the following judgment: "If what I wrote was a true account of myself, I was conceited, heartless, and cautiously malevolent, . . . The damning evidence is there . . . of consistent caddishness. I feel no identity with the boy who wrote it. I believe I was a warm-hearted child" (p. 127).

The truth, however, is otherwise. Friends and relatives repeatedly try to exonerate him but fail. Recent reconsiderations are beginning to acknowledge this. Lane (1981) hesitates somewhat but reluctantly concludes that he was a "misanthrope" who had "walled off his life from the outside world" (p. 41). Jones (1978), speaking of the *Diaries*, puts it more forcefully: "A strong feeling remains that his dominant impulse was to inflict pain or insult and to enjoy grotesque situations" (p. 515). Indeed, both Michael Davie and Mark Amory, the editors, respectively of the diaries and the letters, found it necessary to excise hundreds of references because of the fear of libel suits, particularly in England, where the laws are stringent.

Instances of Waugh's cruelty are legion. Donaldson (1968), who lived next to him at Piers Court for a number of years, says, "He was born with the trick of hurting most devilishly with half a dozen words" (p. xiv) and cites Evelyn's having grossly insulted her father, the writer Freddy Lonsdale, with the result that she "could not forgive him and I loved him less" (p. 82). Another close friend, Nancy Mitford, once asked Evelyn bluntly how he could be so cruel and yet be a practicing Catholic. "You have no idea," he said, "how much nastier I would be if I was not a Catholic. Without supernatural aid I would hardly be a human being" (Sykes, 1975, p. 334). Apparently only a few friends were able to see his cruelty as a defense that he desperately needed. Jollife (1973) speculates on its probable source: "Was it because of the threats, real or imagined, to his sense of security?" (p. 233). MacKinnon and Michels (1971) point out that the paranoid often "searches out loopholes" that "permit him to express some of his aggression, although denying the significance of his behavior" (p. 261). One thinks immediately of the infamous ear-trumpet Waugh affected in later years. According to Fleming (1973), it was another expression of his malice, "a part of his psychological warfare for dinner parties," where he would ask a question, usually impertinent, then wait, trumpet in ear, for an answer. Fleming says at one point she became so incensed with this ploy that she "hit it sharply with [her] soup spoon" (p. 237) to force him to stop using it.

When not discharging this hostility on others, Waugh retroflexed it. According to Sykes (1975), he had "a continuing and distressing psychoabnormality which took the form of a life-long tendency toward self-hatred"; this feeling placed Evelyn in "continual danger of despair, continually subject to a death-wish" (p. 50). Hynes (1972) sees this derivative in Waugh's fiction and considers it his dominant theme (pp. 66–67). The emotional impulses Sykes cites found expression early in Evelyn's life. In a diary entry (July 18, 1921) he confesses, "I think a lot about suicide. . . . I have no really definite cause for killing myself. I suppose it is really fear of failure" (Sykes, 1975, p. 33).

His insight into his motives here is at least partly correct, for paranoids dread adaptive failure and the consequent loss of self-esteem, and Evelyn did make a serious attempt at suicide early in July 1925. It followed his resignation as a schoolmaster in hopes of becoming private secretary to C. K. Scott-Moncrieff, the distinguished translator of Proust. The job fell through, and he again felt abandoned. He walked to the beach, undressed himself, and swam out to sea, presumably to die when physical exhaustion took over. Fortunately, he was stung by a jellyfish and retreated to shore. It is this incident with which he ends his autobiography, adding only these final words: "Then I climbed the sharp hill that led to all the years ahead" (E. Waugh, 1964, p. 229). This attempt at suicide has a number of aspects worth comment. First, even as he reflects upon it forty years later, he once more denies the hostility turned inward: "Did I really intend to kill myself?" Second, with water a common symbol of both life and mother, the mode of his attempt suggests a return to the woman from whom he had emerged. Finally, though he actively swims, his death itself would be passive, in keeping with one aspect of his conflicts. Commenting on the suicide of depressives, Fenichel (1945) elaborates:

> Frequently the passive thought of giving up any active fighting seems to express itself; the loss of self-esteem is so complete that any hope of regaining it is abandoned. 'The ego sees itself deserted by its super-ego and lets itself die.' To have a desire to live evidently means to feel a certain self-esteem, to feel supported by the protectiveness of a super-ego. When this feeling vanishes, the original annihilation of the deserted hungry baby reappears. [p. 400]

Very probably Waugh's hostility and the need to control it led to his early interest in Anglo-Catholicism at age eleven and his ultimate conversion at twenty-seven. One of the most bitter disappointments in his waning years as a Roman Catholic, and one of the greatest sources of anger, was the Ecumenical Movement with its discarding of tradition, particularly the abandonment of the Latin Mass. Speaking of these times, Woodruff (1973) observes, "He had become a Catholic thirty years earlier from a profound conviction of the essential need for authority in religion, and he saw those who should be upholding that authority apparently weakening before the spirit of the age" (p. 131).

It was this authority, presumably, that Waugh had always sought first and foremost. Prior to his conversion, soon after the breakup of his first marriage, he discussed the impending divorce with Alec, ending the conversation by affirming that "the trouble about the world today is that there's not enough religion in it. There's nothing to stop young people doing whatever they feel like doing at the moment" (Phillips, 1975, p. 29). Meissner (1978) details the relationship between paranoia, hostility, and authority. The child's will, he says, is subverted by the parent to believe that one can be unconditionally influenced by another person. The child, in consequence, comes to need the presence of that person or a surrogate and throughout childhood and adolescence maintains an uneasy psychic balance by doing so. "The presence of such a figure serves to organize and direct the pre-paranoid's life and activity. . . . When such an authority figure becomes unavailable, the delusional structure emerges. Its function is to provide the needed maternal influence" (p. 137).

The following incident suggests that for Waugh religion was just such a surrogate. While stationed in Yugoslavia during World War II, his constant companion was Randolph Churchill, son of the Prime Minister. The two were frequently abrasive friends, Evelyn the more so. One day Evelyn made a typically cruel comment about the elder Churchill's *Life of Marlborough*, and Randolph remarked to a third officer present, "Have you ever noticed that it is always the people who are most religious who are most mean and cruel?" To which Evelyn replied with vivacity, and in language strikingly similar to his reply to Nancy Mitford, "But my dear Randolph, you have no idea what I should be like if I wasn't" (Birkenhead, 1973, p. 150). It is difficult not to see the remark as a confession of lack of self-control, his religion expressing his urgent need for external influence.

Along with this hostility, Waugh had a number of symptomatic sexual fears and fantasies. Early in *A Little Learning* (1964), he describes his attitude toward his first name. "I have never liked the name. In America it is used only of girls and from time to time even in England it has caused confusion as to my sex" (p. 27). Not only others, though, but Waugh himself suffered confusion as to his sex. In fact, a fantasy of androgyny permeated Waugh's life and thought. He claimed to dislike his name because of its androgynous quality, yet he repeatedly was given to revealing that he identified strongly with the mother and felt himself to be feminine. And, in keeping with the fact that a paranoid's principal defense is projection, he would often attribute androgyny to others.

His disastrous first marriage, for example, had an element of this fantasy in it, along with narcissism, for he chose a woman with the same first name—Evelyn Gardner, daughter of Lady Burghclere. As Alec put it, "Their having the same Christian name was an amusing bond. They were called 'He-Evelyn' and 'She-Evelyn.' But, of course from every worldly point of view, it was a ridiculous engagement" (1967, p. 184). Though the identical names might be considered merely a coincidence, Sykes (1975) observed this androgynous attitude, declaring that Evelyn "was always liable to entertain, or pretend to entertain, odd suspicions regarding the sex of people he met" (p. 77). He cites an instance when Evelyn, in a letter to Mary Lygan, described a country weekend: " 'There was a pretty auburn-haired girl called Brenda Bracken, dressed up as a man.' He added that he was unable to resist sexual intercourse with this radiant beauty" (p. 114). Here is readily apparent an underlying homosexual fantasy.

Probably the most notorious instance of Waugh's androgynous fantasy was his enduring belief that the Communist leader of Yugoslavia, Marshal Tito, was a woman. His diary entry for July 10, 1944, when he was serving in that country, contains the blunt statement, "Tito like Lesbian" (1976, p. 572). "Thereafter," says Sykes (1975), "he invariably referred to Tito as 'she' and frequently insisted in his talk that in fact Tito was a woman" (p. 261). His colleagues became alarmed that Tito would learn of Evelyn's references and become angry, or worse. Birkenhead (1973) relates that Waugh always called Tito "Auntie" and claimed that "she" swam in a "bathing dress" so there was no doubt of "her" sex; when Tito was stubborn on military matters, Waugh would mutter, "I would think she has come to a rather difficult age for women" (p. 150). Birkenhead became furious and insisted that Tito was a man, but Waugh's only response was, "Her face is pretty, but her legs are *very* thick" (p. 151). Eventually Tito did find out about Waugh's fantasy and confronted him with it. Fitzroy Maclean, Waugh's Mission Commander, relates that this "was the only occasion in his experience when Evelyn was at a loss for a reply" (Sykes, 1975, p. 261).

Almost a decade later, when Tito visited London in 1953, Waugh persuaded Malcolm Muggeridge, then editor of a newspaper, to commission an article by Evelyn on Tito as a woman. Muggeridge refused to print it while Tito was in the city, and the project fell through (Jones, 1978, p. 516). This incident is very likely a foreshadowing of the Pinfoldian delusions Waugh would suffer less than a year later, when he had his most severe paranoid reaction.

Evidence of the concern with androgyny can be found in the fiction in the brother-sister pairs who resemble each other in the middle novels: Basil Seal and Barbara Sothill, Sebastian Flyte and Julia Marchmain. It shows up briefly in *Helena* (1950) when Old King Coel describes his dismay at his daughter's being chosen by Constantius: "I never expected this. You look like a boy, you ride like a boy. Your tutor tells me you have a masculine mind, whatever he means by that" (p. 33). Homosexual attraction on Constantius's part is implied here, as well, and later his son by Helena, the emperor Constantine, wearing a green wig, minces and prances about much like Anthony Blanche in *Brideshead Revisited*.

Waugh's own homosexuality, while acknowledged by his biographer, is usually neglected by critics. This is regrettable, for in the interests of morality or "good taste" we lose insight as to how the ego, in controlling impulses and resolving conflicts, can create literature of high quality. Waugh himself attempted to eradicate references to the trait. Davie, in his preface to the *Diaries* (1976), indicates that Waugh deliberately destroyed the entries for two periods—the homosexual episodes of Lancing and the more extended ones of Oxford. At Lancing, says Sykes (1975), "There was but the mildest element of homosexualism" (p. 31). Evelyn clarifies this in *A Little Learning* (1964): "I was susceptible to the prettiness of some fifteen-year-olds, but never fell victim to the grand passions which inflamed and tortured most of my friends" (p. 135). Within a year, however, having gone up to Oxford, he indulged promiscuously in homosexuality.

> It must be said that at this period Evelyn entered an extreme homosexual phase. . . . the phase, for the short time it lasted, was unrestrained, emotionally and physically. . . . Not long ago I read an article in a magazine written by and for homosexuals in which the suggestion was strongly conveyed that Evelyn remained inclined toward homosexuality throughout life. This is to mis-read him utterly, and in this case probably willfully. Evelyn was never much shocked by homosexuality, even though later in life he became rather prudish in a capricious way about sexual matters. If he took one of his frequent dislikes to a man and found out he was homosexual, then this would furnish him with ammunition. If he liked a man and found out he was homosexual, he would treat the matter with indifference. He was indignant at some police persecution of homosexuals. [Sykes, 1975, p. 48]

This, however, is the indulgent voice of a close friend. Jones (1978) offers a more impartial view: "In later life, once he had become the father of a large family, Waugh's homophile tendencies modified into a hostile vigilance for other homosexuals. According to the evidence of the *Diaries*, Waugh could spot a 'pansy' or a 'queer' where none existed. Tom Driberg, Waugh's fellow pupil at Lancing, has suggested that Waugh's suppression of his bisexual nature contributed to the mental breakdown described in *The Ordeal of Gilbert Pinfold*" (p. 515). When his homosexual impulses were nonthreatening, he could apparently accommodate them within his defenses. On occasion, however, they needed to be projected, as in the case of "Slugger" Urquhart, Dean of Balliol College, Oxford, whom Quennell (1973) admits was "fond of young men" but "innocent" of homosexuality. Yet Evelyn, when in his cups, would chant over and over, "The Dean of Balliol sleeps with men" (p. 37).

After Evelyn left Oxford and traveled to Paris with a friend for the Christmas holidays, he visited a homosexual brothel specializing in young children, where the two "proposed that a youth dressed as an Egyptian girl be sodomized by a Negro, but they could not pay the fee" (Sykes, 1975, p. 66). Both the *Diaries* and the *Letters*, before their editors' excisions, were rife with malicious homosexual imputations, and Anne Fleming, who corresponded with Evelyn for the last fifteen years of his life, observed that "cut-throat razors, 'concs' and catamites played a large part in his letters—concs being concubines, and catamites being homosexuals: references are of course all libelous" (1973, p. 239).

This attraction/repulsion attitude toward homosexuality has its derivatives in the fiction. Evelyn's men are rarely successful in their emotional relationships with women; there is "never a successful love affair leading to a stable marriage" (Stopp, 1958, p. 119). While this might reflect Waugh's own view of marriage, emanating from both his childhood and his personal experience, it is also very probably a derivative of unconscious homosexual impulses which themselves proscribe stable emotional relationships with women. With the possible exception of Barbara Sothill, females come off poorly in his fiction. "The world of Waugh's novels," says Stopp, "is essentially a male world; women gain admittance through being boyish, gamine, and intelligent, or feminine, disreputable and disliked" (pp. 119–120). Sykes (1975) states it even more strongly: "All his attractive women had been [until Barbara] bitches or idiots or both, sometimes, as with Brenda Last, not far off criminality" (p. 208).

Homosexuals themselves figure prominently in some of the novels (Anthony Blanche and Ambrose Silk), less prominently in others (Sir Ralph Brompton), and ambiguously in still others (Sebastian Flyte). Indeed, the literature itself is a repository which shows clearly the relationship between Waugh's paranoia and his homosexual impulses, and it is to that we can now turn.

What emerges from the fiction is a pattern in which families are important but always incomplete or broken, with the children spiritually maimed and desperately craving love. Brother pairs (or their surrogates), which might be expected, virtually do not appear. The sole exception to this among major characters is that of Sebastian Flyte and his older brother, Lord Brideshead. Even sibling pairs are rare. When they do appear, the relationships between them are nonconflictual, the brother-sister pair reflecting the androgynous fantasy discussed earlier.

The dominant family pattern is that of an only son, orphaned like Paul Pennyfeather of *Decline and Fall* or living in a tense, unloving relationship with a widowed father, like Charles Ryder of *Brideshead Revisited*. As Hinchcliffe notes (1966, p. 300), these surviving fathers are nearly all "prematurely senile and grotesquely eccentric." Hollis (1954) adds that these fathers are "uninterested in [their] parental responsibilities," and summarizes his argument with the observation that "Mr. Waugh has clearly a marked aversion to the depiction of his characters as the children of two regular and living parents" (pp. 34–36). Because the family is the essential unit of society, anyone who comes into society from an incomplete family, says Hollis, enters as an incomplete man.

While Hollis would like to see this as a thematic concern of Waugh's, it is probably better to see it as a thematic need. The presence of this pattern everywhere seems to indicate that Waugh's preoedipal conflicts dominated his creative urge. His attempts to resolve these conflicts, via the repetition compulsion, repeatedly produce tales with overwhelming concerns about separation anxiety, loss and abandonment, and betrayal by women. Oedipal concerns of rivalrous, aggressive competition with brothers and fathers never appear.

It is reasonable to assume that in this fictional pattern mothers are dead because Evelyn's own mother was emotionally dead to him, apparently from infancy, and certainly from childhood onward. Fathers are depicted as they are because of Evelyn's own childhood view of Arthur Waugh, and brothers are absent, perhaps because families, as bad as they are, would be better places without them. Their absence in the fiction parallels Alec's infrequent appearance in Evelyn's copious nonfictional writings, specifically the diaries, the letters, and the autobiography. In what follows, familial relationships will be studied in the context of several of his specifically literary works.

A Handful of Dust . . . began at the end. I had written a short story about a man trapped in the jungle, ending his days reading Dickens aloud. . . . Then, after the short story was written and published, the idea kept working in my mind. I wanted to discover how the prisoner got there, and eventually the thing grew into a study of other sorts of savage at home and the civilized man's helpless plight among them. [E. Waugh, 1946, p. 60]

It would seem then that the composition of this novel was the working through of a psychic conflict, one which, by his own account, left him feeling "helpless." It might be suspected, consequently, that this, probably the best of Waugh's novels, is about loss and abandonment. Stopp (1958) has declared that Waugh really has only two themes, which he reworks constantly: "the loss of innocence and expulsion from a haven of refuge" and "the hero going forth to win a kingdom" (p. 201). These themes reflect the childhood conflicts over feeling absolutely unloved and attempting to recapture lost bliss. Tony Last's dream of restoring Hetton and his later search for the idealized City represent these conflicts. The theme of the lost great house, however, did not start with this novel, nor does it end here. One need think only of Anchorage House in the past and of Boot Magna Hall, Brideshead, and Broome yet to come to see Waugh's fascination with this symbol. Carens (1966) believes it to be representative of "graciousness and order," "remnants of a nobler past" (p. 25). While this is true in part, it is also true that the house is a common symbol in literature and dreams for the human body (Freud, 1900, p. 85; pp. 225–226).

This, coupled with the nostalgia that pervades Waugh's characters and is generally attached to their childhood homes—the so-called "nursery theme"—urges us to examine the theme more closely. Many psychoanalysts have commented on the origins of nostalgia. Fenichel (1945), for example, sees its source in separation anxiety and considers it a wish to be united with the preoedipal mother (p. 405). Kleiner (1970) has elaborated on this thesis, noting that when the ego suffers the traumatic loss of objects, it is essentially immature and can neither master the trauma nor mourn properly. Left in a painful state, it attempts to deny the loss, especially by reaction-formation, which leads to the excessive idealization found in nostalgia (p. 472).

Most of Waugh's commentators acknowledge the essentially autobiographical nature of A Handful of Dust, but they see it exclusively in relationship to the traumatic breakup of his marriage five years earlier. Carens (1966) observes that from this point on, "divorce or separation figure prominently in at least five of Waugh's satires; adultery in at least seven" (p. 15). Davie (E. Waugh, 1976), in describing the breakup's effect on Waugh's life, says, "both Harold Acton and Alastair Graham [close friends] found it impossible to comfort him or help him repair what he evidently felt as a deep humiliation; the theme of the betrayed husband recurs constantly in his subsequent novels" (p. 306). It is not that Waugh's divorce was not traumatic; it was. But what this event did was reactivate the original traumatic rejection by the mother. The focus of this novel, for example, is not really the betrayed husband; it is the betrayed child. No one has paid attention to the one truly innocent sufferer: little John Andrew Last, abandoned by both mother and father and dying through negligence on their part.

The "deep humiliation" Davie notes was not only a reactivation of the original trauma but also the precipitant of the first in a series of paranoid reactions. All such reactions result from situations which "share a common element of producing a narcissistic injury" (Meissner, 1978, p. 135) and, as MacKinnon and Michels (1971) observe, "These include the real, fantasied, or anticipated loss of love objects. Closely related are experiences of adaptive failure with loss of self-esteem" (p. 276). Sykes (1975) notes the paranoid element and yet is unaware of its significance. After Evelyn's marriage broke up, Sykes states, "He felt degraded and gave way to an absurd fancy that he had become an object of mockery"; when his friend John Sutro tried to cheer him up by taking him to dinner at the Savoy, "Evelyn persisted in believing that the other diners were laughing at him" (p. 95). Alec (1967) believed Evelyn to be permanently damaged: "He had given himself to She-Evelyn and to his marriage, without reservations. He had trusted her completely; he was vulnerable from every angle. He had no armour against her betrayal of his trust" (p. 192). Alec even attributes his brother's writing block during the last year of his life to his "inability to deal with the painful period of his divorce in his autobiography" (p. 184).

A *Handful of Dust*, which is essentially about betrayal by women, reveals its homosexual undercurrent both in that theme and in the essential passivity of its principal male figures, John Beaver and Tony Last. Beaver, who lives alone with his mother, thrives as a social parasite, waiting by the phone, "hoping to be called up" (E. Waugh, 1934, p. 5). Rather than acting, he is always acted upon. Having left Oxford at the age of twenty-five, he works briefly in advertising, but "since then no one had been able to find anything for him to do" (p. 5). From the beginning of their affair, it is Brenda Last who is the aggressor in the relationship, and even Beaver's mother sees her as somehow able to save him from himself: "I've felt for a long time a lack of something in him, and I think that a charming and experienced woman like Brenda Last is just the person to help him" (p. 75). The mother as betrayer appears doubled here, for John Beaver's mother is instrumental as realtor/decorator in setting up Brenda in her London flat so she can betray Tony. Even when Beaver ultimately abandons Brenda, he does so passively; he must go to America, he explains, because "Mother has taken the tickets" (p. 265).

Tony Last too is a passive participant in the breakup of his marriage. He is childlike, subject to nightmares, still sleeping in the Morgan Le Fay room "within calling distance of his parents" (p. 15). By placing him here, Waugh ascribes a feminine identity to him, since, though the name Morgan seems masculine, it is actually that of the evil half-sister of King Arthur. Tony allows his marriage to deteriorate when he refuses to acknowledge what is going on between Brenda and Beaver and chooses instead to believe she has taken the London flat to study economics at the University. At this point, six-year-old John Andrew begins to feel abandoned by his mother and shows contempt toward his father for not controlling the situation. He inquires when his mother is returning and, when put off and asked if he would like to accompany Tony to the kennels—which he has been aching to do—he prefers instead to paint a picture. A servant points out his previous eagerness to go, and John simply replies, "Not with *him*" (p. 105).

The child is the innocent victim, for a six-year-old cannot be expected to control the lives of others. His parents' negligence leads directly to his death in the hunting accident. Waugh prepares the reader for this in two ways. First, he shows John having difficulty learning to jump his horse, and, second, he uses the theme of the fox, which is introduced early and is repeated in both literal and symbolic form throughout.

John's horse, Thunderclap, has been named for an animal that had killed two riders. When John falls repeatedly in jumping, his Nanny (like the later Nannies Hawkins and Bloggs, emblematic of goodness and wisdom, i.e., proper mothering) informs Brenda of her concern: "It's very dangerous. He had what might have been a serious fall this morning" (p. 24). Brenda promises to speak to Tony and does. "They both laughed about it a great deal. 'Darling,' she said. '*You* must speak to him. You're so much better at being serious than I am' " (pp. 24–25). But Tony never does and even allows him on the fox hunt. Indeed, the night before, he writes to Brenda that "*John can talk of nothing except his hunting tomorrow. I hope he doesn't break his neck*" (p. 135; italics in the original). The father's hostility toward his child is evident.

And he is not alone in the filicidal impulse. The horse that kills John is owned by Miss Ripon's father. He allows his daughter to ride the horse, despite her inability to control it, so that he might exhibit it for sale. "It was like that skinflint Miss Ripon's father, to risk Miss Ripon's neck for eighty pounds. And anyway Miss Ripon had no business out on *any* horse . . ." (p. 139). Despite the parents' contrivance to harm their children, people repeatedly utter variations on Waugh's theme, "It wasn't anyone's fault" (p. 144).

The predatory fox is another refrain that traces the movement in the novel from life to death. Early in the story, when Brenda returns from one of her London excursions, John informs her that "Daddy and I saw a fox just as near as anything and he sat quite still and then went away into the wood" (p. 70). The fox appears again (pp. 133, 146) before the hunt and, in Tony's fever delirium becomes "a mechanical green fox with a bell inside him" (p. 281). Finally, when Hetton itself has become a fox farm, Waugh comments that "the vixen who had lost her brush seemed little the worse for her accident" (p. 308). If this symbolizes Brenda, then the victimizing mother, who has since married Jock Grant-Menzies, emerges unscathed. Meanwhile, in the Brazilian jungle, Tony is reading Dickens to the mad Mr. Todd. Abandoned by Brenda, with whom, like He-Evelyn with She-Evelyn, "he had gotten into a habit of loving and trusting . . ." (p. 172), he has since been abandoned twice more. On the boat he had met an attractive young Trinidadian, Therese de Vitré, who, among other tales, told him of her schoolmate who was abandoned by a lover. She is disliked by the leader of the expedition, Dr. Messinger, who likewise tells him a story of a friend "who had been knifed in a back street of Smyrna, as a warning of what happened if one got mixed up with women" (p. 229). Therese, discovering he is married, abandons Tony. Subsequently, Dr. Messinger also abandons him and drowns, as he seeks assistance for him. Mr. Todd, ironically, is Tony's savior.

Some critics see in Mr. Todd's name the German word for "death" (Lane, 1981, p. 167, n. 34; Phillips, 1975, p. 32), and this view is probably valid. Probable, as well, is Waugh's intention to crystallize the fox motif: Todd is a common English name meaning "fox." (The red-haired Mr. Toddhunter, who puts an end to Basil Seal's child-placement racket in *Put Out More Flags*, is yet to come.) While many believe that T. S. Eliot's "fear in a handful of dust" is embodied in the final grotesque view of Tony reading Dickens to the mad Mr. Todd, the reality is that, paradoxically, Tony's anxiety has in a certain sense been allayed. Stopp (1958) notes, for example, an autobiographical element in the ending: "The works read are those of Dickens; the voice condemned to perpetual reading is a voice from the past, the link with his father's outlook and taste" (p. 216). In other words, after all the betrayals by mothers, the victim is safe, finally reunited with a father figure, both threatening and protective. After failed relationships with women, the homosexual desire once more manifests itself.

Homosexuality is present, as well, in *Brideshead Revisited*. Lane (1981) hesitates in acknowledging its presence. Perhaps, he says, Julia and Charles become lovers "because Julia is really Sebastian's alter ego, and hence appeals to Ryder" (p. 95). Stopp (1958), too, sees this; he notes that Sebastian Flyte is a reflection of Charles Ryder but declares that he is "the 'self-regarding' Narcissus, an aspect of the inner vision of any artist . . ." (p. 118). It is more probable, though, that narcissism is always present in homosexuality and paranoia. Freud (1911) observed in the Schreber case that in paranoia the individual is libidinally fixed in primary narcissism, halfway between primitive autoeroticism and object love. In the former, he takes his own body as object; in the latter, a heterosexual object. Taking one's own body as object, however, leads to homosexual impulses, since one is attracted to bodies exactly like it. These impulses must be defended against, by delusions of persecution, for instance, or by delusions of jealousy in which the love for a homosexual object is shifted to a woman. This shift is the most obvious defense used by Charles Ryder in the novel.

From the start, Ryder relates that "I date my Oxford life from my first meeting with Sebastian" (E. Waugh, 1945, p. 24) and describes him as "magically beautiful, with that epicene quality which in extreme youth sings aloud for love and withers at the first cold wind" (p. 31). The epicene quality reflects entrapment in that intermediate stage, the bisexual polarity of erotic attraction. Charles, like the author, yearns for love. It is absent in his life; there is only his father and himself, and affection between them is nonexistent. Suitably, by novel's end, he will find love through conversion, the love of God the Father. He is attracted, too, to the blatant homosexual, Anthony Blanche, and is at a loss to understand why "all the term I had been seeing rather more of Anthony Blanche than my liking for him warranted" (p. 46). It is Anthony who, before Charles has met her, describes Julia to him in what might be called a quintessential homosexual view of a phallic woman: "My dear, she's a *fiend*—a passionless, acquisitive, intriguing, ruthless *killer*. I wonder if she's incestuous. I doubt it; all she wants is power. There ought to be an Inquisition set up especially to burn her" (p. 54).

When he finally does meet Julia, Charles is stunned. "She so much resembled Sebastian that, sitting beside her in the gathering dusk, I was confused by the double illusion of familiarity and strangeness. . . . Because her sex was the palpable difference between the familiar and the strange, it seemed to fill the space between us, so that I felt her to be especially female as I had felt of no woman before" (p. 76). This is perhaps cryptic, but it becomes clearer when we understand that sex is to be taken literally, i.e., as genitalia, and that the strangeness/familiarity is related to the resemblance or lack of it to his own body. Although Cohen (1971) points to a possible homosexual implication here, he ultimately denies it, stating that the attraction is based upon "family resemblance coloured by nostalgia" (p. 6). The evidence to the contrary, however, is overwhelming.

Sebastian, Charles's original love object, begins to degenerate, both emotionally and physically. His dependency needs express themselves in alcoholism and, as he started in a pseudomaternal relationship with Aloysius his teddy bear, he moves through a pseudohomosexual relationship with the German Kurt and ends up in a passive dependent relationship with God the Father, suffering in a North African monastery. Feeling defectively mothered, like Waugh, he can identify with the helpless Aloysius and the defective, crippled Kurt and attempt to mother them better than he had been: "You know, Charles, . . . it's rather a pleasant change when all your life you've had people looking after you, to have someone to look after yourself. Only of course it has to be someone pretty hopeless to need looking after by *me*" (p. 215). When informed of his mother's death, he responds simply, "Poor Mummy. She really was a *femme fatale*, wasn't she. She killed at a touch" (p. 214).

As Sebastian's life begins to fall apart, Charles shifts his erotic interest to Julia, half aware of its homosexual aspect. "On my side the interest was keener, for there was always the physical likeness between brother and sister, which, caught repeatedly in different poses, under different lights, each time pierced me anew; and, as Sebastian in his sharp decline seemed daily to fade and crumble, so much the more did Julia stand out clear and firm" (pp. 178–179). He says, however, "I had not forgotten Sebastian. He was with me daily in Julia; or rather it was Julia I had known in him, in those distant, Arcadian days" (p. 303).

Each man in this novel resolves his conflict differently. Sebastian, too narcissistic to transfer to a heterosexual object, ends up celibate. Charles tries but fails with Julia. Only Brideshead succeeds; he finds Beryl, a mother surrogate, to care for him. Despite Waugh's sermonizing, it is never really clear why Charles and Julia's love should fail. Perhaps, as Vredenburgh (1957) suggests, Charles is too closely identified with Sebastian and so could not accept Julia because she was too close to Lady Marchmain and so aroused incestuous fears (p. 51).

The last of Waugh's works to be examined is a graphic portrait of an individual whose defenses fail absolutely. The most autobiographical of

Waugh's novels, *The Ordeal of Gilbert Pinfold* (1957a) is based upon a psychotic break the author suffered in 1954. As Pinfold sits musing over his adventures at the end of the novel, he asks himself one key question:

> "What I can't understand is this," he said. "If I was supplying all the information to the Angels [his persecutors], why did I tell them such a lot of rot? I mean to say, if I wanted to draw up an indictment of myself, I could make a far blacker and more plausible case than they did. I can't understand."
>
> Mr. Pinfold never has understood this; nor has anyone been able to offer a plausible explanation. [p. 229]

J. B. Priestley (1957) stumbled across the explanation in a review of the novel. In "What Was Wrong with Pinfold," he imputed madness to Waugh himself and detailed what he believed to be the cause:

> He will break down again, and next time may never find a way back to his study. The central self he is trying to deny, that self which grew up among books and authors and not among partridges and hunters, that self which even now desperately seeks expression in ideas and words, will crack if it is walled up again within a false style of life. [p. 3]

Despite Waugh's reply two weeks later, denying "that I shall soon go permanently off my rocker" (1957b, p. 136), the truth is that Priestley had somehow intuited that Waugh's breakdown was a failure of defenses, his inability to resolve deep conflicts that would continue to trouble him. He was not wrong. Even though Waugh managed to restore stability following the severe reaction depicted in the novel, he was subject ever after to what he called "an odd attack of Pinfold." For example, he was once unable to get home by train because he kept asking for the wrong station and the wrong train (Fleming, 1973, p. 241).

Both Sykes (1975) and Donaldson (1968) have detailed the Pinfold episode in their books, and though Waugh left no diary for this period, the letters of February 3, 8, 12, 16, and 18, 1954 (E. Waugh, 1980, pp. 418–421) show the progression of the conflict clearly. Briefly, the facts are these. Traveling alone to Ceylon, Waugh began to hear voices and, reasoning that they must be coming from somewhere outside him, he believed the wiring in the ship's cabin was acting as a radio receiver. The voices first talked to him, then about him, usually disparaging him as a writer and accusing him, as well, of homosexuality. Successively, he overheard the captain commit a murder, a plot against himself, a serious accident, and an international espionage kidnapping with himself as focus. He believed the plotters, whose leader worked for the BBC, could control his thoughts by means of a device he had heard about before embarking, "The Box," a faith-healing contraption which purported to work by electromagnetic waves.

He wrote to his wife Laura of all these matters, and she became alarmed, urging Jack Donaldson (their next-door neighbor and husband of Frances) to go bring him back. Just then, Evelyn decided to return on his own. When he did, he believed himself possessed by devils and asked a friend, Father Philip Caraman, to exorcise him (Sykes, 1975, p. 364). The priest, however, referred him to a Catholic psychiatrist, Dr. Eric Strauss, who diagnosed his malady as stemming from overdoses of phenobarbitone, taken for his chronic insomnia, and alcohol, which he tended always to overindulge in (p. 48). Dr. Strauss changed his prescription, and the delusions stopped. Three years later, he turned these experiences into a novel.

Because drugs, especially in combination with alcohol, can produce paranoid symptoms, there seems little reason to doubt Dr. Strauss's diagnosis. We can, however, examine both the insomnia and the form of the delusions to see if they are consistent with what has been said so far.

To begin with, the severe insomnia for which Waugh dosed himself with phenobarbitone—and then alcohol—had been a long-standing problem, having begun in 1925 (Sykes, 1975, p. 61). Fenichel (1945) has pointed out that "inasmuch as the voluntary control of motility is lost during sleep, it is first and foremost the fear of forbidden instinctual actions which can assume the form of fear of sleep" (p. 190). He further links the main symptom of orality, depression, to sleep disturbances of this degree. Since we suspect that Waugh's lifelong nostalgic search for the ideal City is connected to his instinctual desire to regain infantile bliss in reunion with a fearful mother, the observations of Orgel (1974) are pertinent: "Permanent re-fusion of subject and idealized victim . . . may be defended against *progressively* by . . . paranoid defenses; or it may be defended against *regressively* in melancholia, or by using such somatic defenses against fusion as insomnia and anorexia" (p. 273). Whatever the reason for it, by the time of these events Waugh's insomnia was of thirty years' duration.

Over the years, Waugh's defenses seemed to have weakened, leaving him even more vulnerable. As Cameron (1974) puts it, "Age brings with it an inevitable accumulation of disappointments; opportunities for new ventures usually fall off in the elderly. Thus a person with compensated life-long paranoid trends may grow less and less able to cope with such losses" (p. 679). Friends have attested to Waugh's extreme disappointment that he never received the public recognition he felt he deserved (Pryce-Jones, 1973, *passim*), and the modernization of the Catholic Church, its dogma and ritual, particularly the changes in the Mass, both upset and embittered him. Knowing that Anne Fleming's nephew had a weakness for firearms, for instance, Evelyn wrote offering "him a bribe if he would go to New York to shoot the Pope" (Fleming, 1973, p. 240). In this overdetermined gesture, we can see Waugh's hostility, cloaked in wit, directed against the Holy Father and, most probably, his own father, long dead.

The Pinfoldian delusions themselves can easily be seen to be full of hostile projections. A seaman, forced to do a dangerous job, is seriously injured in a mechanical accident. The ship's captain slays in his cabin a man accused of making sexual advances to the captain's purported mistress and secretly disposes of the body by slipping it overboard. A spy intrigue, complete with kidnapping and violence, is overheard.

As might be expected in paranoid delusions, sexuality—especially homosexuality—plays a significant part. The plotters, who control Pinfold's thoughts, are members of a family and a group of their friends, all of whom repeatedly accuse him of being "impotent" (E. Waugh, 1957a, p. 174), "a sodomite" (p. 103), and "homosexual" (pp. 96, 105, 121, 147). Bradbury (1973), describing these accusations, declares correctly that they represent "intrusion into himself of the hostile, penetrative forces he fears" (p. 171). Indeed, fears of penetration and anal preoccupation are common among paranoids and "reflect the person's obsessive conflicts and his passive submissive longing for intimacy with his father" (Mac-Kinnon and Michels, 1971, p. 265; Meissner, 1978, p. 50). The mouth and the anus, the major orifices, are usually the focus of concern, and it is fascinating to note that Waugh had curious surgery on both of them. In 1964 he had every tooth in his mouth extracted—without anesthesia—and in 1946 he underwent a completely unnecessary operation to remove hemorrhoids in the interests of what he himself labeled "perfectionism" (Sykes, 1975, p. 304). Perhaps these anal interests help explain an episode in the fiction which many critics feel is, though humorous, overlong and too much embellished: the "Thunderbox" struggle of *Sword of Honor*, a battle between Ritchie-Hook and Apthorpe over a portable field latrine that extends for more than sixteen pages.

The plotters themselves form one of the consistent symptoms in paranoid delusions, that entity which Cameron (1974) has labeled the "pseudo-community" (p. 683). Because it is easier to tolerate a known source of danger than a diffuse, vague persecution, the paranoid organizes the scattered elements into a unified group, viewed as plotting against him for whatever reason. Where once he was puzzled and estranged, he has now out of his anxiety hypothesized the existence of an entity that gives him focus and makes his projections and misinterpretations intelligible.

Although the pseudocommunity is an imaginary organization, it is a composite of real people, misidentified people, and some wholly fictional people. The accusations they make are, of course, Pinfold's own projections; they are castigatory and derogatory because they represent "a relatively harsh and archaic superego" (Meissner, 1978, p. 110). Based firmly in the paranoid's lack of self-esteem, they "are likely to reproduce the content and even the language of the original internal tension quite literally and directly" (Shapiro, 1965, p. 96).

Significantly, Pinfold integrates into the pseudocommunity a family called Angel and a young man he believes to be a member of the family, though the passenger list reveals only a father, a mother, and a daughter, Margaret. Eventually, when he believes the Angels to be reading his private radiograms, he complains to Captain Steerforth and reveals the conspiracy. "What I do know," he tells the captain, "is that the leaders comprise a family of four" (p. 181). It is possible that Pinfold/Waugh's insistence on the family structure here reveals his childhood belief, cited earlier, that the deep bond between Arthur and Alec was a conspiracy against him. Perhaps the presence of a daughter is further indication of Evelyn's feminine identification. If this is so, the imagined sibling, the young man, could represent Alec. It is noteworthy that Evelyn makes him one of his chief persecutors, manipulator of "The Box." In the novel, he is, as well, chief of a BBC team that interviewed him prior to embarkation. (Waugh's first marriage was broken up by his wife's adultery with John Heygate, who worked for the BBC.)

Hinchcliffe (1966), noting that Pinfold calls two of the female plotters Goneril and Regan, observes that Waugh alludes to *King Lear* repeatedly because of the "connected themes of madness, parental grief, and filial ingratitude" (p. 298). He cites Evelyn's own reference to Arthur Waugh's assuming the role of Lear "in deploring the ingratitude of his sons" (p. 298). What Hinchcliffe overlooks, however, is that references to Lear can be considered a recurrence of Waugh's widowed-father motif; especially significant here is the fact that Lear causes much of his own grief by asking the invidious question, "Which of you shall we say doth love us most?" He thus provokes his children to compete with one another for his affection by declaring the degree of theirs for him. Auberon Waugh, in speaking of his father Evelyn as a parent, could criticize him only in one respect: "It was as though he regarded his parental affections as a gift which it was his power to confer or to withdraw. One never quite knew where one was with him" (Sykes, 1975, p. 449). Arthur and Catherine clearly had their lasting effects on Alec and Evelyn.

In addition to the plotters, "The Box" itself must be scrutinized. Since the paranoid's "continuous, rigidly-maintained directedness of himself is a continuous and preoccupying concern with the defense of his autonomy against external assault" (Shapiro, 1965, p. 83), it is understandable that Pinfold would create, as part of his delusion, this external controlling device, consisting, as he believed, "of a glass tube containing two parallel lines of red light which continually drew together or moved apart like telegraph wires seen from a train" (p. 196).

The creation of such a device is consistent with the paranoid's regression to the magical thinking of childhood (MacKinnon and Michels, 1971, p. 271), and is directly related to Tausk's famous "influencing machine," common to schizophrenic thought. As Tausk (1919) demonstrated, the belief that one's thoughts can be known and controlled indicates the regressive loss of ego boundaries (p. 45), and the machine itself is, among other things, a representation of the projected genitals of the paranoid (p. 39). It is both ironic and appropriate that Pinfold believed his persecutors to be primarily members of a particular professional group; he feared he would never get free, as he said, "of those psychoanalysts and their infernal Box" (p. 215). We are left at the end of the novel with Pinfold wondering about his experiences and seeking a plausible explanation. Both Priestley's comment about Waugh's denying his true nature and Tom Driberg's observation that Waugh's suppression of his bisexual nature contributed to his breakdown help to provide this explanation. Analysis of the text substantiates this.

In light of the textual evidence, it is curious to see critics (Lane, 1981; Phillips, 1975) labor to integrate this novel into the canon, an especially difficult task since the work fits into the period of the "Catholic Novels," *Brideshead Revisited* and *Helena*. Phillips goes so far as to call *Pinfold* "a perfect extension of the religious vision which permeates Waugh's later works" (p. 11). That may be. It is, for certain, a perfect logical and psychological extension of the conflicts that troubled Evelyn Waugh from his childhood onward.

It is perhaps appropriate that Waugh was so antipsychoanalytical and antipsychological, though this has disturbed some critics. Stopp (1958) has observed in Waugh's fiction the "almost complete absence of introspective analysis and ironic comment . . ." (p. 181), but Greenblatt (1965) declares, as if in reply, that "one must not ask Evelyn Waugh or any satirist for a deep psychological examination of his characters, for this would be inimical to the satire itself" (p. 25). Lane (1981) excuses Waugh, claiming that his primary interests were clarity and style, with character and motivation secondary (p. 145). Waugh himself openly scorned analysis, advising Stephen Spender in "Two Unquiet Lives" (1951), "Don't analyze yourself. Give the relevant facts and let your readers make their own judgements" (p. 307). Most probably, Waugh was prevented by his conflicts from any deep analysis, either of his characters or of himself, as is any paranoid. "He cannot afford to be intellectually curious about his deeper motives, as he fears that every discovery about himself will only lead to exposure of his badness, with resulting humiliation" (MacKinnon and Michels, 1971, p. 290).

Despite this, it is possible to see Waugh's fiction as significant attempts at self-analysis, as embodiments of the working through of his psychic conflicts. In "On Sarcasm," for example, Slap (1966) differentiates between sarcasm and satire:

> Satire differs from sarcasm in at least two respects: first, satire is a muffled attack and a display of cleverness. There is emphasis on the defensive activity and the talent of the ego at the expense of raw aggression. Second, satire gives the impression of a more or less independent attitude on the part of its user toward his object. One has the feeling that the satirical person has in the past suffered a traumatic disappointment but has at least partially overcome it and attained independence albeit retaining an angry, rueful, or critical attitude toward his object. He seems to polish his target off as if he no longer requires it or has good expectations of it, and would not mind if it disappeared or if he lost its love forever. It may be pertinent that satire is derived from the Latin *satur*, meaning filled with food, sated. [p. 400]

Waugh never used sarcasm in his fiction, only satire. His hunger, as has been seen, was a hunger for love which began early and was never fully satisfied. The representative works analyzed reveal repeatedly the pattern of the search for love—both homosexual and heterosexual—and the victim as hero. Waugh's genius lay in his gift for transforming these manifestations of the unconscious. The works reveal a pattern that would be monotonous in its repetition were not the external symbols for the underlying concerns so rich and varied, the same warp and woof manipulated to produce multiple configurations of different shape, color, and texture. Images of the jungle and desert recur throughout his fiction, for example; they threaten, but they also attract, beckoning the reader to explore the heart of darkness. Bradbury (1973) has noticed that Waugh's primary concern is with irrationality, specifically the chaos *within*. The novels, he observes, are "largely the product of these confrontations with a barbarism and anarchy that is not simply outside and to be resisted; it is also within and to be shaped and organized" (p. 171).

In this shaping and organizing, this working through of his own psychic conflicts, Evelyn Waugh has produced fiction that has made millions laugh and has given us probably the best and wittiest body of satire thus far in the twentieth century.

When Alec came, in his own autobiography (1962, p. 218), to estimate the worth of Evelyn's work, he went even further, proclaiming him "incomparably the finest novelist of our period." Despite this, he apologizes to the reader for not speaking at greater length of his famous brother, begging off with the excuse that he fears getting the "picture out of focus" and does not want to "mislead" readers. He never explains the reasons for these fears, though, and it can only be assumed that they relate to the emotional estrangement of the brothers throughout their lives.

Significantly, Evelyn too, in his autobiography (1964), is virtually dumbstruck when he comes to the subject of his brother. Echoing Alec's words, he admits that "the five years that separated us made, in childhood, a complete barrier" (p. 33). He briefly contrasts himself and Alec, noting that his brother is nomadic, indifferent in religion, gregarious, and athletic. The only similarity he notes between them, astonishingly, is that they are "of the same height" (p. 25).

In truth, however, in addition to their literary talent, Alec and Evelyn had other things in common. Each bonded strongly to a parent, engaged in homosexual activity, had a broken first marriage of a year's duration, relied upon or flirted with drugs, contemplated or attempted suicide, traveled extensively, and served with distinction in battle. Beyond this, as we have seen, they were concerned in their fiction with much the same matters. Although Alec dealt primarily with oedipal conflicts and Evelyn with preoedipal, both created passive victims as the central characters in their novels. Further, both were preoccupied with homosexuality, either overtly or covertly, and both explored extensively unstable emotional relationships, especially those of the family. Fortunately for them and for us, their literary talent enabled them to transform their own personal and familial conflicts into literature of enduring value. It is as Jean Paul Richter wrote, "The words a father speaks to his children in the privacy of the home are not overheard at the time, but, as in whispering galleries, they will be clearly heard at the end and by posterity."

REFERENCES

Birkenhead, F. (1973), Fiery particles. In: *Evelyn Waugh and His World*, ed. D. Pryce-Jones. Boston: Little, Brown, pp. 137–163.

Bradbury, M. (1964), *Evelyn Waugh*. Writers and Critics Series. Edinburgh: Oliver & Boyd.

———— (1973), America and the comic vision. In: *Evelyn Waugh and His World*, ed. D. Pryce-Jones. Boston: Little, Brown, pp. 165–182.

Cameron, N. (1974), Paranoid conditions and paranoia. *The American Handbook of Psychiatry*, 2nd ed., Vol. 3, ed. S. Arieti. New York: Basic Books, pp. 676–693.

Carens, J. (1966), *The Satiric Art of Evelyn Waugh*. Seattle: University of Washington Press.

Cohen, M. (1971), *Brideshead Revisited* and Jaspar Tristram. *The Evelyn Waugh Newsletter*, 5(3):6–8.

Davis, R.M. (1969), The mind and art of Evelyn Waugh. *Papers on Language and Literature*, 3:270–287.

Donaldson, F. (1968), *Evelyn Waugh: Portrait of a Country Neighbor*. Philadelphia: Chilton.

Fenichel, O. (1945), *The Psychoanalytic Theory of Neurosis*. New York: Norton.

Fleming, A. (1973), Yours affec: Evelyn. In: *Evelyn Waugh and His World*, ed. D. Pryce-Jones. Boston: Little, Brown, pp. 235–241.

Freud, S. (1900), The Interpretation of Dreams. *Standard Edition*, 4 & 5. London: Hogarth Press, 1953.

———— (1911), Psychoanalytic notes on an autobiographical account of a case of paranoia (dementia paranoides). *Standard Edition*, 12:3–88. London: Hogarth Press, 1958.

Greenblatt, S.J. (1965), *Three Modern Satirists: Waugh, Orwell, and Huxley*. New Haven: Yale University Press.

Heath, J.M. (1976), The private language of Evelyn Waugh. *English Studies in Canada*, 2(3):329–338.

Hinchcliffe, P. (1966), Fathers and children in the novels of Evelyn Waugh. *University of Toronto Quarterly*, 35:293–310.

Hollis, C. (1954), Evelyn Waugh. In: *A Library of Literary Criticism, Vol. 3: Modern British Literature*, ed. R. Temple and M. Tucker. New York: Ungar, 1966, pp. 305–306.

Hynes, J. (1972), Varieties of death wish: Evelyn Waugh's central theme. *Criticism*, 14(1):65–77.

Jollife, J. (1973), What's in a name. In: *Evelyn Waugh and His World*, ed. D. Pryce-Jones. Boston: Little, Brown, pp. 229–233.

Jones, R. (1978), Evelyn Waugh: a man at bay. *Virginia Quarterly Review*, 54(3):503–517.

Kleiner, J. (1970), On nostalgia. In: *The World of the Emotions*, ed. C. Socarides. New York: International Universities Press, 1977, pp. 471–498.

Lane, C. (1981), *Evelyn Waugh*. Boston: Twayne.

MacKinnon, R., & Michels, R. (1971), *The Psychiatric Interview in Clinical Practice*. Philadelphia: W.B. Saunders.

Meissner, W.W. (1978), *The Paranoid Process*. New York: Jason Aronson.

Orgel, S. (1974), Sylvia Plath; fusion with the victim and suicide. *Psychiatric Quarterly*, 43(2):262–287.

Phillips, G.D. (1975), *Evelyn Waugh's Officers, Gentlemen, and Rogues: The Fact Behind His Fiction.* Chicago: Nelson-Hall.
Priestley, J.B. (1957), What was wrong with Pinfold? In: *Evelyn Waugh and His World*, ed. D. Pryce-Jones. Boston: Little, Brown, 1973, p. 3.
Pryce-Jones, D., ed. (1973). *Evelyn Waugh and His World.* Boston: Little, Brown.
Quennell, P. (1973), A kingdom of Cokayne. In: *Evelyn Waugh and His World*, ed. D. Pryce-Jones. Boston: Little, Brown, pp. 23–38.
Shapiro, D. (1965), *Neurotic Styles.* New York: Basic Books.
Slap, J. (1966), On sarcasm. In: *The World of the Emotions*, ed. C. Socarides. New York: International Universities Press, 1977, pp. 391–402.
Stopp, F. (1958),*Evelyn Waugh: Portrait of an Artist.* Boston: Little, Brown.
Sykes, C. (1975), *Evelyn Waugh: a Biography.* Boston: Little, Brown.
Tausk, V. (1919), On the origins of the 'influencing machine' in schizophrenia. In: *The Psychoanalytic Reader*, ed. R. Fliess. New York: International Universities Press, 1948, pp. 31–64.
Vredenburgh, J. (1957), The character of the incest object: a study of alternation between narcissism and object choice. *American Imago*, 14:45–52.
Waugh, A. (1917), *The Loom of Youth.* London: Geoffrey Bles.
———— (1936), *Jill Somerset.* New York: Farrar & Rinehart.
———— (1952), *Guy Renton.* New York: Farrar, Straus & Young.
———— (1955), *Island in the Sun.* New York: Farrar, Straus & Cudahy.
———— (1962), *The Early Years of Alec Waugh.* New York: Farrar, Straus & Co.
———— (1965), *The Mule on the Minaret.* New York: Farrar, Straus & Giroux.
———— (1967), *My Brother Evelyn and Other Portraits.* New York: Farrar, Straus & Giroux.
———— (1970), *A Spy in the Family.* New York: Farrar, Straus & Giroux.
———— (1973), *The Fatal Gift.* New York: Farrar, Straus & Giroux.
———— (1975), *A Year to Remember: A Reminiscence of 1931.* London: W.H. Allen.
———— (1978), *The Best Wine Last: An Autobiography through the Years—1932–1969.* London: W. H. Allen.
Waugh, E. (1934), *A Handful of Dust.* Boston: Little, Brown.
———— (1945), *Brideshead Revisited.* Boston: Little, Brown.
———— (1946), Fanfare. *Life* (April 8, 1946), p. 60.
———— (1950), *Helena.* Boston: Little, Brown.
———— (1951), Two unquiet lives. *Tablet*, 197:357.
———— (1957a), *The Ordeal of Gilbert Pinfold.* Boston: Little, Brown.
———— (1957b), Anything wrong with Priestley? *Spectator*, 13:328–329.
———— (1964), *A Little Learning.* Boston: Little, Brown.
———— (1976), *The Diaries of Evelyn Waugh*, ed. M. Davie. Boston: Little, Brown.
———— (1977), *A Little Order: A Selection from His Journals*, ed. D. Gallagher. Boston: Little, Brown.
———— (1980), *The Letters of Evelyn Waugh*, ed. M. Amory. New York: Ticknor & Fields.
Woodruff, D. (1973), Judge and jury must decide. . . . In: *Evelyn Waugh and His World*, ed. D. Pryce-Jones. Boston: Little, Brown, pp. 103–132.

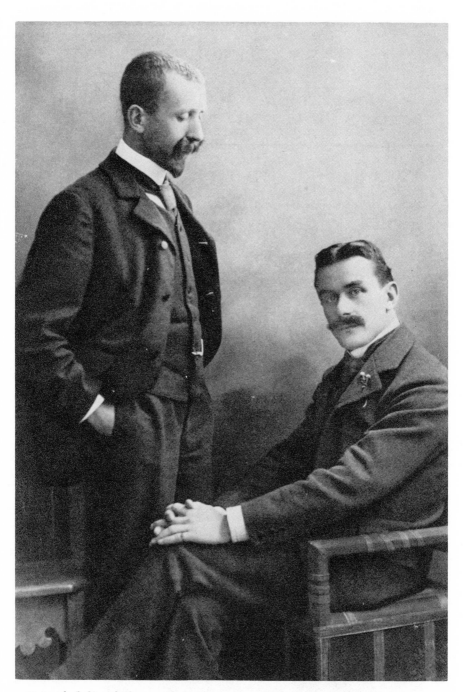

Heinrich (left) and Thomas Mann. Permission: *du: Die Kunstzeitschrift*.

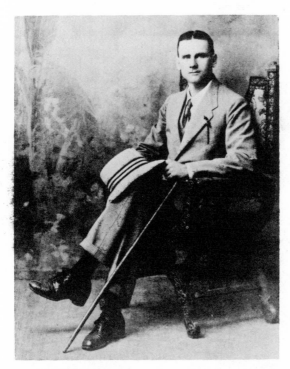

Stanislaus Joyce, Trieste, 1905.

James Joyce, (Zurich, 1917.) From the Harley K. Croessmann Collection of James Joyce, Special Collections, Morris Library, Southern Illinois University.

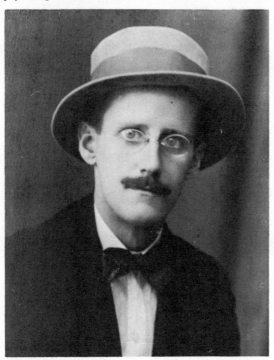

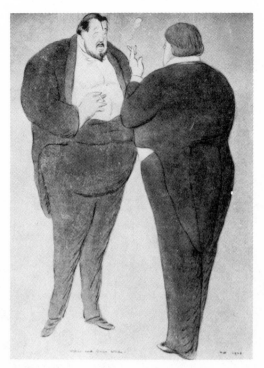

Willie (left) and Oscar Wilde. Caricature by Max Beerbohm. Permission: Humanities Research Center, University of Texas.

Sir Herbert Beerbohm Tree (left) and Sir Max Beerbohm. Caricature by Max Beerbohm. Legend reads *Genus Beerbohmiense, species Herbertica Arborealis, species Maximiliana*. Permission: Mrs. Eva Reichmann.

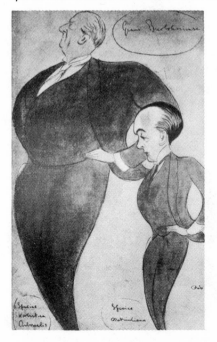

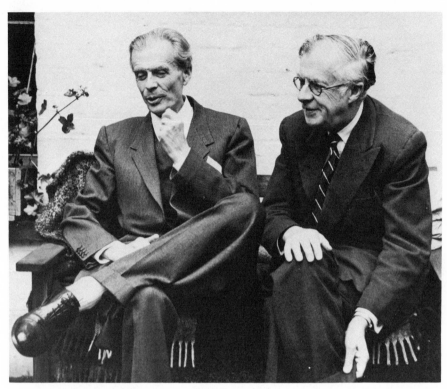

Aldous (left) and Julian Huxley. Photo © Douglas Glass.

Alec (left) and Evelyn Waugh. Photo by Madame Yevonde.

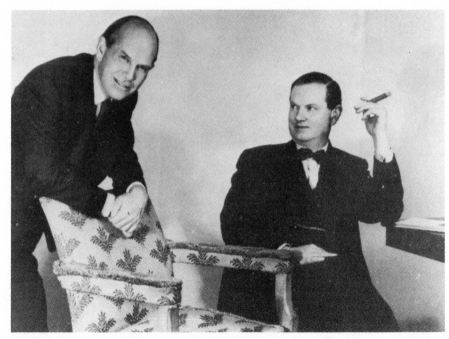

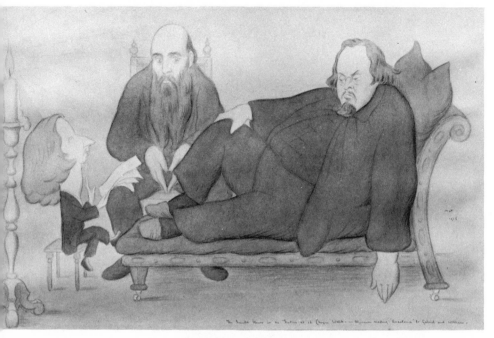

William (left) and Dante Gabriel Rossetti being read to by Algernon Charles Swinburne. "The Small Hours in the 'Sixties at 16 Cheyne Walk"—caricature by Max Beerbohm (1916). Permission: The Tate Gallery, London.

Peter (left) and Anthony Shaffer. "Stirring the 'Pud': Christmas 1979." Photo courtesy of Claudia Shaffer.

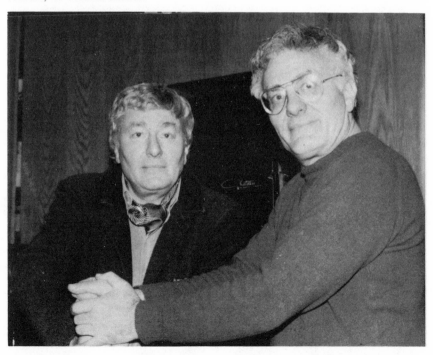

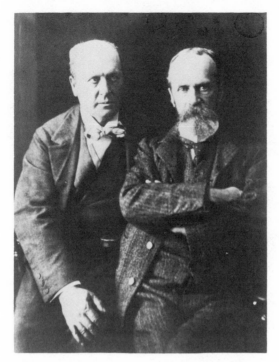

Henry (left) and William James, c. 1900. Photo by permission of the Houghton Library, Harvard University.

James Strachey. Oil painting by Duncan Grant (1910). Permission: The Tate Gallery, London.

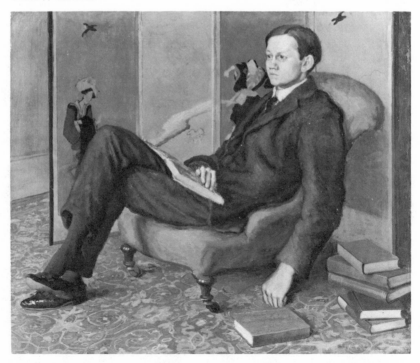

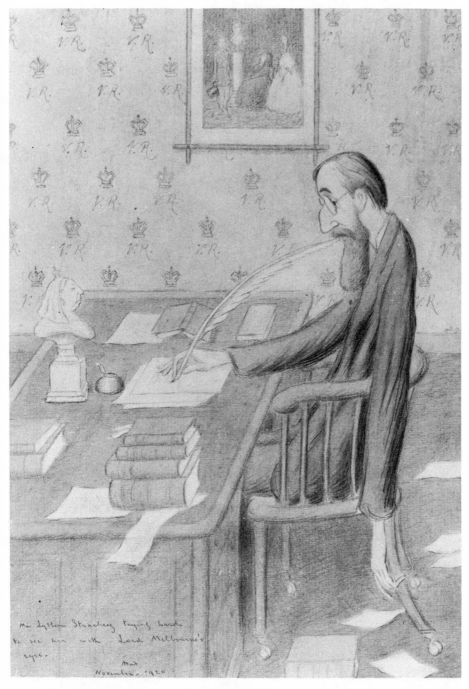

Lytton Strachey, 1920. Caricature by Max Beerbohm. Permission: National Gallery of Victoria, Melbourne, Felton Bequest 1921.

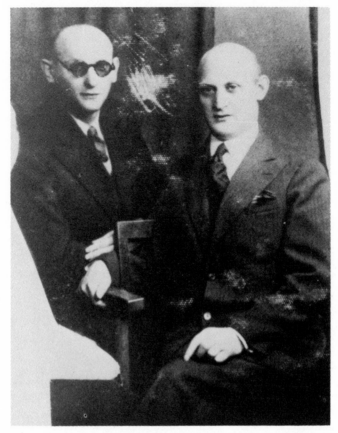

Isaac Bashevis (left) and Israel Joshua Singer, in Warsaw c. 1930.

Lawrence (left) and Gerald Durrell, 1961. Photo by Loomis Dean.

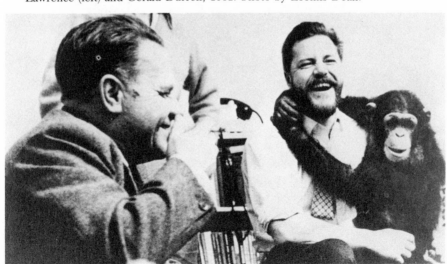

7

His Brother's Keeper: William Michael and Dante Gabriel Rossetti

STANLEY WEINTRAUB

At nineteen, bored by the rigidity of his art studies and absent from classes as usual, Dante Gabriel Rossetti encountered a curious notebook at his free university, the British Museum, at a time when he should have been copying plaster casts in the Royal Academy's Sculpture Room. In April 1847, a Museum attendant named Palmer, noticing that the young man with the neglected hair and clothes was interested in poetry, offered to sell him a manuscript book he had apparently acquired legitimately, crammed with prose, verse, and drawings by a little-regarded eccentric of a generation before, William Blake. The price asked was ten shillings, which Gabriel thought a bargain, considering that Blake, although no darling of the orthodox literati, had written *Songs of Innocence* and *Songs of Experience*. A glance through the notebook showed, his brother William remembered, "outspoken epigrams and jeers against such painters as Correggio, Titian, Rubens, Rembrandt, Reynolds, and Gainsborough—all men whom Blake regarded as fulsomely florid, or lax, or swamping ideas in mere manipulation. These were balsam to [Gabriel's] soul, and grist to his mill."[1]

Gabriel had no money, but applied to William, and the manu-

[1] All quotations, unless otherwise noted, are from S. Weintraub (1977), *Four Rossettis: A Victorian Biography*. New York: Weybright and Talley; London: W. H. Allen, 1978.

script changed hands. **Although Gabriel** held it in reverence all his life, it was not for him a mere **curiosity** for display. Since the pages were a tangle of abandoned starts, **alternative** lines, and cancellations, the brothers decided to copy out what they could, Gabriel taking the poetry and William the prose. The choice as well as the means of purchase would be symbolic of their coordinate lives.

Born in London in 1828, Gabriel was one year older than William. When they were in their teens, Gabriel was already thought of by his father as a literary and artistic prodigy, and sent to the Royal Academy's school to study art. William was literary minded, but no genius. And he was dutiful. At fifteen he had been packed off, unprotesting, to a clerkship in the Excise Office in Somerset House, where he would work until his retirement forty-nine and a half years later. Gabriel, exempted by his genius, would never hold a paying job.[2]

William could afford the purchase. He had just been raised to £90 a year and "put on the establishment"—the permanent staff of the Excise Office, at a desk where he wrote letters to Excise functionaries and to English traders paying duties. The work was dull, and attracted dull types in whom he had no interest. He made no friends there, adopting Gabriel's circle of acquaintances as his own. Gabriel had a way of attracting followers as well as friends, and William's entry into the constantly enlarging group established another feature of the brotherly relationship which would never change. William would work steadily, and Gabriel would count on tapping that source of funds when he needed to. William's literary and artistic interests would largely be reflections of Gabriel's activities and interests. And Gabriel would open his friendships willingly to his younger brother.

Determined that William learn something about art, Gabriel even took him to a session of the Cyclographic Club, where members—young student artists like Holman Hunt and John Millais—according to the rules had to produce a drawing a month as well as critiques of the drawings of the others. William never returned—drawing was not his forte. Yet when Hunt, Millais, and Gabriel Rossetti gave a label to their vague aesthetics about art and nature, and founded their pretentiously named Pre-Raphaelite Brotherhood, Gabriel proposed William as a member. No artist, William had begun attending, at his brother's behest, an evening

[2] The situation was paralleled in the family by the two sisters, Maria, one year older than Gabriel, and Christina, one year younger than William. Victorian women of their class did not work in menial jobs; however, the plain and unremarkable Maria would become a peripatetic teacher of Italian while her poetic younger sister, after some desultory governessing, would be excused by frailty and literary talent from further work. Neither would marry.

drawing class, but he would prove of more use to the group as a compliant model.

The means of all but Millais were limited, and the young men took at least one advantage of their Brotherhood by utilizing each other, whenever possible, to sit for pictures, William soon sitting for the head of Lorenzo in a Millais *Lorenzo and Isabella*. They also began using "P.R.B." on their letters to each other, instead of the gentlemanly "Esquire," and began holding monthly meetings at each other's homes, which meant keeping some form of minutes. Inevitably, William, who could not be expected to do much else, was named secretary, a job he took very seriously, as he valued the entrée that had been made for him.

Under Gabriel's influence, all of them began writing as much, or more, than they painted or sculpted, usually raising the quantity rather than the quality of contemporary poetry. William had been the first P.R.B. to appear in print, as early as September 1848, when a mediocre poem of his appeared in the *Athenaeum,* and he versified at every opportunity, although constant practice never compensated for his thinness of poetic talent. On June 30, 1849, for example, when summer had parted the P.R.B.s more than usual, he dashed off some lines to Frederic Stephens which only proved that although he had nothing to say, and wrote business letters all day at work, the desire to communicate remained insatiable:

> It is now past the hour of 12;
>   Gabriel's dozing in his chair.
> And so this letter I will shelve,
>   As soon as can be, dear Brother.
> Not that I mean to go to bed
>   Quite yet. I have the P.R.B.
> Diary to write up instead.
>   Tho' there is nothing verily.

Before long Gabriel had made a case for a P.R.B. publication to feature their own work. The first entry on the subject in William's journal is dated July 13, 1849—that "in the evening Gabriel and I went to Woolner's . . . about a project for a monthly sixpenny magazine, for which four or five of us would write, and one make an etching—each subscribing a guinea, and thus becoming a proprietor."

The project was one of passionate interest to Gabriel, although he intended to push the real work onto his brother; but when William went off on his annual holiday from the Excise Office, Gabriel set about making his own inquiries to printers. Before he and Hunt had left for France he had tramped through publishers' offices in Paternoster Row and lined up promises of contributions from the P.R.B.s.

By October 4 Gabriel was in Paris, having written a blank verse travel journal en route, which for safekeeping he posted to William, accompanied by a versified letter. William had been working on what he called a "Pre-Raphaelite poem," the application to verse of the principles of "strict actuality and probability of detail," and rushed a copy to his brother for his criticism. Gabriel took hours out of his discovery of new pictures to elaborately praise, criticize, and recommend alterations to the seven hundred lines. Years later it would be published as "Mrs. Holmes Grey"—a verse dialogue about a woman who dies in the home of a man for whom she had conceived an unrequited passion.

Passion, French style, was a shock to Gabriel. The great Rachel, in Scribe's *Adrienne Lecouvreur*, left them "inexpressibly astounded," and the cancan at Valentino's stirred Gabriel to a sonnet of moral indignation which he warned could not be shown to his family. The "frog-hop," he wrote, was

> . . . a toothsome feast
> Of blackguardism and whore flesh and bald row,
> No doubt for such as love those same. For me,
> I confess, William, and avow to thee,
> (Soft in thine ear) that such sweet female whims
> As nasty backsides out and wriggled limbs
> Nor bitch-squeaks, nor the smell of heated q——s
> Are not a passion of mine naturally.

The P.R.B.s and their cronies were remarkably innocent bohemians.

At one meeting it was decided that each P.R.B. (the group had quickly doubled) would write a sonnet for the first issue of their artistic organ, *The Germ*, but as publication time drew near, only William had produced a poem. He knew it was beneath mediocrity, but he had accomplished the requisite number of lines. Early in November he was even mildly encouraged by a phrenologist he had consulted (he had a cautious curiosity) to believe that he had "an artistic development with symptoms of poetry"—but only "symptoms." Nevertheless he noted the fact in his diary.

Despite his being the only member who had a job which kept him occupied all day, the others, having appointed William editor, left everything to him—the negotiations with the printer, the soliciting of subscribers (Gabriel sent him a list of potential patrons), the acquisition of publishable material. But P.R.B. enthusiasm, as their projected December deadline approached, had not turned into finished copy, and William, despondent over its prospects, convinced Stephens that the first number—advertised for January 1850—should also be the last.

Gabriel guiltily dropped his brushes on the seventeenth and resumed writing his trancelike prose tale "Hand and Soul." Woolner was supposed to have completed a poem by the following Monday, but when it did not arrive and William frantically searched for him, he discovered that it was not and would not be ready, nor did Cave Thomas have ready either his promised wrapper design or his article. Fortunately there was a batch of Christina's poems to be mined, and on the twenty-first Gabriel worked all day and into the night on his story, writing the epilogue the next day while William recopied for the printer the undecipherable sections.

On December 28 William corrected the second galley proofs and filled the remaining empty space with an uninspired sonnet of his own. On the last day of the old year, the first fifty copies of *The Germ* came off the press. Fortunately, William had not ordered 4,000 copies, as he had thought of doing in the enthusiasm of October. Of the 700 copies printed, about a hundred were sold by the printers and another hundred by the P.R.B.s and their friends.

Although Gabriel contributed a major work to the second number and convened two P.R.B. monthly meetings in succession at his studio, the reason was less dedication to *The Germ* than desire to remain close to his canvases. *The Annunciation* would be a family production. In William's journal for November 25, 1849, he had written, "Gabriel began making a sketch. . . . The Virgin is to be in bed, but without any bedclothes on, an arrangement which may be justified in consideration of the hot climate; and the angel Gabriel is to be presenting a lily to her." In a full nightdress Christina sat for the Virgin. At first Gabriel used a paid model for the angel, but the day after *The Germ* went to the printer, he told his brother that the model was "useless." On December 30, between other occupations, William began sitting for the head of the archangel. He was loyal but increasingly uncomfortable as a model, for at twenty he was nearly bald, and shy about it. "This, in youth," he wrote, "was anything but pleasant to me. In particular I used to dislike entering a theatre or other public place with my hat on, looking, as I was, quite juvenile, and then, on taking off my hat, presenting the appearance more like a used-up man of forty." People speculated in his hearing that the phenomenon was a symptom of dissipation, for which he could have had little time and less inclination. By the time the second *Germ* was published, Gabriel had completed to his satisfaction all of the Virgin but her hair. And William had become too busy to sit for the angel's arms, compelling Gabriel to invest in a model.

Only forty copies of the second *Germ* would be sold: "The last knock-down blow," William groaned. He was ready to give it up and cut the

P.R.B. losses, but George Tupper saw the journal as a prestige opportunity for his firm, and offered to make good the losses on at least two further issues. On an evening in mid-February, in Gabriel's garret workroom in Charlotte Street, those of the faithful whom William could reach hastily by post gathered to hear Tupper's offer, made before he had received a farthing of their debt. They accepted.

The result was that William, after his hours at the Excise Office, was in effect the unpaid employee of the printers, who promptly renamed the forthcoming issue *Art and Poetry, being Thoughts towards Nature*. As he put it, "I naturally accommodated myself more than before to any wish evinced by the Tupper family." The public remained unpersuaded. The March issue appeared a month late, and the April issue ended the experiment. The Brethren collectively owed thirty-four pounds, seventeen shillings, which William computed, in careful letters to the investors, at three pounds, fourteen shillings and sixpence each. Some of the P.R.B.s squabbled over the bill, and William naturally paid Gabriel's share.

Perhaps William realized that despite the depressing, unremunerative work he had put into *The Germ*, only for him was the publication worth anything. With it he had served his apprenticeship as editor and critic, two occupations he would retain—along with the Excise Office—all his working life. The *Guardian* had observed that "some of the best papers [in *The Germ*] are by the two brothers named Rossetti." And several poets—notably Arthur Clough, Coventry Patmore, and William Allingham—commented appreciatively on William's criticism. Further, the Rossettis' friend, Major Calder Campbell, who had contributed a sonnet to *The Germ*, had shown an issue to Edward William Cox, a barrister who edited the *Critic*, then a modest rival to the *Athenaeum*. The result was an offer to William to become the magazine's art critic. The post paid no better than *The Germ*, but it was a chance to champion P.R.B. causes and a respectable entrée into London critical journalism.

Despite financial problems and professional frustrations, the remaining P.R.B.s and their cronies continued to see each other regularly, and Gabriel often worked his old magic in giving them cause to remain together. William, as a critic, now had access to review copies of new books, which gave him a new importance. Publicly Gabriel was outgoing and optimistic, although he lived largely on "loans" from William and gifts from his aunts, and was even reduced, in mid-1850, to hiding his shabby clothes under his painting smock. From Newman Street one morning he sent an urgent appeal to William at the Excise Office. "I know not whether you have to go anywhere tonight, but . . . you have put on the only pair of breeches in which it is possible for me to go to the Opera tonight.

Unless you *do* want them yourself, I wish if possible you would manage to be at home by five, in order that we may make a transfer. . . ."

At least once in the frustrating summer of 1850 Gabriel was even embarrassed by poverty not his own. The tenant of his building, the proprietor of a dancing school from whom he subleased the rooms above what he called the "hop shop," defaulted on his rent and Gabriel's goods were seized. (His books were saved because William managed to smuggle them to Madox Brown's.) Why Gabriel had to be in hiding, since he was not the guilty party, is not clear, unless his sublease made him doubly liable; but Christina wrote cautiously to William from Brighton, "If his whereabouts is to be kept secret, pray do not let me have his address." This time it was Aunt Charlotte who bailed Gabriel out of what he described to her as "the late unlucky pickle." He paid his rent and sent Margaret Polidori a sketch of his *Kate the Queen* as evidence of his application to his work. He would soon be hiring models again, he told her. Yet he was already planning to put the work aside, explaining dubiously to William that it could not be completed in time for the next annual exhibition.

He was more frank about his brother's work, pressing him to write more lucidly. "I have just read your review in the *Critic*," Gabriel observed, ". . . many parts of which I do not understand. What do you mean by the 'enforcement of magnificence having a tendency to impair the more essential development of feeling'?" But although Gabriel could urge his less talented brother to work, William regularly put in a day's labor at a regular job before he began his after-hours writing. Gabriel might write hortatory letters, but was doing less painting than before, or at least was not carrying anything to completion, returning more to the unremunerative solace of composition and translation.

Gabriel did not wish to fulfill himself, in proper Victorian fashion, in work for its own sake. Carlyle had proclaimed that "all work, even cotton-spinning, is noble; work is alone noble." But even William, Gabriel knew, did not profess to be exhilarated by his hours at the Inland Revenue. The cult of work no more appealed to Gabriel than the cult of moral earnestness, and to lower the implicit pressure on him to become a wage earner, he devised an appropriate gesture. After preliminary publicity at home, he betook himself to Nine Elms Station (on the South Bank of the Thames east of Battersea) to investigate a position as a railway telegraph operator. He examined the apparatus and explained courteously to the authorities, as he did afterward to his family, that he could never understand telegraphic code or the complexities of the device. Then he left, having fulfilled, for the rest of his life, his obligations to salaried employment.

Outwardly he evidenced no distress. As Madox Brown recorded, Gabriel had "thrown up" his pictures, but "his head and beard grow finer every day, and he had . . . some designs which were perfectly divine . . . but paint he *will not*. He is too idle." He "purports to keep himself," Madox Brown noted shrewdly. "I had thought for some time there had been some estrangement between Rossetti and his brother, and I asked Deverell. . . . He said no. That he believed they were as good friends as ever, but that he supposed his brother did not call on him oftener than he could help because he was ordered peremptorily to hand over all the cash he had about him." Somehow William's relationship to his brother survived such episodes, but they were seeing less of each other. William worked all day, and Gabriel often stayed evenings at the Red Lion Square studio, where his (and Deverell's) landlord, concerned about the young women who entered alone and remained for hours, stipulated in his lease that models had to be "kept under some gentlemanly restraint, as some artists sacrifice the dignity of art to the baseness of passion."

The P.R.B.s were always looking for interesting faces and figures to paint, William Rossetti writing in his journal on December 7, 1850, that he had encountered Millais, Hunt, and Charles Collins (painter brother of novelist Wilkie Collins) "parading Tottenham Court Road . . . on the search for models." And when they found "one or two adaptable for Millais—the best being in the company of two men"—their courage failed, as they worried that addressing her would bring "the likelihood of a cry of 'Police.'"

Deverell first told Hunt about the "stupendously beautiful creature" he had found plying her needle in a milliner's shop in Cranbourne Alley. It was then March 1850, and Academy submissions were a month away. "By Jove!" he had gone on; "she's like a queen, magnificently tall, with a lovely figure, a stately neck, and a face of the most delicate and finished modelling. . . . Wait a minute! I haven't done; she has grey eyes, and her hair is like dazzling copper, and shimmers with lustre. . . ." She would be at the Red Lion Square studio the next day to pose in page's garb for Viola in Deverell's *Twelfth Night*.

So was Gabriel, who sat for the head of the Jester in the picture. "To fall in love with Elizabeth Siddal," William Rossetti afterward wrote, "was a very easy performance, and Dante Gabriel transacted it at an early date."

How much the family knew by 1851 is not certain. None of the Rossettis but William as yet had seen Lizzy,[3] who as Madox Brown put it, could be "beautifully dressed for about three pounds, altogether looking like a queen," and spoke with a soft voice which belied her origins. At worst William assumed that she would be no added drain on his own finances.

As the family's income had declined, William's had improved. He had confided to his diary about work as an after-hours critic that he would "certainly be glad to do for something, and with better prospects, what I am now doing for nothing," and he did get an offer to write art criticism for the *Spectator* from its proprietor, Robert S. Rintoul. It paid relatively well—£50 a year, which in addition to William's £110 from the Inland Revenue (its later name), made him, as he put it, almost a capitalist among the P.R.B.s. (Only Millais earned more, selling his paintings easily, regardless of critical disapproval.) But William made the brotherly mistake of inducing Rintoul to offer assignments he could not handle himself to Gabriel, who should have needed the money. Yet he would not bestir himself to earn it. Writing about an art exhibition he was to review while William was away visiting Bell Scott in Newcastle, Gabriel lazily informed his brother, "I am not well enough to stir out tonight . . . but will write an article from recollection and catalogue—which Brown has got. This I suppose will be sufficient. The P.R.B. business will not lose. . . ." But it was, and had been, losing. William's contrary opinion in the *Spectator* remained almost the only exception to the general humiliation.

By August 1852, Gabriel was planning complete removal from the family; in order to be with Lizzy he wanted a domicile of his own, which he explained to his mother (the prospective "lender" of the money) as a place for William and himself. William in fact had to sign as cotenant, at £40 annual rent, since Gabriel was jobless and could not guarantee the sum. On November 22, 1852, the move was accomplished. At twenty-four, with almost no income, and a mate to support as well as the rent to find, Gabriel was on his own.

Three days after his move to the three-room upstairs flat at 14 Chatham Place Gabriel wrote William, "I have Lizzy coming, and of course do not wish for anyone else." He was referring, he quickly added, to a possible visit from Hunt, and indeed offered William dinner if he came over after his Friday at the office, but the implication remained. William evidenced no feeling of being put upon.

The atmosphere was often foul at Chatham Place, the pilings of which

[3] *Lizzy* is the writer's choice of Elizabeth Siddal Rossetti's nickname. Both Rossetti brothers used *Lizzie* and *Lizzy* interchangeably, and in quotations the spelling of the name may differ from one citation to another.

were awash in sewage when the Thames was at high tide; but the pic-
turesque location near Blackfriars Bridge, looking out over the river, kept
Gabriel there. When summer 1853 came and the air was especially
bad—he attributed some of Lizzy's chronic bronchial illness to it as
well—Gabriel borrowed a carpetbag and "ten or twelve pounds" from
Aunt Charlotte through the good offices of Maria and went off to visit Bell
Scott in Newcastle, telling his aunt that he needed the sea air at Tyneside.
And from there he pressured William—who slept at Blackfriars sometimes—to pay the rent.

Despite deficiencies in talent or in its application, Gabriel from the
start reigned among his friends like Arthur among his knights. In Elizabeth Siddal he had his Guinevere and at Chatham Place his Camelot.
The charisma would persist all his life, one of his last young followers,
Philip Bourke Marston, writing to a friend, "What a supreme man is
Rossetti! Why is he not some great exiled king that we might give him
our lives to try to restore him to his kingdom!" Even the unsentimental
Bell Scott wrote afterward that he began then "to feel some sort of fascination about the personality of D.G.R." that made one "accept certain
peculiarities in him. I found all his intimate associates did so, placing him
in a position different from themselves, a dangerous position to a man
whose temperament takes advantage of it." It gave Gabriel, Scott felt,
"a sort of supremacy." His deep-set dark eyes, his rich voice, his combination of Latin grace and Anglo-Saxon wit, deflected skepticism and
induced the impecunious to lend him money, the cautious to trust him
with their wives and mistresses, the wary to offer him friendship, the
discreet to confide in him, and the cynical, despite themselves, to admire
his poetry or his painting. And like any king worth his scepter, Gabriel
supported his royal style by taxing his willing subjects, living off subsidies
from his mother and his aunts, his brother and his friends, eventually,
too, his admirers and his patrons. Whatever the matter of service, somehow those Gabriel used found in it a kind of fulfilment, and in a subliminal
way the cult of medievalism to which his circle responded may have
acquired new force.

Although William gave his daily hours unstintedly to the Inland Revenue,
his life was really elsewhere. Literary and artistic journalism took up those
of his evenings and weekends not devoted to Henrietta Rintoul. Tight-
lipped and high-cheekboned, she looked even more imperious than she
was, and William counted himself fortunate to be on the verge of moving
up in the English caste structure by marrying into her family. But *she*
would not set the date. In the meantime he courted her decorously and
continued to write for her father's journal.

William was also London correspondent for the American art journal the *Crayon*. He was to be further involved with America through William Bell Scott, who sent him a copy of Walt Whitman's *Leaves of Grass* early in 1857. "Obliterate utterly with the blackest ink half-a-dozen lines and half-a-dozen words, ignore the author altogether, and read as one does the books that express human life like the Bible—books that have aggregated rather than been written—and one finds these *Leaves of Grass* grow up in a wonderful manner. The book is very like opening into a quite new poetic condition." Bell Scott had given a better gift than even he knew. In 1868 William Rossetti would become, implicitly following his astute friend's instructions for discreet expurgation, Whitman's first editor abroad.

Gabriel, irresponsible even to his own work, was a poor risk through which to live the surrogate life of a genius. Yet William was trapped by family fealty as well as by the gut feeling that Gabriel's potential—and even his reality—made the sacrifice little sacrifice at all. William's talents were confessedly modest, and without the Gabriel component even his private life was dull. His brother seemed that rare creative spirit with genius in literature as well as art, who could command the friendship and service of all manner of interesting people, and the love of beautiful women. William knew his talents were limited, that his most attractive friends were his largely because he was Gabriel's brother, and that his own prim and unresponsive fiancée hardly measured up to his brother's "stunner." Vicariously through Gabriel, William hardly dared breathe to himself, he was living almost a double life; and it was worth the investment. Yet he was not without pride, though without creative impulse, and sought in such editorial labors as he would perform for Whitman's reputation, and later for Shelley's, the safe harbor of a reputation all his own.

During the August doldrums, when there were no exhibitions to review or interesting new books to criticize, William took his annual holiday from the Excise Office and went to his favorite watering place. On the Isle of Wight, Tennyson—who lived there—looked William up and invited him home. William also kept up with Tennyson's peer, Robert Browning, who was living in Italy. Though interested in Gabriel's poetry, Browning realized that if he wanted his English interests looked after competently, William (whom he also knew) was the more prudent and businesslike of the brothers. To his publisher Browning wrote, "We have many artistic friends in London generous enough to care about our concerns and help us in such a matter: but I think William Rossetti is our man just now."

On holiday William had visited with Henrietta and her mother, but that long-standing engagement was no closer to ending in marriage than was Gabriel's with Lizzy. Although Robert Rintoul's health was sufficiently frail, and his years advanced, to induce him to relinquish the *Spectator* —to which William then ceased contributing, in December 1858—Rintoul was still not eager to relinquish his only daughter. Reviewing for other journals, William did not at first miss his regular appearances in the *Spectator*, but the end of the relationship gave him fewer opportunities to press his suit with Henrietta, as the publication's offices were still below the flat in which the Rintouls lived when in London.

Since Gabriel knew that his mother and sisters could get along without William's income, he badgered his brother regularly for money, on the last day of the year confessing shame at plaguing William for another ten pounds. He was doing his best to keep at work at Chatham Place, he insisted, but was being driven mad by bill collectors. He had tried vainly to sell something to Charles Eliot Norton (a Ruskin acquaintance) across the Atlantic at Harvard, and tried through his aunt Charlotte to sell drawings to Lady Bath and a Miss Baring. Averting further recourse to William or to the pawnbroker (his "uncle" in their parlance), he made a sale to Miss Baring and another—two drawings for seventy guineas—to "Old Plint." Temporarily he was solvent. His income as an artist—sometimes in advances on work never delivered—was actually much higher than William's by the late 1850s, but he also spent more extravagantly.

In 1860 the long engagements into which the two Rossetti brothers had entered both ended, only one of them with a marriage. The unexpected element was not only that it was Gabriel who was marrying, but that the bride was the long-suffering Lizzy Siddal, with whom he had lived and loved for so long without benefit of clergy. At Hastings she appeared again to be dying, and Gabriel, at what seemed his final bedside watch, felt his guilt acutely. He renewed his abandoned offer. "Like all the important things I ever meant to do," he wrote his mother on April 13, "—to fulfil duty or secure happiness—this one has been deferred almost beyond possibility. I have hardly deserved that Lizzy should still consent to it, but she has done so, and I trust I may still have time to prove my thankfulness to her. The constantly failing state of her health is a terrible anxiety indeed; but I must still hope for the best. . . ." Then he explained lamely that improved "money prospects" made marriage possible when it had been impracticable before.

William immediately dispatched a congratulatory message, to which Gabriel responded with a brotherly letter rare in that it did not ask for money. "I am not short at present," he noted, "though I only have it as an advance on work to do." But he had forgotten his money when he rushed to Lizzy's side, and had to return to London to fetch it when a long stay in Hastings seemed at least as likely as a funeral and more likely than a wedding trip. (He had already made what seemed to be the essential purchase for Lizzy's rallying, a marriage license.)

William's hopes had risen when, after seven years of waiting for Robert Rintoul to assent to his daughter's marriage, Rintoul died in 1859. But Henrietta pleaded the needs of her ill and aged mother. Then, in October 1860, when William was in Italy with the Brownings, Mrs. Rintoul died. Returning home, William proposed, and the next month—William wrote discreetly in his memoirs—"the lady announced to me that, consequent upon her grief for her mother's death, she viewed with dismay the idea of forming any new ties, and she preferred that the engagement should be regarded as at an end. Against myself no sort of complaint was made or suggested. I was unable to consider this second rupture of the engagement entirely reasonable. I submitted to it, and determined to remain a bachelor." He was diplomatic. Henrietta had agreed to marriage—but on her terms. She proposed a sexless union, and William refused. Four years older than the thirty-one-year-old William, she may have feared a pregnancy at her age, or, after a life spent in cautious suppression of the primal urges, she may have feared them altogether. He never saw her again.

Gabriel's marriage would not be as long-lasting as his "engagement" had been. The oft-told story of his infidelities and Lizzy's apparent suicide (via an overdose of laudanum) in February 1862 belongs to another narrative, although not its aftermath. Madox Brown told William that his brother had found a note pinned to Lizzy's lifeless body—"Take care of Harry." The faithful Brown had put it in the fireplace and withheld the information from the inquest, which reached a verdict of accidental death. Harry was Lizzy's somewhat retarded brother, and the note (hardly an affectionate farewell) seems an implicit accusation of neglect on Gabriel's part, as well as the expression of a natural impulse toward her helpless brother. The guilt-ridden Gabriel did indeed take care of Harry Siddal, and for years after Gabriel's death William dutifully continued his brother's ghostly penance. "At intervals," William's daughter Helen remembered, "a bent and rather dilapidated man would call at our house and my father always welcomed him into his little library and there for a while remained with him in talk, reaccompanying him to the front door with his wonted courtesy. On one occasion, happening to be entering the house myself at the moment, my father said to me, as he closed the door behind his visitor, 'That aged man is a brother of Gabriel's wife, Lizzie.'

And then he told me that for many years he had helped him with a small allowance."

Burial was at Highgate on February 17. For nearly a week Lizzy's body had reposed, in an open coffin, in Chatham Place, and just before the lid was closed, Gabriel, unseen, deposited a manuscript book of his own poems, which had already been advertised as forthcoming in his *Early Italian Poets*, next to Lizzy's pale face, concealing it with her golden hair. To Brown, Gabriel confided what he had done. "I have often been writing at those poems when Lizzie was ill and suffering, and I might have been attending to her, and now they shall go." Realizing that not all of the poems in the calfbound manuscript book existed elsewhere in publishable form, Brown appealed to William to help change Gabriel's mind. But the renunciation of possible poetic fame had its impact upon the usually cool and unsentimental brother. "Well," said William, "the feeling does him honour, and let him do as he likes." With the Siddal and Rossetti families present, and a few other mourners, the coffin was lowered.

Gabriel never slept at Chatham Place after Lizzy's death, but while in temporary rooms, he worked at convincing his brothers and sisters that they could all settle together with him in a new house, along with such friends of his as he felt might provide him useful companionship—in particular, the eager Swinburne. The idea was hardly practical, although William was agreeable and Mrs. Rossetti easily convinced, and Gabriel went ahead to lease the large property at 16 Cheyne Walk, Chelsea, with its pre-Embankment grounds sloping down to the Thames, and Battersea beyond. He relinquished Chatham Place, but the objections to his moving the family wholesale, to assuage his own increasing fear of solitude, grew. Not only was a family of women involved, including the aged Mrs. Rossetti and the near-invalid aunt Margaret Polidori, but Maria, who continued to go out to give lessons in Italian, would have been remote from her pupils in still-suburban Chelsea. Also, to have the pious, reclusive women in the same house with the blasphemous, noisy, often-inebriated Swinburne would have created more problems than it solved.

William agreed to pay part of the £100 annual rent, advance Swinburne's out of his own pocket, and stay overnight at least three days a week at Tudor House, so named because it was reputed to have been part of the red-brick pile to which Queen Catherine Parr had retired after the death of Henry VIII. The women gratefully agreed to abide where they were.

At Tudor House, Gabriel was more harassed by claims upon his canvases and his cash than ever before. The small army of tradesmen who had furnished him with everything from paints and frames to animals and port wine continually pressed for payment. The burden of meeting his debts and his artistic obligations affected both Gabriel and his work, both often becoming coarsely commercial. As his biographer Doughty (1960) put it, "Consequent over-work, inevitably often inferior painting, mental and physical fatigue, financial worry itself, and lack of exercise, all gradually wore down his morale, encouraged his tendency toward neurotic anxiety previously induced by his natural disposition and unhappy past." The resulting insomnia wrecked his nights and defeated his days.

William slept well. In 1867 he was promoted to Committee Clerk at the Excise Office, putting him in direct working contact with one of the Inland Revenue Commissioners. A "larger and better-looking house" was in order, especially since he now expected to house indefinitely his mother and sisters and surviving aunts Eliza and Charlotte. For £125 annual rent he settled upon 56 Euston Square (afterward renamed 5 Endsleigh Gardens), with a front vista of the tree-lined square. Late in June 1867, the family moved into their new quarters, and William was again able to spend his evenings at literary work, which did little more than pay the rent but was a way of maintaining his contacts with the less dull world in which he would rather have moved.

For William it could have been a full-time occupation to be his brother's keeper, and some days, and even weeks, it was. Haunted by what William called "poignant memories and painful associations" related to the death of Lizzy, Gabriel "was prone to think that some secret might yet be wrested from the grave." Seeking that secret in hope of allaying his own sense of guilt, Gabriel became an easy mark for the occultists. Although without religion, he was superstitious even to worrying over thirteen at the dinner table. Early in October 1865, Bell Scott noted in a letter a piece of gossip he had picked up from William—that Gabriel claimed that his wife was "constantly appearing (that is rapping out things) at the seances in Cheyne Walk—! William affirms that the things so communicated are such as only she could know. No reasoning seems to have the least effect with these absurd people. I am going to be present on Friday evening, but expect nothing but rubbish." Although the most thorough skeptic of the four Rossettis, and the natural person—as brotherly confidant—to supply the antidote, William had found himself unable to furnish it.[4] He wanted to experience the phenomenon himself, in another setting than at his brother's house, in order to confirm his unbelief. But when he encountered the allegedly occult his curiosity was only whetted,

[4] William kept a special seance diary apart from his regular notebook, indicating the sensitivity with which he treated the matter. Extensive quotations from it appear in my *Four Rossettis* (1977). The notebook itself is in the University of British Columbia library.

and his growing inability to remain an unbeliever helped undermine Gabriel's tenuous hold on himself. Suspicious of his own reactions, Gabriel leaned heavily on his brother's coolness and unflappable nature. When William's fascination with the seeming manifestations of Lizzy's presence suggested to Gabriel that there might be something to them, his guilty feelings toward her shade intensified.

After William's first table-turning he wrote to his literary friend Anne Gilchrist, "I must avow, at the risk of seeming very absurd, that I am a believer—i.e., things do actually take place which I cannot account for by any physical hypothesis, or any deception of the senses, & which would be adequately accounted for by the spirit hypothesis, which therefore, till something better offers, . . . I feel no hostility to." While for him the investigation was an attempt to get to the bottom of such phenomena, each seance would contribute further to Gabriel's neurotic disintegration. The brothers, each for his own reason, would attempt other seances over the months, some with tantalizing intimations of Lizzy, others with no results. Still, the need of both Gabriel and William to conjure Lizzy up remained powerful. Finally, near midnight on August 14, 1866, with the gaslight lowered at Cheyne Walk, William, Gabriel's assistant Treffry Dunn, and Fanny Cornforth (Gabriel's "housekeeper" and occasional model) sat at a sturdy round table in the upstairs studio, while Gabriel stood by in the adjoining room. Quickly, strong rapping and tilting began, and "ER" identified herself. Gabriel came in. "Are you my wife?" "Yes." "Happier than on earth?" "Yes." "If I were to join you, should I be happy?" "Yes." "Should I see you at once?" "No." "Quite soon?" "No." "Tilt the table to the person you like best." The table tilted toward Gabriel, who then asked whether she liked Fanny. "Yes." "But some while ago you used not to like her?" "No." "Did you pull her hair on a particular occasion?" (William recalled being present when Fanny felt her hair being mysteriously tugged.) "Yes." It was two in the morning when the "manifestations" ceased. Whether Gabriel slept any the better is unknown. It was not the last time he sensed the presence of his dead wife, but it was the last of twenty seances William recorded. By that time Gabriel was in the throes of chronic and deepening insomnia, and was having serious problems with his vision. Finding daylight painful, he further curtained his rooms, and seldom left Cheyne Walk until after dark. Lizzy had never lived at Tudor House, but her psychological presence there, whatever the truths of table-turning, seemed undeniable.

On rare occasions Gabriel forgot his anxieties. William Allingham remembered one evening at Tudor House when his host read aloud new poems by the blind young Philip Marston, after which "the talk turned on early memories; and the two Rossettis reminded each other of childish things; how Dante made drawings of his rocking horse, at the age of 4; how Christina, in those days had such a dreadful temper; how they all talked Italian and English both. . . . At last, about 1 A.M., [Gabriel and William] opened the hall door and showed the moonlight shining on the river, through the lofty iron gates, between the ancient elms: and . . . I said Goodnight. . . ."

Gabriel, it was clear, was in one of his happiest moods, and all was right with the world. For the second time in his life he had found himself deeply in love, in a relationship which had nothing to do with his continued need for the vulgar amiable Fanny, yet everything to do with his marriage to a young woman, since dead, his duty to whom—he now thought—had prevented a lifelong idyll with Jane. Nearly thirty and the mother of two girls, Jane could have discouraged Gabriel, but her marriage with William Morris, despite his great artistic and literary gifts and his affection for her, had been unsatisfactory. A many-sided genius to others, to her he was a loud bore whose enthusiasms she tolerated by retreating into silence and her embroidery. Insensitive to people in many ways, Morris understood that with Gabriel his wife was happy. Reluctantly, he condoned the sittings, and hoped they were nothing more, for Gabriel offered him every opportunity to join Janey at Tudor House, where he passed the time by teaching himself Icelandic and completing the first volume of *The Earthly Paradise*.

Gabriel's letters to Jane were full of passionate declarations not meant to be hidden from her husband. "Top" understood. Janey's large, sad eyes were

> . . . most times looking out afar
> Waiting for something, not for me.

In May 1868, Gabriel had turned forty. The past could not be undone and relived; yet his rapture with Jane Morris restored both his painting and his poetic enthusiasms, and what he wrote suggests that Janey—for a time, at least—reciprocated his passion. Fanny, on such occasions, could be bribed and banished briefly; but Lizzy could not be so eliminated. His entombed sonnets to her, resting under her golden hair in the grave, Gabriel knew mostly by heart. They rang hollowly next to his impassioned new verses to Janey. No wonder his nights were sleepless, and that Janey—too late—began a cautious retreat into the assumed safety of protestations of ill health. The meetings continued, and Rossetti's sensuous, if not sexual, worship of Janey during his days were recompense for his literally dreadful nights.

William understood the anxieties which pressed upon his brother, yet accepted the hysterical eye trouble Gabriel had begun complaining of as organic and his sleeplessness as related, although both brothers had sat through seances at which Gabriel probed his own disquietude in the way one returns to a throbbing tooth.

There was still the appearance of normality at Cheyne Walk. Gabriel was producing pictures and replicas at a record rate, although some seemed never to be near completion. For once he even found himself able to aid William, who was in financial difficulties, having had his money stolen from his luggage while vacationing in Verona. To Venice Gabriel sent his penniless brother £30.

In 1868 Gabriel spoke of being blind by Christmas, and hinted to William of an end to his troubles that suggested the example of Lizzy. "He talks of making a deed of gift of all his property to me; so that, whatever may befall himself, I may be empowered to do the best for all parties concerned." By "all parties" he meant Fanny and Janey, and William understood. Gabriel also talked of forbidding the "posthumous exhibiting of his collected works," and William tried to divert his brother from "these gloomy anticipations," as did two physicians, one of whom bought a *copy*—not the original—of the *Bocca Baciata* for 150 guineas. Gabriel promptly renamed it *La Bionda del Balcone*.

Rest, and distance from Chelsea, was the prescription. While Gabriel recuperated away from home, William finally extracted from Moxon, the publisher of the famed illustrated *Tennyson*, a contract to do an edition of Shelley's poetry with a prefatory life. It had long been his ambition to rehabilitate his literary hero, and the work on it helped create an atmosphere in which Gabriel not only offered his editorial assistance but furnished conjectural emendations which William diplomatically put aside out of a concern which he kept to himself that Gabriel's notoriety might cause the edition to "fall into disrepute." But his brother was, at least, now thinking in poetic channels, and in his journal for November 27, 1868, William noted that Gabriel, "being still, from the state of his eyes, unable to resume painting, has been looking up his poems of old days ["raveled rags of verse," he deprecated them to Allingham], with some floating idea of offering some of them to *The Fortnightly Review*, and at any rate with a degree of zest which looks promising for *some* result with them." Dunn continued executing replicas to pay Gabriel's bills, and in mid-December William noted that his brother had "just written a series of four sonnets—*Willow-wood*—about the finest thing he has done. I see the poetical impulse is upon him again."

The Morrises were about to revisit Cheyne Walk, so that Gabriel could resume his carefully choreographed courtship by straining his still-weak eyes at the recumbent figure of Janey. The Willow-wood poems and their successors recorded his mood. He hinted of long-divided love now freed, "alive from the abyss," and "the shades of those our days that had no tongue" were exorcised in a flood of ecstatic new poetry unleashed by the brooding, half-mystical sexuality of his best friend's wife. Only months later Christina wrote "An Echo from Willow-wood," using a line from her brother's poem as epigraph, and describing "hungering hearts" which knew the "bitterness" of "craving each for each," which although "one moment joined," would have to "vanish out of reach." William, much later, suggested in print that the reference was to Gabriel and Lizzy, then cryptically ventured that a "wholly different train of events" was in Christina's mind. Were they both alluding to Janey? William would protect his brother by such guarded comments even at the expense of private scoffing from his friends and public skepticism from his critics. The scaffold he would erect about Gabriel's reputation would inevitably enclose his own.

Although William had heretofore handled all of his brother's difficult errands, in September 1868 Gabriel returned from Scotland to complete arrangements for an event about which William knew nothing. Because their mother could have legally prevented the enterprise had she found out about it (Lizzy's burial plot was Mrs. Rossetti's property), Gabriel had kept his negotiations with the Home Secretary a secret. On an evening in early October, hoping to exorcise the ghost of Lizzy by publishing the poems he had buried with her—Gabriel had even thought her spirit had appeared to him in Scotland in the shape of a nearly tame finch—he sat with Kate Howell in Brixton while, by light of torches and a graveside bonfire, workmen spaded the soil from a coffin. Charles Howell stood by with a physician whose task it would be to dry and disinfect the manuscript book if it were salvageable. Howell lifted the lid as soon as it was clear, extricated the volume after making sure it was not the Bible also buried with her, and resealed the coffin.

With the deed done, Gabriel could write to William, explaining painfully on October 13—he could not bring himself to do it in person—that "no mistrust or unbrotherly feeling" was involved, but that

> the thing is done. All in the coffin was found quite perfect; but the book, though not in any way destroyed, is soaked through and through, and had to be still further saturated with disinfectants. It is now in the hands of the medical man who was associated with Howell in the disinterment, and who is carefully drying it leaf by

leaf. . . . It was a service I could not ask you to perform for me, nor do I know anyone except Howell who could well have been entrusted with such a trying task. . . . I have begged Howell to hold his tongue for the future, but if he does not I cannot help it. . . . I suppose the truth must ooze out in time. It is very desirable, as you will think with me, that our family should not know of it.

The devoted William replied as expected. "Under pressure of a great sorrow you performed an act of self-sacrifice: it did you honour, but . . . you have not retracted the sacrifice, for it has taken actual effect in your being bereaved of due poetic fame these seven and a half years past: but you now think—and I quite agree with you—that there is no reason why the self-sacrifice should have no term." To Swinburne, who had adored Lizzy, Gabriel acknowledged, "I have undergone so much mental disturbance about this matter." It told in many ways, from his persistent sleeplessness to a "constant shaking of the hand . . . with corresponding internal sensations." He had to convince himself further that he had done the right thing, and the renewed presence of Janey as he painted, and prepared new poems for the printer, was consolation. His letters to her took on a constant lover's plea, for she would sometimes withdraw herself on excuse of illness, and Gabriel no longer worried about caution. "To be with you . . . ," he wrote, "is absolutely the only happiness I can find or conceive in this world, dearest Janey; and when this cannot be, I can hardly now exert myself to move hand or foot for anything." Another letter between "sittings" emphasized that "places that are empty of you are empty of all life."

Well before the end of the year he was able to utilize the exhumed manuscript book, although (as Bell Scott, then back in London, wrote Alice Boyd), "It was so decayed through the *middle* parts of the pages that he has had to *copy it himself*. A queer sensation it must give him." Undoubtedly it did, for as Gabriel confided to William (in a letter its recipient drastically expurgated for the *Family Letters*) it also had "a dreadful smell—partly no doubt the disinfectants," and was in the handling an "unpleasant job."

The new *Poems*, Gabriel confided to William, would be dedicated to him because the other "possibility"—presumably Jane Morris—was "out of the question." The dedication would thus become a left-handed compliment to William, and William had not been spared that truth. Yet the strains on the relationship did not show, although Gabriel's renewed heartiness to visitors at Tudor House was often supported by brandy, and he soon began limiting his breakfasts to sherry. William later denied Gabriel's dependence on alcohol, except as his brother used whiskey—neat—to wash down the sleep-inducing chloral; but he had no idea of the extent of Gabriel's craving for palliatives to his burden of anxieties. Not all of Gabriel's concerns were communicated to William.

Before he left for Barbara Bodichon's farm at Scalands, Gabriel wanted William to dine with him to discuss strategies for insuring appropriate publicity for the new book. In particular he wanted to outmaneuver Robert Buchanan, a prolific (and mediocre) poet and reviewer whose tastes were conservative at best, and who seemed eager to settle old scores against what he called the Rossetti coterie. Years earlier, William had dismissed him as "a poor but pretentious poetaster." Buchanan had evened the score by denouncing William's *Shelley* in the *Athenaeum* that January, provoking Gabriel to refer to the journal in a letter to Swinburne as the "Arse-inaeum." He fancied, he told Ellis, elaborating on the metaphor, that Buchanan has "his natural organ of speech hitched up for an utterance," and hoped that it would be "a silent emanation" which would leave him "nothing but the smell to enjoy." But the bawdy wit belied Gabriel's concern.

Although William had publishing problems of his own in the late 1860s and early 1870s—his Moxon "Popular Poets" series had become a dry well, with six volumes issued and no payment—his real publishing problems arose from Gabriel's poems. The new (1870) edition was attacked on grounds of sensuality. As Robert Buchanan wrote, "Animalism is animalism, nevertheless, whether licensed or not; and, indeed, one might tolerate the language of lust more readily on the lips of a lover addressing a mistress than on the lips of a husband virtually (in these so-called "Nuptial" Sonnets) wheeling his nuptial couch out into the public streets."

It was no secret that his wife had been dead for ten years, and it was not claimed by Gabriel that all, or even most, of his published poems were written about, during, or prior to his luckless marriage. What nuptial couch, then, was he wheeling out into the streets of London? Did Janey's face and figure emerge too conspicuously in his poetry, despite the cosmetic alterations? Whatever his actual lifestyle, Gabriel had not acquired a public reputation for bohemianism, or worse, and in fact needed the respect of respectable people in order to elicit purchasers for his paintings. His way of life, he thought, was being threatened. Through the spring of 1872, according to William, "His fancies . . . ran away with him, and he thought that the pamphlet was a first symptom in a widespread conspiracy for crushing his fair fame and hounding him out of honest society."

As Gabriel would see criticism even in the most innocent writings, William would have to contend with Gabriel's paranoia as well as with the results of attempted antidotes—drugs and drink. In "Lewis Carroll's"

Hunting of the Snark, for example—despite Charles Dodgson's friendship of a decade's standing—Gabriel "found" a veiled personal attack. Toward the end of May his emotional state began alarming William, who nevertheless had other things on his mind and could not take wild talk of secret conspiracies seriously when Christina was "exceptionally low" and again confined to bed. Gabriel had to be left to his delusions. On Sunday, June 2, when William was again able to go to Chelsea, he found his brother so agitated that it was unsafe to leave. Bell Scott came by to help. The day should have been further improved by the arrival of a representative of the firm of Pilgeram and Lefevre, who was to pick up, and pay for, the just-completed *The Bower Meadow*, the background for which Gabriel had painted at Sevenoaks (as *The Meeting of Dante and Beatrice in the Garden of Eden*) twenty-two years before. Obsessed with treachery, he took the high price he was willingly paid—£735—as evidence that he was being cheated, and that night was racked with paranoia. The next day, "so far as office attendance allowed," William noted in his diary, he remained with Gabriel: "Scott, Dunn, F[anny] also about him: & in the evg. he & I went rd. to Brown's. Some table-turning the evg. rather earlier at Chelsea: the table moved very consider[abl]y, but not violently, & some messages came, purporting to be from Lizzie. Nothing very marked in these, unless one can so consider the answers that she is happy, & still loves G.—Initials for her young brother, H.S., given correctly. G. was, I fancy the only person at the table who knew of the 'H': I did not—or rather had wholly forgotten."

That Gabriel had to again "summon" Lizzy indicated the extent of his anxiety, and that "H"—the subject of her suicide note—was again alluded to, could only have reinforced a guilty conscience which had, at least since the exhumation, seemed dormant. On Wednesday June 5 the postman arrived at Cheyne Walk with a parcel. It was a presentation copy of Browning's new *Fifine at the Fair*, with a personal inscription: "To Dante Gabriel Rossetti from his old admirer and affectionate friend. R.B." "This is very handsome of Browning, very handsome!" he commented to Madox Brown, and rushed off an acknowledgment. "My dear Browning. Thanks once more for a new book bearing your name loved as of old. And even before I read it, let me say, Thanks. . . ."

Walking up and down in the studio after posting his letter, Gabriel began leafing through *Fifine*, first becoming startled, and then horrified, by what he began imagining as a sly undermining of his reputation. Since Gabriel's senses were at times confused by sleeplessness, whiskey, and chloral, Madox Brown assured him that no personal allusion was possible, but Gabriel's anger only increased, and he threw the offending book into the fire. Brown quickly rescued it, but Gabriel would not take it back.

As William remembered it, "My brother looked into the book: and to the astonishment of bystanders, he at once fastened on some lines at its close as being intended as an attack on him." Very likely he saw his "Jenny" and "The Blessed Damozel" lampooned, his guilty conscience about his dead wife ridiculed, and himself alluded to as a sensual seeker-out of lewd women. The Epilogue—which Rossetti may have glanced at first, if he thumbed the pages back-to-front, confronted him, in the ghost-haunted widower, with a mirror-image of himself:

> "What, and is it really you again?" Quoth I:
> "I again, what else did you expect?" quoth She.
>
> "Never mind, hie away from this old house—
> Every crumbling brick embrowned with sin and shame!
> Quick, in its corners ere certain shapes arouse!
> Let them—every devil of the night—lay claim,
> Make and mend, or rap and rend, for me! . . ."

Browning probably did have, at the least, "Jenny" in mind when he wrote *Fifine*, and was far less enthusiastic about Gabriel's "scented" poetry when apart from the poet than he was in person; but he could not have imagined the result, especially since two decades of widespread turning and rapping had left the Epilogue allusion a personal reference only to paranoiacs who fit the description.

From William, who "no doubt . . . knew more than we did," Bell Scott learned some details which he wrote to Alice Boyd. Browning, Gabriel was sure, "was his greatest enemy, determined to hunt him to death." In the process, he decided, the walls of Tudor House were "mined," as well as "perforated by spies," and everything he did and said "was known to the conspirators." While in the literary journals London critics confessed bafflement at *Fifine*, at an old brick house in Cheyne Walk where a rapping session had evoked a dead wife two nights before, one reader, at least, understood every obscure passage. Delusional conspiracies closed in darkly about Gabriel, and from Euston Square William hurried to Chelsea. That night, shaken, he closed his diary with the concern that it might be his last entry. "This diary work," he confided, "is becoming too painful now if important matters are to be recorded, & too futile & irritating if the unimportant are made to take their place. I shall therefore drop it. Perhaps a great change may have come over the face of things when—or if—I next resume it: or there will have been as Swinburne says, 'An end, an end, and end of all,' & no resumption of it."

Gabriel's paranoid delusions impelled his doctors, Thomas Marshall and

Thomas Hake, to send for an eminent specialist in nervous disorders, Henry Maudsley; but on his arrival at Cheyne Walk, Gabriel accused him of falsely posing as a doctor in order to further the conspiracy, and Maudsley hastily bowed out. Since Hake had been a literary friend, his words were more persuasive. He sent for a cab, urging Gabriel to go home with him to Roehampton. Again Gabriel argued about conspiracies, but when the cab came he agreed to climb into it with Madox Brown and William.

Darkness comes late on a London June evening, but it was already night when the cab arrived at Hake's house overlooking Richmond Park. It had been a harrowing journey. Gabriel kept insisting that a bell was being rung on the roof of the cab to annoy him, and he even berated the cabman, as they alighted at Hake's house, with "Why did you ring that bell?" The cabman looked blank. Gabriel's auditory delusions, present earlier in Cheyne Walk, would continue.

Gabriel may have taken his nightly dosage of chloral before going to bed, but if so it had no useful effect, for he lay awake and heard (he later told William) "a voice which twice called out at him a term of gross and unbearable obloquy." What voice, and what term, William would not repeat, but what followed may be the clue. Feeling unable to escape his persecutor, Gabriel "laid his hand upon a bottle of laudanum which, unknown to us all, he had brought with him, swallowed its contents, and dropped the empty bottle into a drawer."

No one awakened Gabriel on Sunday morning, June 8. He always slept late. When morning turned to afternoon, and Hake looked in and saw his guest sleeping with unusual placidity, he decided it was a turn for the better. Toward four o'clock he changed his mind. Gabriel's appearance seemed "no longer satisfying to a medical eye." William rushed out for a neighboring doctor to confirm Hake's worst fears, and the two physicians agreed that the cause was probably "an effusion of serum on the brain," and that Gabriel was "already past all hope." It was William's grim duty to inform his mother and sisters, to whom Hake extended the hospitality of his home. Accompanied by young George Hake, William went off to Euston Square, stopping first at Madox Brown's in Fitzroy Square, for his good friend was a combination of surrogate elder brother and father-figure. Refusing to consider the case hopeless, Brown rushed off to locate John Marshall, who had been Gabriel's doctor for years. William went on to Euston Square, seeking first his tough old aunt Eliza, who had an apartment in the house. Someone would have to take care of Christina, who was bedridden; and William also wanted assistance with him when he broke the news to his mother and Maria. Aunt Eliza, who had served in the Crimea with Florence Nightingale, was an indomitable and useful lady.

Long after dark Mrs. Rossetti and Maria arrived with William at Roehampton, followed closely by Brown and Marshall. Gabriel was still alive. Taking William aside, Hake produced the empty bottle he had found, clearly labeled "Laudanum—Poison."[5] Marshall ordered strong coffee force-fed to Gabriel as antidote, and directed that he be massaged to keep his circulation and respiration active, not leaving until he saw some signs of returning consciousness.

The next day Gabriel gradually revived. He was passive and despondent, and suffered from partial paralysis in one leg, from the hip down, brought on, Dr. Marshall suggested, "by his remaining so long in a recumbent position, under the benumbing influence of the laudanum." A colloquy of friends and relatives was necessary. Planning a funeral would have been easier than planning for Gabriel's convalescence. He could not be left in Cheyne Walk, with its attendant memories, and Marshall flatly rejected that possibility. The Rossettis felt unwilling to impose upon Hake any longer than necessary, but the other alternatives, including a private asylum, were few. "In my own house," William noted, "with Christina on a bed of sickness, perhaps of death, three other female inmates (not to speak of servants), and myself daily called away to a Government office, Gabriel would just then have caused the most wearying anxiety." The anxiety was felt most by William, who realized that if word got out of Gabriel's incapacity, or—worse yet—of his removal to an asylum, creditors would descend upon Cheyne Walk in hordes. His brother's finances at the best of times were chaotic and debt-burdened. Now everything might be seized, and sold at a fraction of its value, with Gabriel's further emotional collapse assured. Brown and Scott suggested moving all of Gabriel's pictures, finished or in progress, to Scott's house nearby. With Dunn's help the transfer was hurriedly accomplished, and the collection of rare blue china removed as well. Then the asylum plan fell through.

Despite William's entreaties, Gabriel insisted on returning to his own house. Realizing that he had lost control of the situation, William was perilously near breaking down himself. The responsibilities pressing upon him, with Christina possibly dying, and Gabriel worse than dead, were more than he could bear any longer. Seeing as much, Madox Brown proposed the experiment of taking charge of Gabriel himself at Cheyne Walk. Gratefully, William agreed, and leaning on a stick, Gabriel hobbled to a cab and went off with Brown to a house stripped of all his working canvases. Sunk in depression, William went home. He had not consciously

---

[5] Mrs. Rossetti and her daughters were never told of the laudanum, nor that the illness was the aftermath of a suicide attempt. "They finished their days," according to William, "in ignorance of the facts."

balked at helping Gabriel yet again, but body and spirit had faltered. There was often more loyalty than exhilaration in being Gabriel's lieutenant.

Passive and despondent, and still subject to delusions, Gabriel seemed not to notice that his occupation was gone. William was kept away by Brown with assurances that there was "improvement" and "the most perfect quiet & reasonable behaviour," and that a joint checking account was being set up so that William could handle Gabriel's finances. All the principals, Fredeman (1970-1971) wrote in his exhaustive chronicle of the summer of 1872,[6] seemed "determined to send optimistic reports to William," whom Scott described to Alice on June 14 as "getting into a more composed state," and no longer looking upon his responsibilities as "overwhelming."

Acting for William, who had finally returned to daily business at the Excise Office, Brown made arrangements to sell Gabriel's china and to settle the matter of what to do with the Cheyne Walk servants. He also opened all of Gabriel's mail, and found an offer from William Graham of one of his country places in Scotland. Arrangements were made quickly. George Hake, then between terms at Oxford, would stay with Gabriel, and he, Brown, and Gabriel's manservant Allan, left for Urrard House, Perthshire on June 20. There Gabriel turned to matters of immediate concern, as the walls at Urrard House could not be expected to conceal conspirators. To his mother went a letter assuring her that the only one in the party not in the best of health was Allan, who had not yet adjusted to Scotland; and to William went two letters, one asking him to secure in his name the furniture and goods in Fanny's house at 36 Royal Avenue, to put off prying creditors, and the other a formal one in which he consigned all the goods in Fanny's house to William in payment for loans made over the years, and asked that an appropriate legal stamp be affixed to the document. If technically William's property, Gabriel's assets could not be seized. Loyal to Fanny, although he seldom if ever now utilized her sexual services, he wanted her taken care of. William hardly needed that worry.

Reports on Gabriel's condition went largely to Madox Brown, who wrote Scott on July 6 that he and Hake "did quite right not to send your letters to William [as] he is not in a state to bear them." At least one other agony was spared William as Christina, able again to travel, went with her mother to Glottenham in Sussex, where, languid and listless, she wrote William of her hope to return in September "to keep house with you, as in old days, in much harmony."

---

[6] Fredeman quotes from or refers to 206 letters and other documents relevant to the months of Rossetti's breakdown and recuperation.

However depressed by his family's circumstances, William had its business to attend to. "Not a day passes," he wrote Scott, still then at Stobhall, "—& sometimes not an hour or two consecutively—without my being called off to write some letter, run some errand, receive some visit, offer some information . . . regarding Gabriel or his affairs, so that the pull upon my working faculties & my spirits continues not small. . . ." Having his brother in a remote place in Scotland made matters worse, for diagnoses of his condition were made by nonmedical companions to physicians hundreds of miles removed from the scene, and the remedies suggested applied the same way. Added to Gabriel's discomforts was the swelling of his chronic hydrocele, which made sitting uncomfortable but at least stimulated his desire to walk. Dr. Hake thought the hydrocele "a useful reality among his fancies," but in the end it was relieved by a local doctor. Still, Scotland had proven no solution to the basic problem, and William was not being consulted. Brown wrote to Scott that William was "rather more composed but by no means fit to hear discouraging reports as yet."

Sending his accounts to William on August 11, George Hake emphasized the progress that had been made, but did not suggest that William visit. The brothers had not seen each other for nearly two months, but William had earlier noted that he could not leave Somerset House for any extended period during August and September. He had been referring to the possibility of his being needed to accompany Gabriel abroad, and it was the excuse to keep him away altogether until it was certain that his own emotional state was sound. Perhaps the least of William's anxieties was that sooner or later his brother would demand to see Jane Morris, and the Pandora's box of problems would reopen. Several letters had arrived from Janey earlier, asking for information about Gabriel and even hinting that she might be in Scotland and could visit. None of the inquiries were mentioned to Gabriel. The subject came up, finally, from Gabriel himself on August 12. First he announced that he felt prepared, henceforth, to open his own mail. Then he wrote a long letter to Janey, the effort—or the contents—upsetting him sufficiently to disturb his sleep. "On waking this morning," Dr. Hake wrote to William, his brother "spoke unpleasantly about the conspiracy for the first time this fortnight."

Hake was in a quandary about how to handle the letter to Mrs. Morris. Finally he decided that it had to be mailed, but sent at the same time his own tactful letter to Janey, with a copy to William:

> As a medical man, and viewing you and Mr. Morris as among Rossetti's dearest friends, an anxiety arises in my mind to learn whether his letter exhibits any sign of delusion. If so it must be inferred that there are still remains of his disorder; if happily it does

not, a more favourable view may be entertained—for there is a certain wilfulness about our dear friend in his present state which may even make him say certain things for the sake of consistency partly, and in part to attain some indulgence as to whisky &c, when it is advisable to oppose him—

May I further take the liberty of asking you to be very guarded in your reply to him—telling him only amusing and cheering facts, not noticing in the slightest degree his delusion if he has manifested any to you—

I am sure you will appreciate my motive in thus writing. . . .

To William, Mrs. Morris responded that Gabriel's letter "showed no sign of his late distressing illness," and to Hake she reported the same thing, the discreet doctor writing to William that he burned the letter "together with all yours and all other letters on the subject of this illness." Since Gabriel was beginning again to direct his own affairs, Hake was already making cautious plans to withdraw, his confidence bolstered by Gabriel's writing to Treffry Dunn for painting supplies, and renewing correspondence with William and Christina. He suggested his own release from captivity—that it would be useful for Gabriel's rehabilitation "to have an exchange of prisoners by substituting Dunn for me. . . ."

Dunn's leaving Cheyne Walk for Scotland first alarmed Gabriel. It meant abandoning the house to the servants. He wrote Fanny to lock the studio and keep the key. He was also sufficiently worried about "poor Fanny" to ask William to look in on her and to have her call at Somerset House if he had no objection. (The picture it raises, of the florid, buxom Fanny calling, in her best cockney, upon the staid, gray-bearded Assistant Secretary, defies description.) Now that he was somewhat improved, Gabriel thought better of William's zeal in paying off the most pressing creditors with funds realized by the sale of the Cheyne Walk china and some of the pictures, and in cutting costs by disposing of the garden menagerie. With the implied reproof came instructions to "pay away as little as possible"—that it was not necessary "to have made payments at midsummer to those who received good instalments at Xmas. . . ." The old Gabriel was indeed reviving.

To his mother on September 12 he wrote that the interruption to his work had been "a heavy evil," and that it remained to be seen whether he could resume it. But he was already planning to do his painting at Kelmscott, where he had lived the happiest months of his life. Once the good Dr. Hake had left, Gabriel found no compensations for the remoteness, and with the replica delivered to Graham, he was ready to leave. Rejecting William's offer to provide companionship at Kelmscott he wrote that what he needed most of all was to be left to himself. "Wherever I can be at peace," he wrote, "there I shall assuredly work. But all, I now find by experience, depends primarily on my not being deprived of the society of the one necessary person."[7] He was aware of his "somewhat morbid state of mind," and was still limited by his lameness, but late in September, accompanied by George Hake, he boarded a third-class carriage for London, en route to "the one necessary person."

Gabriel celebrated what would be nearly two years at Kelmscott in his sonnets. It was one of the most curious of idylls, in that Gabriel's partner in felicity was—and remained—the beautiful wife of the man who had once been his best friend, and who now abandoned the country house he loved to let someone else usurp his marriage. Left alone in Kelmscott at the close of the secluded summer of 1871 the year before, Gabriel had written a sonnet describing his desolation with intense physical imagery:

> What of her glass without her? The blank grey
>   There where the pool is blind of the moon's face.
> Her dress without her? The tossed empty space
> Of cloud-rack whence the moon has passed away.
> Her paths without her? Day's appointed sway
>   Usurped by desolate night. Her pillowed place
> Without her? . . .

"I cannot tell you," Rossetti explained to Hall Caine ten years later, in a voice choked with sobs, "at what terrible moment it was wrung from me."

Reunited with Janey four hours after he had left London, Gabriel counted his blessings. "Here all is happiness again," he wrote William the next day, "and I feel completely myself. I know well how much you must have suffered on my account, indeed, perhaps your suffering may have been more acute than my own dull, nerveless state during the past months. Your love, dear William, is not less returned by me than it is sweet to me, and that is saying all."

He began a new, brooding *Proserpine* with Janey, had his brother for a visit in October, William sleeping in Morris's vacated bedroom, and—when Janey was to be away—invited his mother and sisters, explaining that another visiting model was likely to be about, but that Miss Wilding was "quite ladylike." After a silence of nearly five months, on his return from Kelmscott William noted in his journal for November 3,

---

[7] When William published Gabriel's letter he discreetly omitted the second sentence.

1872, "I resume this diary under much less gloomy circumstances than when I left it off, altho' all causes of distress & anxiety are by no means removed. . . ." William had found his brother "in very good trim, although occasionally something showed in his mind some trace of lurking suspicion. . . ."

At Kelmscott, with George Hake remaining with him as factotum, Gabriel felt removed from conspiracies against his reputation, yet his living there at all while Morris conducted The Firm at Queen Square was enough to set tongues in London wagging. To Aglaia Coronio, Morris, in a stream of letters, poured out his bitterness at being kept from his "harbour of refuge." Rossetti's presence at Kelmscott, he complained, was "quite selfish business," and "a kind of slur on it: this is very reasonable though when one thinks why one took the place, and how this year it has really answered that purpose [of Gabriel's]." His meeting Gabriel when necessary had become "really a farce," but Janey was back again: "Her company is always pleasant and she is very kind and good to me." Like Proserpine, Mrs. Morris at intervals returned to her husband.

William was ready for a vacation, and receptive to Bell Scott's invitation to join him, his wife Letitia, and Alice Boyd on a trip to Italy. But rather than become the chaperone for his friend's *ménage à trois* William invited Lucy Madox Brown to join the party, using the Scott threesome for purposes of decorum. "Old Scotus seems quite sulky about it," Gabriel told William, adding that he did not want the remark to get back to Scott. But William was determined to have her along. "For several years . . . I had had a warmly affectionate feeling for Lucy Brown," he wrote in his memoirs. "She was the mainstay of her father's house; I always saw her [as] sweet, gentle, and sensible; she had developed ability of no common order as a painter." Also, like William, she was freethinking in religion; and she was far more attractive than one might have expected of a woman of twenty-nine who had yet to elicit an offer of marriage.

During their travels in Italy, William wrote later, "I decided that I would not again part with Lucy, if I could help. I proposed marriage to her, and was accepted." At their ages—William was forty-three—they had no need to consult their parents, but in any case secured the cordial approval of Mrs. Rossetti and Madox Brown. He had told Lucy from the moment that they began considering marriage, William assured his mother, that he would continue living with her and his sisters, and that his wife would have to accommodate herself to that arrangement. But as a modest gesture in the direction of Lucy's need for a room of her own, William offered her "one room or other" to be turned into her studio. It seemed—to him—an adequate compromise. It would not last. They would soon have their own home.

William and Lucy were married on the last day of March 1874, minus a church ceremony and with a minimum of guests. Gabriel predicated his attendance on "a few real intimates," since after two years' absence from the social gatherings he used to love, and often staged himself, he confessed, "I am not equal to it, now that solitude is the habit of my life." At the wedding breakfast were, other than William and Lucy, only old Mrs. Rossetti, Christina, Gabriel, the Madox Browns, and the Morrises.

Late in 1876 Maria, by then an Anglican nun, died of cancer, the first of the four Rossettis in birth and in death. But William's augmented family had been shattered by an earlier death, that of Lucy's nineteen-year-old half-brother Oliver, a year earlier. The two months' nursing of Nolly left Lucy exhausted, and Gabriel, who had worried earlier about Lucy's susceptibility to "colds and such-like," confided to Dr. Hake what he could not have told William—that her health seemed to him "destined to be a permanent cause of anxiety." After the marriage he began, as a wedding gift, a portrait of her in which she appeared in the full bloom of health, but it was completed before Nolly's illness and death. In its full-lipped exaggeration, William conceded, it hewed "somewhat too much to the known [late] Rossettian type to be an absolute likeness." A more accurate likeness, he thought, was done two years later by Madox Brown, showing Lucy and her first-born daughter, Olivia. Named for Nolly Brown, she was born on September 20, 1875, and to the anguish of the elder Rossettis at Euston Square she was not baptized.

In February 1877, William's second child, named Gabriel Arthur Madox Rossetti, was born. Again Lucy used a borrowed cradle, William writing Anne Gilchrist some months later, "I religiously hope . . . there will not be a[nother] new baby to put into it. Our two children are a great pleasure and interest to us both: but at my present age, 48, & with income dependent on my continuing to be alive in this world, we both think two of them enough, if only Destiny will so permit." Despite such pious organizations as the British Union for the Discouragement of Vicious Advertising, antidotes to Destiny were available in many forms; but William and Lucy would have three more children, including twins. The cradle would continue to be rocked.

In the mid-1870s Gabriel was restricting his walks to a narrower and narrower compass, because he assumed paranoiacally that anyone else who happened to be in the street was scrutinizing him. As William later described his brother's agoraphobic strategy, defending him from stories of pathological reclusiveness while indirectly corroborating them, Gabriel "did not go to and fro in the streets, in a casual sort of way, to any extent worth mentioning; but he went out constantly—I believe only occasionally missing a day—in the late evening. His habit was to enter a fly from his own door with George Hake, and drive to some airy spot, very often the Circles of Regent's Park. There he got out, took a longish walk with this companion, and then reentered the fly, and drove home. I am far from saying that this was a wholly rational proceeding, or that it did not bespeak a certain exaggerated craving for seclusion; but it is a very different thing from [Bell Scott's allegation of] 'living within the house, and never going even into the street.' " In Cheyne Walk it was the life as before, although Gabriel assured his friends, not without hints of annoyance, that he was taking only a third of the quantity of chloral he had needed before his most recent calamity. Less would be useless, he told Brown testily. "Any man in my case must either do as I do, or cease from necessary occupation. . . ." Still, his ability to paint unflaggingly was itself a restorative, and he declared that he was not dead yet. He even advised Lucy Rossetti on her painting, suggesting to her a way to lay on a white ground "more crisply and brightly," and even sending her a tube of his favorite paint. Lucy until her marriage had considered herself a professional painter, but since had been hampered by ill health and child rearing (her third child, Helen Maria Rossetti, was born in November 1879). Gabriel's willingness to interest himself in her work was another sign of his restored equilibrium.

For William these were years of disappointment. He conceded himself as trapped in the Inland Revenue, and found new solace in the work he had been doing since 1874 as art critic for the *Academy*. As a young man he had brought zest to his criticism because it had been possible "to strike a stroke or two for the 'Praeraphaelite' painters in the days when they were ringed round with foes, and to carry the battle into the enemy's camp." But nearly twenty-five years later, even though he had accepted the assignment, "it was stale to me, and to a great extent monotonous, and moreover it often diverted me at inconvenient moments from my regular work at Somerset House. I had to run out to an exhibition when I had more than enough employ at my office-desk." In an unguarded moment he had said as much to Charles Appleton, the *Academy* proprietor, and had quickly added the equally hazardous comment that "as I was now a family-man, and not justified in throwing up any source of regular income, I was fully minded to continue my function as art-critic." Appleton bided his time, but one evening in 1878 William received a message from him that the duties of art critic had been transferred, effective immediately, to a young journalist, James Comyns Carr. William was shocked, but was able to keep his hand in artistic and literary matters by using Gabriel's lawyer-friend Theodore Watts as intermediary with Norman MacColl, editor of the *Athenaeum*. Soon William was reviewing books there occasionally.

To Lucy, Gabriel once confessed, "I must seem as bad an uncle as the one in the *Children in the Wood* almost," and William recalled that Gabriel's almost complete seclusion self-limited him after 1877 to rare visits to his family. "He saw our eldest child Olivia twice or thrice in her earliest infancy; the other four he never saw at all. And yet he took an interest in all of them, and was pleased to hear any little details of how they were going on. This was assuredly a rather curious state of things, as affecting two brothers who had always been and always continued to be extremely fond of one another." But there was one day in 1880 William did not recall (perhaps he was never told of it) when Lucy decided on her own to take her children, including Gabriel's young namesake, to Cheyne Walk to brighten her brother-in-law's day with their high spirits. From the poet as he sat in the studio in his shabby painting coat there was a reluctant, momentary effort at welcome, and the elder children responded dutifully. After that he ignored them, and unaware of any snub they romped happily up and down the stairs and through the corridors until their mother took them home. Gabriel never saw his nieces and nephews again.

For William alone, Gabriel was always at home. Among other things, to his brother he was eager to talk of his renewed interest in spiritualism, although without any further desire to experiment with it himself, and of his conviction, after years of skepticism, in the immortality of the soul. He needed William to share such confidences. With the handful of intimates not always available, one pathetic appeal to William (who had just visited) was, "I am so low and lonely that it would be a great boon if you could come up for an hour or two this evening. I know it is a tax on you, but tell Lucy, with my love, that I hope she will not mind." Very likely William followed soon behind the servant who brought the note.

Gabriel continued to rely on his small band of friends, who, usually by arrangement, came at least one each evening, William taking the Monday evenings, staying to dinner and often overnight. Shields added the enthusiasm the increasingly careworn William lacked, and Watts supplied efficiency and vigor. His wig looking increasingly too large for his face as age shrunk him, the tall, dour Bell Scott still made regular calls, but Madox Brown, dignified in old age by a long white beard, lived now in Manchester, where he was painting frescoes for the town hall, and could only look in when in London.

Isolation had its compensations, for in solitude Gabriel plodded on with both pictures and poems, reading new lines to his visitors and unveiling the evidence that his painter's hand had not lost its cunning. But as he wrote to Christina early in 1881, "With me, Sonnets mean Insomnia." Whatever the restless agonies of his nights, he still managed, most days, some brushstrokes worthy of his better years, and his friends usually found him genial in the evening, coiled on a sofa and ready to talk spell-bindingly about writers and writing, or to declaim, from memory, long stretches of poetry in a voice as deep and rich as ever. But at Christmas 1880 his health was again undermined by the toxic effect of the chloral he craved, and he was too ill to visit his mother, now lodged at Torrington Square. The weather was too foul for her, despite a long sealskin coat, to travel instead to Cheyne Walk; but William and Lucy, sensing his need, left their children long enough to see that Gabriel was not alone on the day that meant much to him.

On his visiting evenings after Somerset House, William had begun con-fiding to Gabriel his unsuppressed desire to write poetry, although he knew he did not have the creative powers of his brother and sister. The traditional sources of inspiration, Gabriel knew, had not moved William to verse, and he suggested instead a Whitmanesque series of "Democratic Sonnets," which would give his brother an opportunity to versify the political events of his own lifetime. The idea intrigued William, for in better days he had argued happily for hours with Swinburne on such subjects, and although Gabriel for years had put Swinburne off, William had kept up their friendship and often came to the poet's aid. Nearly dead from drink in 1879, Swinburne had been rescued by the indefatigable Watts, who cared for him at Watts's pretentiously named "The Pines" in Putney and limited him to a daily glass of ale. Swinburne had become very deaf, making exchange of conversation difficult, but his letters to William were filled with the old political fire, including an unceasing regicidal fervor, and may have pushed William's sonneteering into more radical channels.

More businesslike than inspired, William had mulled over Gabriel's idea and decided that a hundred sonnets were "a proper number; fewer than this would not make a batch producible as a small volume." From January 28 to February 8, 1881, when he was away lecturing in Newcastle and Glasgow, William produced at least a sonnet a day, sending one on Garibaldi to Gabriel. "I rejoice to see so fine a sonnet," he wrote William, "and shall await the others with great interest. You may be the family bard yet." Encouraged, William sent more, on Mazzini, the Corn Laws, the French Republic, and Louis-Philippe, and Gabriel expressed concern that William was "doing them rather fast." A veteran of childhood *boutes-rimés* competitions with Christina as well as Gabriel, William could turn out lines that scanned properly whether or not they were poetic in feeling, and as someone who lived a systematic life he had begun by making a chronological list of a hundred subjects for sonnets and crossed out the subjects he had versified. Gabriel criticized each one he received, recommending changes, and on March 6, after William's forty-fifth sonnet, warned Lucy, "I should think that [absence from work with a] sore throat must have resulted in two sonnets instead of one daily on William's part. I hope the ailment does not make his political poetics quite inexorable."

After seeing sonnets titled "The Red Flag," "The Commune," "The Red Shirt," and "John Brown," Gabriel was roused to protest, feeling, like Dr. Frankenstein, that he had created a monster beyond his power to control. The family might be embarrassed by the radical slant of the sonnets. Gabriel, shut inexorably into his reclusiveness, worried about unwanted attention called to himself, that his own forthcoming *Ballads and Sonnets* could be hurt. William's government job might itself be put in jeopardy. Pressing the latter motive, Gabriel decided to confront William indirectly, through Lucy. On April 12, 1881 he wrote her:

> Several of William's truest friends, no less than myself are greatly alarmed at the tone taken in some of his Sonnets respecting 'Tyrannicide,' Fenianism, and other incendiary subjects. It seems to me and to others that the consequences are absolutely and very perilously uncertain when an official (as William is) of a monarchial government allows himself such unbridled license of public speech. . . . The least evil I should apprehend, were William to persist in including such subjects, would be the certainty of his never attaining the final step of the Secretaryship in his office which he so well deserves. But very much worse consequences than this seem to all of us but too likely; and my object in writing this letter is to awaken your mind to the clear possibility of absolute ruin, in such a case, for my dear brother, and his family whom he loves so well. The very title, Democratic Sonnets, seems to me most objectionable when coming from one who depends on the Government for his bread. . . .
>
> It is extremely painful to me to trouble you on this subject, while in your present delicate state;[8] but I really can keep silence no longer, the series being so far advanced; also I do not venture to speak to William direct, lest his first impulse should be to resent

---

[8] Lucy was in her final month of pregnancy. The twins Michael Ford and Mary Elizabeth were born on April 22.

it as an encroachment, and so frustrate all attempts to avert what
I and others view as a great danger. . . .

The same day, thinking better of his approach through Lucy, Gabriel
wrote "a short propitiatory note" (as he described it to his mother) to
William, in which he explained what he had done, ascribing his reaction
to "the absolute call of brotherly love," and hoping that it would cause
"no kind of division" between them.

For the "brotherly letters," William sent his thanks, while tactfully
upbraiding Gabriel for any anxiety he may have caused Lucy. Then he
set out his own position. As a government official he was "prepared to
encounter criticism" and to "brush [it] aside with equanimity." He realized, too, that if he were in line for the Secretaryship at what was by
then the Inland Revenue Office of the Treasury, his published radical
opinions might be held against him, but he regarded his chances of succession as "not a little" dubious. Beyond that, he thought, there was little
cause for alarm. Democracy coexisted with monarchy in England, and
freedom of expression was his right. Although he was "not wedded" to
his title, he saw none better and he intended to be his own man:

> Any idea of my undertaking to write verse about the public events
> of my own time, & yet failing to show that I sympathize with foreign
> republics, & detest oppression, retrogression, & obscurantism,
> whether abroad or at home, must be nugatory. To set me going is
> to set me going on my own path. . . .
> As you evidently don't agree with the tone of the sonnets, I shall
> drop my idea of dedicating them to you—unless you revive the
> proposal; & shall abstain from reading [to] you new items of the
> series, if you don't ask for them. . . .

Rejecting Gabriel's concern about the subversive nature of his verses,
he nevertheless accepted his "affectionate solicitude," and there was no
acrimony. Gabriel even offered to continue to read and criticize any new
sonnets, while insisting that it had been his duty to warn William of the
implications of the project. "Of course," he added, "much as I should
prize the dedication to me of a work of yours, I think now that I will ask
you for some other than this one." William persevered with his project
into the autumn, completing seventy-two of his hundred. "Some of them,"
he thought later, "which I wrote with real interest for the subject, and
an inclination to have my say about it, show a sufficient measure of force
and ardour, both in thought and in diction—somewhat less in poetic
accomplishment. Several others, which I produced merely as being ger-

mane in theme to the series, are the reverse of good. This therefore was my essential reason for leaving off."

Long afterward they were published, with a dedicatory sonnet "To the Memory of Dante Gabriel Rossetti." By then the radicalism had little but historical interest; but even so "The Red Flag," "Chartism," and "Tyrannicide"—to which Gabriel had particularly objected in 1881—were excluded.

Part of Gabriel's apprehension had concerned the possible impact of William's verse upon press reaction to his own new volume of verse, which, through the spring, he was preparing. *Ballads and Sonnets* would contain forty-seven sonnets written since the 1870 collection, which nearly doubled the group constituting *The House of Life*, and narrative poems he labeled as ballads. Asked to go through the proofs, William made voluminous notes on his objections and recommendations, Gabriel acknowledging on May 20, "I read all your notes with interest and some with advantage." Translated, it meant that he incorporated some of the suggestions, and rejected others.

To William's relief, Gabriel had begun the 1880s with a live-in secretary-companion-disciple, young Hall Caine, but his recuperative powers were not what they once were. Late in 1881 he confessed to being "very ill," and his few letters suggested little desire to hang on to an existence where his only pleasure was the nightly blotting of consciousness. The "calm presence of William" helped, but he could see few of his old friends who wanted to congratulate him on his new book as a way of seeing him for perhaps a last time. He brooded over his imminent inability to provide even for himself, and William assured him that his brother's home would always be his own. A nurse, Mrs. Abrey, was called in to oversee his needs, and as the obvious signs around him gathered he surprised his rationalist brother by asking to see a priest for confession and absolution.

Canon Burrows called at Christina's suggestion, but Gabriel insisted to Bell Scott, "I can make nothing of Christianity, but I only want a confessor to give me absolution for my sins." None was sent for. Gabriel spent most of his days prostrate on a sofa, where with friends around on Sunday, December 11, he suddenly exclaimed that his left side felt paralyzed. Hall Caine and Westland Marston carried him to bed and summoned Dr. Marshall, who placed a newly qualified young doctor in the house and tried to wean Gabriel from chloral by substituting morphine and diluted chloral; a week later the chloral was stopped altogether, and only a token amount of whiskey permitted. By Christmas 1881 the paralysis was restricted to Gabriel's left hand and arm, but he was too ill for visitors, and only William left his Christmas dinner to come to Cheyne Walk. Late in January 1882, Gabriel's old friend, the architect John Seddon, offered a cottage near Margate to remove the patient from the gloom of Tudor House, and despite Gabriel's vow never to leave London again, uttered only two months earlier, he left via Victoria Station for Birchington-on-Sea on February 4, with only Mrs. Abrey, Caine, and Caine's twelve-year-old sister Lily as companions.

Birchington was dreary, even stormy, with brief intervals of sunshine. Too feeble to walk about outdoors much, he lounged about in his old, nearly threadbare painting coat, paid tender attentions to Lily, and complained of cold and discomfort, often removing a black glove he now wore on his partially paralyzed hand to warm it at the fire. His easel had been set up to continue work, but he could apply himself barely long enough to set up brushes and paints, and looked forward instead to visitors. Because of Gabriel's shifting moods, William saw a new crankiness in one of his brother's letters, and Christina, who had to deal with him far less, replied, "It is trying to have to do with him at times, but what must it be TO BE himself?"

For William it was difficult to keep his mind on the bureaucratic routine at Somerset House, since by almost every post came news of Gabriel's further deterioration. One letter, at least, was unexpected. He was invited to act as the junior examiner for Italian literature and language for a scholarship in the Taylorian Institute at Oxford. The academic distinction felt good to a bald graybeard who had left school at fifteen to become a clerk. William accepted.

At a time when Gabriel was nearly past caring, plaudits were becoming commonplace. Laudatory articles about him were appearing in journals formerly hostile, or even vicious, and twelve thousand copies of *Ballads and Sonnets* had been sold within a month of publication. Even the cranky Buchanan—perhaps looking for publicity—had dedicated his newest book to "An Old Enemy," with apologetic verses in which he confessed having wronged "an honoured head," and now offered "peace and charity." Visiting Gabriel just before the retreat to Birchington, William had seen Buchanan's bathetic apology, and observed that it was "a handsome retraction of past invidious attacks." Gabriel was more cynical. Twenty years later, Buchanan died, and the *Morning Leader* inquired whether William would write an obituary notice, assuming that he would have nursed his brother's grievance through the intervening years and might now be expected to affix an eye-catching diatribe onto Buchanan's grave. William declined. It was not his style.

Free from chloral in the raw, final weeks of winter, Gabriel's mind was clear but his body ravaged. He surrendered to pain by taking to his bed, remaining chatty and animated when friends called, but giving in to depression about his condition when Christina arrived with her mother. To William on March 24, Christina reported that Gabriel was "going back apparently rather than going forward, and is so comfortless and sinking and so wasted away that at last this morning I urged him to see a local Dr. . . ." Diplomatically, Dr. Harris concluded that Gabriel's state was "*not* irremediable," but it was. On April 5 Christina delivered to William his revised opinion, that Gabriel's kidneys were seriously diseased. Nephritis had been almost inevitable once his liver and kidneys had finally been overwhelmed by chloral abuse, and the uremia was irreversible. William had traveled to Birchington the previous weekend, finding Gabriel "barely capable of tottering a few steps, half-blind and suffering a great deal of pain," but he was rational and had even managed to dictate two weak sonnets to Caine, who dutifully set them down. William planned to return the following weekend, which would begin with Good Friday, but he was recalled a day early by telegram.

Although drowsy most of the time, Gabriel was able to make his will with the assistance of Watts, a necessary precaution as William realized that the testament still in force left everything to Lizzy, and that her brothers might be the beneficiaries. She had urged Gabriel with her dying words to take care of Harry Siddal, and had he died before making a new will that object might have been achieved with a vengeance. The residue of the estate after payment of debts and testamentary gifts and expenses was to be divided equally between Mrs. Rossetti and William, while William was declared sole executor. Following that, Gabriel's desire to live failed altogether. He permitted the rector of Birchington, who had been denied admittance weeks before, to see him and pray at his bedside with Watts and Mrs. Rossetti. Throughout the night as Saturday passed into Easter Sunday, April 9, Christina and Mrs. Abrey kept vigil beside the barely conscious figure, and twice during the day, in a calm voice much clearer than his usual indistinct speech, Gabriel said, "I believe I shall die tonight. Yesterday I wished to die, but today I must confess that I do not." Although a rigid unbeliever, William, perhaps thinking about staging a dignified end, tried to read to his brother sections of Ecclesiastes. Gabriel objected. That evening, as preparations were being made for another night of waiting for the end, Gabriel cried out twice, writhed convulsively, and then lay still. It was 9:31 P.M.

Although William recorded in his diary late on Easter Sunday, 1882, that "the pride and glory of our family" had died, that was all the time he had for sentiment. He had to try to keep the death secret long enough to permit the last check Gabriel signed—for £300—to be cashed, so that local funeral expenses could be met, and so that creditors, and Fanny, could be held off. Watts was to delay the obituary notice in the *Athenaeum* until the day of the funeral, and William wrote to his wife's brother-in-law, Franz Hueffer, *The Times'* music critic, to postpone the appearance of a death notice. In tiny Birchington the news was too big to be suppressed, and it leaked quickly to London. Then Fanny read the death notice in *The Times*, and rushed a letter to William, who prevented her mourning in person by not replying until it was too late. "Your letter of the 12th only reached me this morning about 9," he wrote coldly on the day of the funeral. "The coffin had been closed last evening, and the funeral takes place early this afternoon—there is nothing further to be done."

The burial took place on Friday afternoon, April 14, at Birchington churchyard. The *Standard* reported the next day that a "public funeral at Highgate, where the wife and father of the deceased are interred," had been thought of, "but for family reasons . . . was abandoned." It had never been a possibility, Gabriel fearing to the end the posthumous wrath of Lizzy.

Despite the secluded burial spot, interest in Gabriel's death was intense, and *The Times* marveled that a painter who almost never exhibited his work, and avoided press publicity to an extent unprecedented in the modern history of art, "should on this principle have achieved a reputation scarcely inferior to that of the most popular favourites of the day."

William had little time to dwell upon such effusions. After hours at Somerset House he had the business of settling his brother's chaotic and debt-ridden estate. He employed Dunn at a pound a day (for nearly four months) to make watercolor sketches of the familiar rooms in Cheyne Walk before everything was inventoried and dispersed (and to complete some of Gabriel's unfinished replicas), invited the friends and relatives named in Gabriel's will to choose as directed from drawings and books and personal effects, and began fending off claims against the estate, one of the earliest of them a bill for £52 from a pharmacy in New Bond Street for chloral Gabriel had furtively acquired in addition to his open purchases from another firm.

Bargaining adroitly, William privately sold what he could from Gabriel's effects before a two-day auction was held at Cheyne Walk on July 5 and July 6. According to the Liverpool *Mercury* the attendance was "enormous," while in London the *World* carped that the sale of Gabriel's belongings "must be considered a high festival of the relic *cultus*. One understands the interest attached to the easel of a distinguished painter, or the writing-table of an eminent poet; but an ordinary-minded person finds it difficult to understand an enthusiasm which runs up window-curtains and occasional chairs to four times their value." William may have been especially pleased that four unbound issues of *The Germ* went for six guineas, and that the Blake sketchbook for which he had "lent" Gabriel ten shillings, was sold for one hundred and five guineas. The sale raised nearly £3,000. Although William thought that the amount was about equal to Gabriel's debts, and that the sale of Gabriel's own paintings would bring in a handsome inheritance, there were many more debts still to be claimed, especially those resulting from undelivered commissions for which advances had been paid. Still, prospects appeared good that Gabriel's estate could cover its obligations.

William was now deep into the business of guarding and enhancing his brother's reputation. Watts called often at Somerset House, where William now freely conducted his family's business as well as the Queen's, and proposed a memoir, which William agreed would have more credibility coming from a non-relative. He began to collect Gabriel's letters to his family to fill out the volume, Christina copying out for her mother those passages their "monitory blue pencil" left as fit for print, rather than furnishing William the originals. Even before the family was at work there was another memoirist in the field, Hall Caine, who wanted to do a book of his recollections and Gabriel's long letters to him. The proofs William and Watts read were largely innocuous. Caine, however, claimed more intimacy than his few months with Gabriel suggested was possible, put the story of the exhumation of the poems into print, and quoted voluminously from Gabriel's purported conversations with him. Reluctantly, Caine insisted on revealing the exhumation, rebutting William's plea: "I should be grieved to give pain to your mother, but my first duty is to truth as I know it." By mid-autumn the book was out, and Christina pronounced it "neither unkind nor unfriendly," understanding "the circumstances under which his experiences occurred."

Handling Gabriel's posthumous business required hard bargaining by William, especially with Fanny, who had acquired letters, drawings, and paintings, and with Gabriel's patrons, who were owed sums for undelivered work. They had to be settled out of the earnings of the estate, as long as enough remained to pay the death duties.

Assembling Gabriel's manuscripts and letters, William saw editorial projects looming once Watts completed his memoir, but Watts gave no sign of even working on it, and William restively approached Gabriel's publisher, Ellis, about a collected edition of the works. Something had to be thrown into the breach to keep Gabriel's reputation alive. Skeptically, Ellis pointed to the many copies of *Ballads and Sonnets* he had remaining. A few months later, however, he impulsively retired from business in favor of his nephew Gilbert Ellis, who reconsidered in favor of a collected edition of the poems to be followed within a year—he hoped—by Watts's and William's joint volume.

Hearing that William was contemplating a study of Gabriel, and an edition of his letters, Bell Scott wrote to urge reasonable candor. "The personality of Gabriel with all its weaknesses and delusions was a perfect individuality, and the most fascinating I have met. . . . The place he must take . . . makes it certain that a true picture of his nature as exhibited in his life, is necessary to avoid the lies and revelations that have been poured out by half-enlightened writers about Shelley, Byron, and others and warrant[s] such a treatment. If your dear mother wd. dissent from this, delay your work. But to give only one side of him by letters to his family [alone] you must see is only like Mrs. Stowe's *Sunny Memories* with alas! the infernal unrevealed story beneath. . . ." But William was not about to let loose infernal unrevealed stories, and counted upon Watts's dilatory biographical muse to be equally discreet. In the meantime, there were the unpublished poems.

Not concerned about textual variants, William came home from Somerset House each evening to work on reordering Gabriel's published pieces and sorting through unpublished material for additional writings worthy of the ones Gabriel had passed for publication himself. The unpublished matter was to be the project's chief claim to attention, and William had to be less than fastidious in order to find enough new copy, selecting, he confessed in a preface, "only such examples as I suppose that he would himself have approved for the purpose, or would, at any rate, not gravely have objected to." Uncollected, out of Victorian timidity, was the sonnet "Nuptial Sleep," because Buchanan had found in it "merely animal sensations," and "After the French Liberation of Italy," which used the imagery of a prostitute's embrace. And there were more problems. William worried about giving precise dates of composition of individual sonnets in *The House of Life* because—he noted in his diary—there were "considerations" to dissuade him. He knew which poems were prompted by a passion which *followed* the death of Lizzy Siddal, and wanted to inhibit any biographical reading of the sonnets.

Cautiously, William blurred the chronology by omitting dates, and in a preface he carefully blended fact with reticence. Lizzy's death, and the retreats to Kelmscott, were unavoidable realities, but William saw no reason to do more than acknowledge them. Yet he also conceded that his brother had found himself in difficulties by "loving, if not always practising, the good." When the edition finally saw print in 1887 the notices were favorable. Those of William's (and Gabriel's) friends who supplied a number of them were very likely relieved by William's skillful combination of fairness and propriety. For a time the preface stood as the major biographical source regarding Gabriel.

By the mid-1880s Lucy Rossetti was shut indoors for long periods, and her chronic bronchitis seemed a euphemism for what neither she nor her doctor were willing to name. Finally, in mid-November 1886, Lucy and the two elder children left for San Remo, while the two younger ones were housed with the Browns and the Hueffers. When William could take a holiday he followed his family to Italy.

William's commitment to Gabriel's reputation continued to direct his life. With Watts back-pedaling from a life of Gabriel, William predicated his willingness to do a Keats monograph in Eric Robertson's "Great Writers" series on the inclusion of his brother, his ultimatum being that "if Gabriel were omitted, greatly postponed, or treated contrary to my feelings, I am at liberty to resign Keats entirely." Joseph Knight was commissioned to do a *Rossetti*, and William agreed to make materials available to him if Knight would submit the manuscript for examination. He did, and William—especially concerned about the Lizzy Siddal section—found "the spirit in which the facts are treated" satisfactory.

Well into the year of the Golden Jubilee of Queen Victoria—1887—Lucy returned to England, seemingly improved. William returned gratefully to Somerset House, from which he was still managing his brother's estate, managing the government business which came his way, and writing a biography of Shelley. Since biography absorbed him, he should have realized that public lives are difficult to expurgate, and that his caution in seeing that a safe life of his brother were written would have as much success as had Shelley's relatives in their attempts. A review of the hapless Joseph Knight's *Dante Gabriel Rossetti* by Oscar Wilde in the *Pall Mall Gazette* in April 1887 attacked William by inference. The best that could be said of the book, Wilde observed, "is that it is just the sort of biography Guildenstern might have written of Hamlet. Nor does its unsatisfactory character come merely from the ludicrous inadequacy of the materials at Mr. Knight's disposal. . . . Rossetti's was a great personality, and personalities such as his do not easily survive shilling primers."

In 1888 William took on a new assignment at the Inland Revenue, in addition to his usual duties, which had become monotonous and easily reassigned. Lord Iddesleigh asked him to undertake, for the Board of the Inland Revenue, the reviewing of lists of art works received in probate matters in order to provide an opinion of the prices estimated. It would become one of the happiest of his occupations, as it took him to stately homes to review the works themselves, and brought him anew into an art world not encompassed on four sides by Gabriel's pictures. Lucy was less and less well, gradually giving up the children's education to the governess. Enforced inactivity exasperated her, but by 1891 she was usually too exhausted for anything else. When, in April 1892, she got up from her bed to attend, with William, the funeral of Tennyson at Westminster Abbey, her appearances in public had become rare. Now forty-nine, she was weak and wasted from tuberculosis.

By the summer of 1893, Dr. William Gill was urging Lucy to return to Italy. On September 29 William drew a check to her to pay the next month's rent, and another to Christina to pay her the half-share due on Gabriel's royalties. Drained by medical bills, and down to £67 in his account, he planned to sell some of his few investments in order to finance Lucy's stay abroad, although it appeared likely to be brief. Early in October she left, spared by three days the shock of her father's death, at seventy-two. Cautiously, William prepared her for it by sending letters intimating Madox Brown's serious illness. In any event, she could not return.

After settling the affairs of his brother's old friend, and his father-in-law, and securing leave from his post, William prepared to follow Lucy to Italy but, he wrote in his memoirs, "she preferred that I should not do so." On March 19, 1894, he received a telegram that Lucy was sinking rapidly, and he and his eldest son, Arthur, rushed to San Remo. She rallied, but there was no hope. William was at her bedside when, in the early morning of April 12, Lucy died. They had been married twenty years.

When William returned to London a widower in April, he had little desire to return to the routine of Somerset House. Under Civil Service rules he was due to retire at the beginning of the month of his sixty-fifth birthday, September 25, 1894. He was only a few months from that date. To the Board of the Inland Revenue he applied for leave until the date of his official retirement, August 31. It was granted. He had given forty-nine and a half years of service to his department.

His sister Christina died in the last days of 1894. Early in 1895 William poked around in the hushed house in Torrington Square, pondering how to make the accumulations of three generations of Polidoris and two generations of Rossettis intelligible to the inheritance tax appraiser. Then he had to decide what he wanted to retain and what would go to the auctioneer, although some articles were disposed of by sale or gift to

Christina's friends, and William unwisely let some of her poetical man-uscripts go for small sums as well. For a while, too, his memoir of Gabriel occupied his days, until on April 28 he noted its completion "with a sense of thankfulness and relief."

The companion volume of family letters had first been planned to have only a few letters from Gabriel to persons other than William, but Chris-tina's death brought William all of the surviving letters from Gabriel to their mother, to Christina, and to the Polidori aunts. With so much material, he could choose the most attractive and the most significant letters, discreetly excising references—and even allusions—to Fanny Cornforth or Jane Morris; indiscreet or unreasonable remarks about Ga-briel's long-suffering and impatient patrons, friends, and relatives; and even most of the paragraphs about the borrowing of money. What would be printed would be scrupulously dated and annotated, but the result was a duller and more high-minded Dante Gabriel Rossetti than the facts might have shown. "A brother neither is nor can be the best biographer," he admitted in his preface, and added frankly, "Some readers of the Memoir may be inclined to ask me—'Have you told everything, of a substantial kind, that you know about your deceased brother?'—My an-swer shall be given . . . without disguise: 'No; I have told what I choose to tell; if you want more, be pleased to consult some other informant.'" His reticence would be accepted as exactly that, rather than as whitewash. When the volumes appeared late in 1895 William was rewarded by the assumption of his biographical integrity, for which he was willing to take the criticism that his prose was stuffy and inelegant.

Grand schemes for producing, in five volumes, a compilation of letters and documents that would combine the history of the Rossettis in England with the history of Pre-Raphaelitism filled William's days in the later nineties. First he methodically bundled all his raw material into segments representing each projected book, then put everything into chronological order. Even five months spent in Switzerland were no handicap, as he took the appropriate bundle with him, finishing the first volume of 1,368 manuscript pages (which would become *Pre-Raphaelite Diaries and Let-ters*) late in 1896.

For a man in retirement he remained as busy as before. What treasures and memorabilia had been accumulated only became clear to him as through 1898 and 1899 he catalogued the museum which his muffled rooms at St. Edmund's Terrace had become. The hoard was awesome in quantity. There were "834 drawings &c by Gabriel or connected with him; 1015 by the Family (Lucy, Lizzie, &c) or connected; 4358 miscel-laneous; 159 Japanese. . . ." He was amazed at the total.

The English-reading audience was already glutted with cautious com-
pilations of Rossetti papers. Mackenzie Bell's earnest biography of Christina, supervised by William, brought its author only £34 in its first year
of publication. Disappointed, William persisted on his family projects,
editing and translating, between attacks of rheumatism and gout, his
father's versified autobiography, editing Madox Brown's diary, his own
P.R.B. diary, John Polidori's diary about the Byron-Shelley circle, and
Rossetti papers bringing the story beyond Lizzy's death. His typist, Ethel
Dickens, granddaughter of the novelist and one of the innovators of the
secretarial service concept which the typewriter made practical, was earning more from William's projects than was William himself.

Living in his family's past was not always of William's own doing.
Correspondents were constantly asking him to sell or give away memorabilia of Gabriel or of Christina, evidence to him that there was an
audience for Rossetti books. Readers wanted notes, autographs, scraps
of manuscripts and letters, even locks of hair; and some shrewdly asked
also for a memento associated with William. Where the object was available and of no great commercial value, he generally offered it without
charge, making up his postage deficit by charging overly modest prices
for books or letters, in the process scattering Rossettiana around the
world.

Not all his reminders of the glorious past were so pleasant as to enable
him to pass the emptying hours in the study at St. Edmund's Terrace in
blissful nostalgia. In 1899 Harry Siddal and his brother James were reduced to the poorhouse. The brothers had remained close, James looking
after "his rather half-witted brother," who had "never been able to take
up any definite occupation," and carrying on a cutlery business—the trade
long in their family—until both were too enfeebled and indigent to remain
out of the Kennington Workhouse. When William discovered their plight,
he extricated them and gave them a regular allowance, but they found
the workhouse easier than maintaining themselves, and returned. When
out again, they turned to William, once offering him a faded watercolor
of Lizzy by Gabriel. He bought it for eighteen pounds, sold it to Fairfax
Murray for more, and gave Siddal the extra money.

As late as 1908 there was a knock on the door from James Siddal. Harry
was dead. William no longer would have to carry out Lizzy's deathbed
entreaty. Yet at seventy James Siddal could not survive outside the workhouse without help, and William agreed to pay him £25 a year in quarterly
installments. Later Siddal managed to secure an old-age pension, but
since it was too small to live on, William continued a portion of the old
allowance as a supplement. A long life was expensive. He had inherited

what remained of the Rossetti and Polidori estates, but also their obligations.

For the most part William's work, at eighty, was done, except to continue to be the watchdog of the Rossetti reputation, and he was under no illusions about his own fame when writers came to call, or—as William Rothenstein did—to draw his portrait. He knew what his current literary worth was, for when he made out his annual income tax return on May 4, 1910, he discovered that only one percent of his income of nearly £2,000 (including his pension) was earned by his own writings. He had produced £19.5.1. by his pen. Now and then he wrote letters to the editor, correcting biographers and memoirists who alleged things about Gabriel or Christina or Madox Brown which William felt were erroneous, even correcting, in painstaking detail, his nephew Ford, in the *Outlook*, when Hueffer published his *Ancient Lights and Certain New Reflections*. The future Ford Madox Ford had faint regard for accuracy.

Troubled by rheumatism and gout, as well as by continuing publishing frustrations—for no publisher wanted his three later volumes of Rossetti papers—he confessed early in 1912, "I feel of late very aged and feeble, but am not *ill*: my literary career is no doubt closed." As the executor for Gabriel and Christina he was still consulted regularly on matters concerning them, but his chief consolations had become his pipe and his first phonograph, with its huge horn of a loudspeaker. His life remained orderly and benign. He methodically docketed his papers and letters, preserved book catalogues he received, attached labels to everything in the house connected with Christina or Gabriel in order to validate its provenance, and managed the sale of photographs of his brother's pictures. When William discussed his own role in the past it was as much without ornamentation as without vanity, as he recognized his limitations and understood his role. Reading William's long and unsuccessful poem "Mrs. Holmes Grey," Richard Curle noted aloud that two lines in it appeared superior to the rest. Unperturbed, William said simply, "These were the only lines in the poem written by Gabriel."

At St. Edmund's Terrace he puttered in his study, wrote letters daily, and worried over dwindling royalty income and increasing prospects of a European war, which he worried that the Germans would win. Early in 1914 he received a telegram from May Morris: "Mother died suddenly here yesterday." He had not been in touch with her in many years, and had even hesitated sending her Gabriel's *Collected Works* a quarter century earlier, fearing to remind anyone—even Janey—of the relationship he would barely mention in his books about Gabriel. His eyesight was failing badly, and even with new spectacles William found it difficult to read the small print of the newspapers at just the time that war news was filling so many columns.

By 1917 he was living entirely downstairs, where, to spare his feeble legs, his bed had been moved. The war deprived him of small comforts, and the old age he hated deprived him of other small pleasures. He characterized his eighty-eighth birthday as "that dismal anniversary," for, he scrawled in his diary, he was now "half-seeing," and could only write "a wretched scrap." The memorabilia on the study walls had grown hazy. The last letter he wrote was dated October 13, 1918.

To Curle he had once said, "I should regard it as a disaster if I were to live to be ninety." During the winter of 1918–19, just after he was cheered by the end of the war, he suffered a severe chill, and took to his bed. With none of the painful melodrama which had accompanied the end of his brother and sisters, William Michael Rossetti died at three o'clock in the afternoon on February 5, 1919. He was eighty-nine.

The last of the four Rossettis, he had lived long enough to be nearly forgotten. And he was, J.C. Squire wrote in his weekly book column, "not the kind of man about whom anecdotes clustered." He had been the chronicler of the Pre-Raphaelite movement for nearly seventy years, and had been involved in its origin. He had been instrumental in rescuing Blake from neglect, Whitman from opprobrium, Shelley from textual emasculation. Posterity has looked kindly on men for much less.

Although his own role had been modest, William Rossetti had been part of something which had shaken and shaped his times. After a prudent, unadventurous career he had lived on to inherit the lot of the survivor. Not for him the melodrama—nor the achievement—of his brother's life, nor for him the hidden desperation masked by the outward piety and serenity of his sisters' lives. His family had left an imprint upon English writing and English art which his own contributions—as well as his censorship of the family documents—could only enhance. The family letters, diaries, pictures, and manuscripts were William's. And also his, for more than two decades, had been not only his civil service pension but the accumulated bank accounts of the long-lived Rossettis and Polidoris, Englishmen and Englishwomen despite their names, though none as tenacious of the years as he. Publishing their histories and their life-records had not been acts of personal immodesty, nor attempts to turn a profit. Nor did he appear jealous of a fame he had not earned.

It is not every man's fortune—or fate—to have a king as brother. It was William's, and from childhood he had been ennobled rather than embittered by his role. As, too, with the poetic Christina and the prosaic

Maria, sibling support rather than sibling rivalry was routine in the more Italian than English closeness of the family. Whistler had protested, from his own deathbed, "You must not say anything against Rossetti. Rossetti was a king." Earlier, a disciple during the *annis mirabilis* at Oxford had cried out, "Why is he not some great exiled king, that we might give him our lives to try to restore him to his kingdom!" Whether or not William, who knew him best, believed that, he died still in his king's service, keeper at times, liege always.

REFERENCES

Doughty, C. (1960), *A Victorian Romantic: Dante Gabriel Rossetti*. London: Oxford University Press.

Fredeman, W.D. (1970–1971), Prelude to the last decade: Dante Gabriel Rossetti in the summer of 1872. *Bulletin of the John Rylands Library* (Manchester), 53.

Weintraub, S. (1977), *Four Rossettis: A Victorian Biography*. New York: Weybright & Talley; London: W.H. Allen, 1978.

Rarely does the student of the creative mind possess sufficient knowledge of a special family configuration, and its influence on the personality, to accurately surmise the characteristics of artists from such families, or to determine their influence of these traits on their creative acts. We are fortunate, then, that a multitude of documented psychoanalytic studies has provided us an understanding of the way twins frequently think and feel.[1] And when we discern the traits that twins commonly possess in many of the protagonists in plays by twins, we know that fate has provided us the means for a study of creativity.

In this chapter I will describe the familial interrelationships commonly present with twins and their influence on them. I will then demonstrate that some of the characters of the twin playwrights Peter and Anthony Shaffer behave as if they were twins, even though they are not presented as twins on the narrative surface. Much of the excitement and drama of these plays stems from these twinlike interactions. Since most of us find our-

8

Twins in the Theater: A Study of Plays by Peter and Anthony Shaffer

JULES GLENN

[1] Abraham (1953), Arlow (1960), Burlingham (1952), Cronin (1933), Demarest & Winestine (1955), Gardner & Rexford (1952), Gifford et al. (1966), Glenn (1966), Glenn & Glenn (1968), Hartmann (1934–1935), Joseph (1959, 1961, 1975), Joseph & Tabor (1961), Karpman (1953), Lacombe (1959), Leonard (1961), Lidz et al. (1962), Maenchen (1968), Mesnikoff et al. (1963), Orr (1941), Peto (1946), Wiedeman (1973).

selves remarkably enchanted by twins, curious about them, and stimulated or even titillated by their presence, it is not surprising that disguised twinship holds our interest and stirs our passions.

But first let me outline the known facts (Wakeman, 1975; Myers, 1976; Herbert, 1977; Vinson, 1977; Klein, 1979; Reilly, 1980) about Anthony Shaffer, the author of *Sleuth*, and Peter Shaffer, who has written such well-known plays as *Five Finger Exercise, The Royal Hunt of the Sun, Equus*, and *Amadeus*.

Anthony Joshua and Peter Levin Shaffer are fraternal twins born in Liverpool on May 15, 1926. Anthony was born five minutes earlier than Peter. Their parents, Jack, who worked in real estate, and Reka, were Jewish. A younger brother, Brian, is a biophysicist. After moving to London in 1936 and then relocating repeatedly from 1936 to 1942, the family established itself in London, where the boys were educated at St. Paul's School. Peter and Anthony were both conscripted as coalminers from 1944 to 1947 and then attended Trinity College, Cambridge, where they were graduated in 1950. Both showed literary ability and served as magazine editors at Cambridge.

Anthony then worked as a barrister, journalist, ad man, and television producer, but also wrote plays, screenplays, and novels, the first with Peter in 1952. He is married to Carolyn Soley and has two daughters. Peter, after graduation in 1950, worked for a New York bookstore and then the New York Public Library acquisitions department from 1951 to 1952. He was employed by Boosey & Hawks, London music publishers, from 1954 to 1955. He was the literary critic for *Truth* from 1956 to 1957 and music critic for *Time & Tides* from 1961 to 1962.

Although the twins' lives diverged at many times, a marked convergence is obvious. Brought up in the same household, they shared the same room and dressed alike for a few years. As is generally true of twins and siblings, they played together and attended the same schools.

In 1951 Peter wrote a novel entitled *The Woman in the Wardrobe*, using the pseudonym Peter Antony.[2] The pair used this same pseudonym when in 1952 they wrote the novel *How Doth the Little Crocodile?* together. In 1955 they published *Withered Murder* under their actual names of Peter and Anthony Shaffer.

Peter turned to playwriting first and has produced an impressive body of work: *Five Finger Exercise* (1958), *The Private Ear* and *The Public Eye* (1962), *The Merry Roosters' Panto* (1963), a sketch in *The Establishment* (1963), *The Royal Hunt of the Sun* (1964), *Black Comedy* (1965), *White*

---

[2] According to Vinson (1977), the two brothers collaborated on the novel, but Klein (1979) and Schwartz (1973) say Peter wrote it alone.

Lies (1967, produced as *White Liars* in 1968), *A Warning Game* (1967), *It's About Cinderella* (1969), *Shrivings* (1975) (an unproduced play modified from a play entitled *The Battle of Shrivings*, 1970), *Equus* (1973), and *Amadeus* (1980). He received the Evening Standard Award in 1958, the New York Drama Critics Circle Award in 1960, 1975, and 1981, and the Tony Award in 1975 and 1981.

Anthony Shaffer's first produced play was *The Savage Parade* (1963) followed by *Sleuth* (1970) and *Murderer* (1975). He has written a number of screenplays: *Black Comedy, Forbush and the Penguins,* and *Absolution* in 1970; *Frenzy* in 1972; *Sleuth* in 1973; *The Wickerman* and *The Goshawk Squadron* in 1973; *Masado* in 1974; *The Moonstone* in 1975; *Evil Under the Sun* in 1976; and *Death on the Nile* in 1979. For *Sleuth* he received the Mystery Writers of America Edgar Allan Poe Award for Screenplay in 1973. He also wrote the television play *Pig in the Middle* and is the author of two novels—*The Wicker Man* with Robin Hardy in 1978 and *Absolution* in 1979.

Early in their careers, then, Peter and Anthony Shaffer wrote two detective novels in which their shared characteristics appeared in the jointly produced content and, in the case of *How Doth the Little Crocodile?*, was symbolized by the condensed pseudonym, Peter Antony, a combination of their first names. As they proceeded with independent authorship, they retained certain similarities but diverged as well.

Most of Peter Shaffer's plays are of epic scope. They deal with broad philosophical problems and compelling historical issues. Peter Shaffer compares primitive and civilized man and wonders which is superior. He explores the borderline between passionate creativity and destructive psychopathology and notes that normality can connote banality and dull existence. He struggles with the question of whether idealistic activism can prevail in a world of unleashed aggression. He ponders the sources of creativity and the envy of the merely talented for the genius.

Anthony Shaffer's plays concentrate on the enjoyable rather than the profound. Like his brother, he is interested in the interrelationships of people, but historical and philosophic contexts are not essential to the humorous and exciting interplay in his stagings. Tragic elements are diluted by wit, and wisdom is hidden in humor.

Anthony Shaffer's settings are more or less naturalistic, but can be imaginative and imposing, especially in the film version of *Sleuth.* Peter Shaffer, while not eschewing reality entirely, can create a sense of pageantry and grandeur, and often relies on symbolism and stylization. In *Equus* the set consists of a series of benches which create a clinical atmosphere. Men play horses on which men may ride. And in *The Royal*

Hunt of the Sun the audience is engaged in the rituals of an ancient people.

Despite the disparities between the plays of Peter and Anthony Shaffer, certain similarities of theme and characterization appear. These, I suggest, can be attributed to a great extent to the twinship of the authors.

The milieu in which twins reared together grow up is unique indeed. Two individuals of identical or similar appearance live in close proximity and proceed through the various developmental stages in unison. As infants they learn to give up symbiosis and become individuals together while clinging to each other. They hear each other babble and babble to each other. They seek mutual comfort through sounds, speech, sight, and touch, through verbal reassurances, hugging and playing together. They protect each other from loneliness when their parents are absent, but also compete for the grownups' attention and care. If both infants are hungry, mother may find herself allowing one to cry while she feeds the other.

These complicated, confusing, and contradictory life circumstances tend to create certain personality configurations seen in twins generally, whether identical, fraternal same-sex, or fraternal opposite-sex. The twins, growing up in close proximity and gratifying each other, will often develop a special love for each other. Their games together may be un-usually intense and pleasurable. But, as competitors for parental care, they will often find themselves angry at each other and at their depriving parents. They will have to seek means to dampen their conflicting feelings of love and hate—for example, through fusion of the love and hate into a sadomasochistic compound, or through an extreme insistence that they be treated equally. What one acquires the other should get in exactly the same quality and quantity, lest rage at deprivation get out of hand and lead to fear they may hurt their beloved sibling, who is experienced as part of the self.

As the twins grow up, their proximity and similarity often interfere with their feelings as individuals. One twin may call his identical sibling "the other John." If the parents dress them identically, or if on occasion friends, teachers, and strangers fail to differentiate them, this tendency will be accentuated. They may be further encouraged to picture them-selves as a unit by being called "the twins," by their being considered special as a pair. The fun in being twins—in confusing adults and friends and through warding off anger and anxiety by emphasis on their identical or similar state—will facilitate their picturing themselves as a unit.

Learning, as they do, how twins are formed will reinforce their feeling of being a unit and their fantasies that they were split into two identical parts. Identical twins, of course, are in actuality formed from a single fertilized ovum which divides so that each twin has the same genetic structure. But the cognitive immaturity of the children when they first learn about the formation of twins leads them to ignore the subtleties of this actuality and to imagine a gross and later splitting. Not only identical twins, but fraternal, even opposite-sex twins, frequently believe they were a unit divided into two parts in the womb or after birth.

Their later, more complicated fantasies draw on and incorporate their earlier and continuing feelings of love, hatred, and unity. Not only were the twins once one; they must also return to oneness, must join each other in loving unity. Their fantasies resemble Plato's description of lovers. Originally, he said in the *Symposium*, every person possessed two heads, two bodies, four arms, and four legs joined into a single body. These double beings then split and separated. Love consists of the reunion of the halves into the original double state, a fantasy shared by singletons but more potent in and characteristic of twins.

Frequently a twin unconsciously imagines he has been robbed during the split, deprived of half his body, or even more. He may wish revenge and want to steal back the missing part, but may fear that in the retaliatory theft he will be further injured. In the normal course of development, the child's narcissism—his primitive love for himself and those he feels part of, his mother in particular—recedes and becomes more mature as he enters the oedipal period; he comes to love his parents and others more and to recognize and appreciate them for their actual traits to a greater degree. The special narcissism of the twinship will often influence his relationship with his parents in destructive ways. Resentment against parents as deprivers, or as favoring the other twin, may remain dominant features in the child's relation to his parents even in adulthood. Further, the parental imago may become infused with representations of the twin. For example, a twin who pictured himself and his brother as defective half persons also viewed his parents as deficient. He emphasized certain "double" images related to his mother, the double letters in her name Sally, for instance, as if these somehow conferred twinship on her. He then selected a girlfriend whose name contained the same double letters, Ellen.

The special organization of love and hate found in many twins includes intense drives that require discharge and forbidden elements. The love is often taboo in that it contains a strong homosexual element and a powerful primitive narcissistic core. The hatred is dangerous in that it is directed at the twin, who is considered part of the self, and the parents, who must care for the child. In addition, incestuous love and hatred of parents and twin are forbidden by the developing conscience. As is true of all children, the child must develop defenses to deal with his forbidden urges, but twins use certain defenses to an unusual degree. The resultant adult traits are often typical.

Twins, in common with humanity in general, repress their forbidden feelings and related thoughts, relegating them to the unconscious part of the mind, from which they may emerge in disguised form. Hence the twins are unaware of much of the ideation already described. In addition, as they utilize the mechanism of displacement to hide the objects of their affection and anger, they unconsciously deal with their friends and acquaintances as if they were twins. They picture the world as filled with twins and, by that means disguise and dilute their feelings toward their actual siblings. One twin patient, for instance, wanted to give me his clothes so I could dress like him. He also pictured his wife as a twin who would try to rob his possessions, just as he wished to steal hers.

Projection and identification are defenses typical of twins because their tendency to confuse self and object facilitates their formation. Projection consists of the attribution of one's own characteristics to others, while identification involves the feeling that one possesses another's traits. Both imply a temporary or partial dissolution of ego boundaries. A twin assumed that because he was extremely logical so too were others, an example of projection. He also thought the same things that made him angry made others angry. Another twin imitated her twin sister and, feeling like her, married a man with similar artistic interests. Twin girls, seen separately in consultation, wanted to know what the other twin did during her session with me so that she could carry out the same activities.

Many twins denounce and deny their feelings that they are like their siblings. Instead they want to be different from their siblings and thus preserve their identity. To accomplish this, and also to avoid the competition and antagonism that can be so painful to twins, they may enter different, even opposite, fields of endeavor. At the same time, their complementary traits may promote their feeling that together they comprise a single whole person.

Twinship may cause difficulties but can be rewarding as well. It can facilitate empathy and creativity based on empathy. A twin's ability to understand others through identification and projection—especially if reality testing is intact—can help him create moving literary characters. A twin's closeness to and love for his sibling can lead him to write with the conscious or unconscious intention of pleasing his twin and the audience that, through displacement, represents him. Greenacre (1957) has discussed the artist's creating for an audience of "collective alternatives," and Meyer (1972) has suggested that the fantasied reader or viewer is a "secret sharer" (see also Glenn, 1974c).

The need to discharge libidinal and aggressive tensions originating in the twinship, the need to defend against forbidden wishes, and the need to master difficulties inherent in the twinship may help shape the form of the literary creation and determine the characteristics of the protagonists. We may expect at least sometimes to find characters with traits typical of twins, characters who interact as twins do. This will result from the adaptive interplay of projection and displacement in the creation of literary characters.

In the plays of Peter and Anthony Shaffer, we frequently find that the protagonists are twins in disguise. Often there are two protagonists who are in some way similar, but who also complement each other. As the play proceeds, they imitate and identify with each other, become more alike. They become close to one another to the point of appreciation and love, but also compete, envying and attacking one another and often a parent surrogate such as God. They may picture themselves as half persons, or the author may display his interest in halves, doubles, mirror images, pairs, and opposites by introducing these concepts into the play.

I will discuss two plays by Anthony Shaffer, *Sleuth* and *Murderer*, and then two by Peter Shaffer, *Equus* and *Amadeus*, in order to demonstrate how the twinship enters these dramas.

Sleuth

Andrew Wyke, a writer of mysteries, invites Milo Tindle, his wife's young lover, to his house in order to punish him for the affair. Pretending to be friendly, Andrew's plan is to convince Milo that the two should cooperate in stealing Wyke's jewelry. Milo would then have money from the sale of the purloined valuables, while Andrew would receive the insurance money. Milo would run off with Mrs. Wyke, of whom Andrew has tired. Milo is at first mistrustful, but soon agrees. They run through the sham burglary; when it is finished, Andrew reveals that he intends to shoot Milo as a thief. Milo is terrified. He begs for mercy as Andrew attacks him verbally and finally pulls the trigger.

It appears that Milo has been killed, but in the second act Andrew reveals that the pistol had contained blanks, and that Milo had run off after being sadistically humiliated. It had all been a game. Inspector Doppler, a police officer who is investigating the disappearance of Milo, now appears. He frightens Andrew by producing circumstantial evidence that Andrew had murdered his wife's lover, and then reveals that he is actually Milo in disguise, returned to make things even by humbling his opponent. After Andrew recovers from his panic, he rejoices in admiration for Milo. He observes that Milo's methods are the same as his, and adds that when he, Andrew, had tricked Milo he "wanted to get to know you—to see if you were . . . my sort of person." Milo asks, "A games-playing sort of person?" (p. 101), and Andrew agrees, adding that such a person is "a complete man" (p. 102). The affection between the two men becomes clearer as Milo jokes, "Where would you find homosexual woodworms? . . . In a tallboy" (pp. 100–101). Andrew compliments Milo as his sort of person and admits, "At bottom, I'm rather a solitary man. . . . I've never met a woman to whom the claims of the intellect were as absolute as they are for me" (p. 102).

The men admire, even love, each other, but their competitive antag-onism returns to the fore. Milo tells Andrew that his game was "superior to mine" (p. 103). Like a twin who needs to make things equal, Milo says, "My only duty now is to even our score. That's imperative" (p. 104). Andrew asserts that they are indeed equal—"It's one set all" (p. 104)—but Milo insists on further evening the score.

Adamantly, Milo proceeds to exact further vengeance, again through a charade. He states that he strangled Andrew's mistress, Téa, after he had made love to her. He tortures Andrew by proving to him that he has buried the woman in the garden and has planted evidence incriminating Andrew. The police, he says, are about to arrive, and Andrew's only hope is to discover this evidence by finding the answers to riddles which Milo poses and then to destroy the clues. As Andrew excitedly rushes about trying to find the evidence, the sadomasochistic interplay between the two men, with its loving and hating aspects, stands out in relief.

> MILO: The thought that you are playing a game for your life is practically giving you an orgasm. [p. 113]
> ANDREW: You sadistic bloody wop! [p. 114]

When Andrew retrieves the evidence just as the police are supposedly about to enter, Milo reveals that this too is a hoax and that he has hu-miliated and tricked his opponent once more. The two protagonists agree that things are now squared. Indeed, Andrew's love for Milo is so great that he asks him to stay rather than go off with Marguerite, Andrew's wife. He urges him not to "waste it all on Marguerite. She doesn't ap-preciate you like I do. You and I are evenly matched. . . . I just want someone to play with" (p. 120).

But Milo is determined to leave and thus upsets the balance once more. He now firmly intends to possess the older man's wife. He starts to leave, Marguerite's fur coat in hand, but Andrew, enraged at Milo's deserting him as well as the inequity of the situation, shoots him. The mystery writer has apparently achieved the revenge he sought in the first act. The actual arrival of the police tips the balance once more. Milo's dying words, "Game, set and match" (p. 125), reveal that he considers himself the winner, although each man has destroyed the other.

We begin to realize that *Sleuth* contains material especially revealing of the author when we observe that Andrew, like Shaffer, is a writer of mysteries. But even without this clue there is much in the play pointing to the author's twinship.

In a direct reference to twinship, Andrew imagines himself an identical twin accused of having committed a crime. Robbery, a prominent preoccupation of many twins (Lacombe, 1959; Glenn, 1966), is a dominant theme in the play. The "logic" behind the tendency of twins to cheat and steal is this: I have been robbed of half my body (or more) and of love and supplies by my twin. Therefore I will steal back that which I lost; but if I do my twin or parent (or twin surrogate or parent surrogate) may attack me. Thus Andrew seeks revenge because Milo has stolen his wife. Later Milo even takes Andrew's mistress, at least in fantasy. The two men plan a robbery in the first act, while the final encounter between them involves the feigned theft of a fur coat. Andrew, of course, is well prepared for illegal activity, since he earns his living inventing and solving crimes.

There are many references to doubles and halves. Milo's father is half-Jewish and Andrew jokes that "some of my best friends are half-Jews" (p. 21). One of the clues planted by Milo for Andrew contains the phrase "For any man with *half* an eye" must see "what stands before him" (pp. 109–110). A second clue, referring to a pair of shoes, begins, "Two brothers we are, / Great burdens we bear" (p. 113). When Milo selects a name for himself as the inspector, it is "Doppler," meaning "double" or "Doppelgänger." This name suggests, in addition to twins, the inept inspector in Andrew Wyke's mystery stories, being almost an anagram of his name, Plodder. Thus Milo becomes identified with Andrew's creation, introducing clearly the shifting identities and role reversal of the protagonists. Throughout the play Milo imitates and identifies with Andrew in his attempt to even things between them. Although he is first presented as a rather dull young man, he becomes transformed into a person capable of playing Andrew's intellectual game.

The men, in their struggle to win the games, are constantly reversing roles, playing now the aggressor and now the victim. These identifications with the aggressor serve to reverse matters. The identification is a reflection of the poor distinction in twins between self- and object-representations. And there are libidinal and defensive elements as well, the identification signifying a type of pleasurable union of the two, a union which may succeed in quelling hostility through the triumph of affection.

Further, identification may diminish the twins' mutual antagonism through keeping things equal. The pressing need to establish equality is the motivating force behind both Milo's and Andrew's behavior. This preoccupation with equality is closely linked with the fantasy that one twin is half a being, that one is deprived by the other. There may be an attempt to make up for this deficit by being near the twin, by having close contact through types of activity engaged in as children, including games and storytelling.

These games may be sexual. A latent homosexual attraction is more than hinted at in the relationship between Andrew and Milo, especially in Andrew's attempt to exclude women from their lives. Andrew unquestionably prefers the male Milo to women in general and to Marguerite in particular. He explicitly asks Milo to stay with him rather than run off with his wife. Despite his boasts, it turns out that Andrew is not potent heterosexually; rather, his energies are directed toward games. He jokes that "sex is the game and marriage the penalty" (p. 80). His attachment to Téa, whom he describes as a goddess, is sadistic rather than tender and mature. Milo appears to function on a more advanced level, but he soon becomes caught in the gamesmanship with Andrew, and regresses to childlike play.

We can see here the tendency in twins to regress from the oedipal to the preoedipal twinning experiences. Oedipal loves and rivalries are expressed in twin terms. Marguerite and Téa appear to represent the mother for whom the twins compete. The preoedipal mother becomes the mother of the Oedipus complex, and the other twin can substitute for the father, the later rival. Milo is thus both the twin fighting his brother and the child competing with his father.

It has been observed that twins, once they have entered the oedipal phase, have difficulty resolving the Oedipus complex. Deficiency in superego formation may result. Certainly the morality of the protagonists in *Sleuth*, who are willing to steal, trick, torture, and murder, can be said to reveal a weakness of conscience.

Murderer

The twin theme is more hidden in Anthony Shaffer's *Murderer* (1979). An artist, Norman Bartholomew, disenchanted with his efficient, Prussian-bossy gynecologist wife Elizabeth, with whom he is impotent, engages in an affair with Millie. Significantly, Millie resembles his wife physically.

As he had with his wife early in their relationship, Norman plays murder games with Millie. He acts out killings previously committed by well-known criminals, pretending he is laying the groundwork for the actual murder of Elizabeth. Millie is getting wise to him and believes he is too weak to commit the crime that will allow him to marry her.

Returning from an artists' party, Norman finds Millie in the bathtub, pretending to be his wife come back early from a trip. Thinking she is Elizabeth, he kills her. When the real Elizabeth returns home and finds the corpse, she thinks Norman has inadvertantly killed his mistress in one of his games and convinces him to pretend she has died accidentally. The price of saving him from a murder charge is that they remain together without threats of divorce. But when she realizes Norman had in fact meant to kill *her*, she quickly reneges on her bargain. In anger Norman strangles her until she becomes unconscious. He then plans to finish off the job by asphyxiating her with gas. He will pretend she had come home, found Millie in her bath, killed her, and then committed suicide. Elizabeth awakes before he carries out his plan, stabs him in a rage and then kills him deliberately with a scalpel. As she murders him she says, "Well, darling, tell me—does it represent a mirror image of man's potential to realise bliss?" (p. 93) and then "Norman . . . Norman . . . listen to me. . . . It's worth listening to, because you see you've finally made a convert. . . . Do you know what story I'll tell the police when they get here. I'll say I came in and found your mistress in my bath. In a sudden, uncontrollable burst of passion I drowned her and then killed you. It will be *my* murder" (p. 93). The play continues:

> NORMAN (very weak): What!! . . . you can't do that. I killed. It was *my* murder.
> Elizabeth *smiles a wicked smile at him and slowly shakes her head as she takes away from him all he has left.*
> ELIZABETH: No, I think not. Did you really think that an inept little man like you could challenge the great moral laws of this universe. Mediocrity, my darling, has no theological status. . . . I will have what you have always wanted—a true and abiding notoriety. [pp. 93–94]

When the crime is discovered by Sergeant Stenning, he says, "I told him he didn't know the game he was playing. I told him it was the victim who looked for the murderer" (p. 95), and Elizabeth adds "he didn't have to look very far. We made an appointment—years ago" (pp. 95–96).

The primary twins in disguise in *Murderer* are Norman and Elizabeth. They are quite different at the start of the play—he is the imaginative game-player who pretends to be a murderer, and she the down-to-earth, efficient doctor. It turns out that early in their relationship they had shared the game-playing, but she found it boring. By the end of the play she has imitated her husband and become like him, inventing, playing, and acting out murder games.

But Elizabeth is better at committing a successful murder than Norman. She competes and beats him at his own game. She, not he, will gain notoriety. As in *Sleuth*, we see their differences, their complementary characters, their identification, their growing similarity, their competition with one surpassing the other. As also in *Sleuth*, other indications of twinship are the sadomasochistic relationship in which the sadistic and masochistic roles are alternated; the affection between the pair as they seal their deal; and mutual hatred. Other such indications in the story include the reference to the mirror, the physical similarity between the two women, and the suggestion of rivalry for a parent, here disguised as a theological competition.

Equus

In *Equus* (1973), Dr. Martin Dysart, a psychiatrist, reluctantly undertakes the treatment of Alan Strang, a seventeen-year-old boy, only to discover himself engaged in a compelling but ambivalent relationship. Alan is hospitalized because he had blinded six horses with a hoof-pick, a kind of metal spike.

Alan's parents, although peripheral to the therapeutic interplay between doctor and patient, provide background material that helps us understand the boy. Alan's mother, a devout Christian, stimulates her son's religious interests by preaching and reading the Bible to him. His father opposes Mrs. Strang's child-rearing methods. He is a stern, moralistic, but anticlerical socialist who proclaims work and asceticism as ideals, and pleasure an evil. When Alan was twelve, Mr. Strang angrily removed from the boy's room a picture of a chained and beaten Jesus walking to Calvary. The boy, who had purchased and prized the portrait, had cried unconsolably until his father replaced the picture with a photograph of a staring horse. To his horror and dismay, Mr. Strang, some months before Alan's hospitalization, discovered Alan bowing before the picture of the horse while flagellating himself and verbigeratively chanting Bible-like sentences: "Prince begat Prance . . . and Prance begat Prankus . . ." (p. 58), etc.

Alan, retaining a mythopoeic bent, had turned from a love for Jesus to a fascination with horses. A number of experiences adumbrated this preoccupation. Mrs. Strang had repeatedly talked of her grandfather's attachment to horses, and of his daily morning ride "on the downs behind Brighton, all dressed up in bowler hat and jodhpurs!" (p. 37). She had given her son a book about a horse, Prince, which only one boy could ride; Alan read the book "over and over." He recalled with excitement the time when he was six and a horseman, after his steed had nearly trampled the boy, lifted him to his shoulders and raced the fleet-footed animal. Further, his mother told Dr. Dysart that Alan had been preoccupied with the word *equus*, which he used as a generic name for horses, "because he'd never come across [a word] with two U's together before" (p. 38). She told Alan stories of when Christian cavalry first appeared in the New World: the pagans thought "horse and rider was one person" (p. 36) and must be a god. She related to Alan passages in the Book of Job about horses.

Gradually, Alan had displaced his passion for the picture of the tortured Christ to that of the staring horse. He got a part-time job as a stable-boy which enabled him to ride horses, secretly and in the nude, at night. As he cantered, he imagined Equus saying to him, "Ride me. Mount me, and ride me forth at night . . ." (p. 77).

Psychotherapy is difficult and marked by resistance: Alan refuses to talk. Instead, he repeatedly sings the television commercial, "Double your pleasure / Double your fun / With Doublemint, Doublemint / Doublemint gum" (p. 27). Eventually Alan agrees to respond to the psychiatrist's questions if Dr. Dysart answers his turn for turn. In accordance with this agreement, Alan asks the doctor whether he has intercourse with his wife. Like a vulnerable patient, and true to his multiple-punning name, Dr. Dysart is infuriated and calls a halt to the session. The answer, we later learn, is no. This revelation of the doctor's sexual difficulties anticipates Alan's description of his own potency problem.

We come to see other similarities between the two. Dr. Dysart is engrossed by Greek mythology, while Alan has developed his own mythology. And, just as the boy is impelled to injure horses, so the psychiatrist is plagued by aggressive impulses toward people. He describes a dream in which he, as a sacrificial priest, surgically removes children's hearts. Indeed, the physician views his treatment of patients as destructive; he fears that he will deprive Alan of something vital by removing his symptoms, curing him. Nevertheless, he proceeds to treat him.

As the therapy progresses, the patient enacts his ecstatic desire to ride the horse and to fuse with Equus. Alan imagines himself saved by Equus. As the horse bears him away, he shrieks, "Two shall be one" (p. 76). . . . "I want to be *in* you! I want to BE you forever and ever!—*Equus, I love you!* Now!—Bear me away! Make us One Person!" (p. 85). The horse is both a substitute for Christ and a father surrogate to whom he is attracted, whom he loves and hates.

As the audience becomes entranced by the stylized, mystical, but nonetheless clinical milieu of the play, the viewers learn of the exciting, frightening, shocking events which led to Alan's stabbing the horses. Alan recalls how Jill, the twenty-one-year-old girl who had obtained the job in the stable for him, had seduced him. First Mr. Strang had discovered the pair at a pornographic movie to which Jill had taken Alan. Alan was terrified at being caught watching the film by his father but was also amazed and disillusioned at his father's attendance at the obscene show. He and Jill then went to the stable. He was excited and frightened.

In a vivid flashback, the audience sees Jill take Alan into the stable, where he insists that the horses be locked out lest they see him having intercourse with the girl. Alan and Jill undress and attempt intercourse as the sounds of the horses are heard in the background. The boy tells Dr. Dysart that he enjoyed superbly successful sexual relations. But when the psychiatrist contends that he is lying, Alan admits to his impotence. He feared the horses' gaze and impulsively stabbed a sharp grooming instrument into their eyes, shouting, "Equus . . . Noble Equus . . . Faithful and True . . . Godslave . . . Thou—God—Seest—Nothing!" (p. 121). Alan then collapses as he stabs at his own eyes.

This intensely dramatic abreaction leads the psychiatrist to predict that the boy will soon be cured. In a final soliloquy, Dr. Dysart expresses his dissatisfaction. Alan will now be free of pain, be normal. But he will have lost his passion and his poetry. The physician feels he has harmed his patient. He characterizes his treatment: "I stand in the dark with a pick in my hand, striking at heads" (p. 125).

Before applying our knowledge of the psychology of twins to the understanding of *Equus*, we must note the complexity of the story and the overlapping of themes. First, the play can be viewed as the story of an adolescent's pathology and his therapist's countertransference (Glenn, 1976), but we will not focus on these aspects here.

An oedipal theme is clear as well. As with Anthony Shaffer's *Sleuth* and *Murderer*, the reader versed in psychoanalysis may first be struck by the oedipal motif. Over and over again, we observe Alan's anger at his father for interfering with his pursuit of pleasure, including his undisguised wish for intercourse with an older girl. (In *Sleuth*, a younger man tries to elope with an older man's wife, and in *Murderer* the triangles involve Norman, a police officer, and a mistress on the one hand, and the two women and Norman on the other).

Alan and his mother share a passion for religion. This is, indeed, a vehicle for Alan's enjoyment of his mother's Biblical readings. When his father interferes, Alan circumvents him and develops a fervent interest in horses which substitute for Christ and Christianity. Early in the play, Mr. Strang objects to his son's watching television and later, to his attending a pornographic picture. Finally, he interferes with Alan's sexual relations with Jill. Here, displacement from father to horse leads the boy to feel the piercing, prohibiting, Godlike equine eyes observing and inhibiting his intercourse. In a fury, Alan attacks the horses' eyes, and then, like Oedipus, guiltily attacks his own.

But behind the oedipal theme, overlapping and contrasting, we find the twinship motif. As in *Sleuth* the two protagonists are male. The drama centers on their interaction. They behave like twins in their similarity, mutual identification, and ambivalence toward each other. They are opposite and complementary in some ways—one is a patient and the other the physician—but their basic similarities dominate. Each is motivated by desires to destroy: Alan has blinded horses; Dr. Dysart, who conceives of psychotherapy as a destructive process in which the patient is hurt, describes a dream in which he removes children's hearts in a sacrificial ceremony. Each has sexual difficulties: Alan is impotent with Jill; Dr. Dysart has refrained from sexual intercourse with his wife. Each is fascinated by mythology: the boy, long been interested in Christianity, has created the religion in which he worships Equus; Dr. Dysart has read avidly about Greece and has imagined himself a priest.

The two are not merely similar. They grow even more alike as they identify with each other. The boy forces a role reversal; he presses the doctor to act like the patient as he, psychiatristlike, asks penetrating and distressing questions. Dr. Dysart's identification with his patient when he says that he stands "in the dark with a pick in my hand, striking at heads" (p. 125) brings the play to a powerful and impressive conclusion.

As twins envy each other for their opponent's supposed superiority, so the physician envies Alan for his more active and passionate participation in the mythopoeic process. Dr. Dysart regrets that he merely reads about imaginary Greek creatures while Alan acts the centaur, even becomes the centaur, as he rides and feels fused with Equus.

The mutual ambivalence of the protagonists is openly displayed. Dr. Dysart becomes fed up with Alan and decides to end the treatment, only to change his mind and engage in a session at night. The doctor's belief that he is hurting his patient, although intended by the author as a realistic probability which gives philosophical force to the play, can be seen as a derivative of a reluctant wish to harm him. Alan is suspicious and hostile toward the physician he thinks will trick him.

It is not all hatred, however; Alan's revelation of his secrets would be impossible without trust and affection. Dr. Dysart's love for the boy is fully exposed when, after Alan's intense abreaction, he tenderly covers his spent patient; he is remarkably sympathetic with Alan's wish to remain creative and unconventional at the price of staying ill.

The antagonism characteristic of twins can be dampened by making things even. For a twin's hostility arises to a great extent from his fantasy that he is but half a person deprived of his double, the other twin who is similar to him. In the play, this preoccupation with doubles and a desire to keep things even are prominent. Alan gets Dr. Dysart to answer his questions like a patient, thus placing them on a more or less equal plane. The treatment at this point consists of the two taking turns questioning each other.

The twinlike interest in doubles openly appears twice during the play. The reader will recall the jingle that fascinates Alan: "Double your pleasure / Double your fun . . ." (pp. 26, 27). We also learn that one determinant of Alan's interest in horses is the existence of the double U in the word "equus." It may be suspected that an unconscious pun has manifested itself here, a twinlike image of two adjacent "you's."

Twinship again appears in Alan's imagined fusion with Equus as he rides the horse. In addition to a heterosexual imagery in the centaurlike state, we may suspect, in accordance with psychoanalytic observations, the existence of fantasies of fusion derived from early infantile desires for symbiotic union with the mother. However, we are emphasizing the twin-imagery of fusion which appears intertwined with the other fantasies.

Twins, we have seen, unconsciously feel that they were originally a single organism but were later split in two. They wish to join together once more to undo the loss of half a body as a result of the division. The fantasy of fusion may be sexualized, as in *Equus*, but in any case it defends the individual against the fury at those involved in the imagined deprivation, usually his sibling and his mother. Fused and one again, Alan is joyous and complete. He shrieks: "I want to be *in* you! I want to BE you forever and ever!—*Equus, I love you*! Now!—Bear me away! Make us One Person" (p. 85) or again, "Two shall be one" (p. 76).

Amadeus

Peter Shaffer has observed that *Amadeus* (1980) contains the elements of an opera, featuring arias, duets, a trio, and a quintet (Schoenberg, 1980). The play starts with a duet. Two men called Venticelli, little winds, proclaim that they don't believe the rumors that Antonio Salieri killed

Wolfgang Amadeus Mozart. The Venticelli serve as gossipy fellows who gather information for Salieri throughout the drama, echo his sentiments, and at one point join the action by engaging in a sexual game with Mozart's fiancée. They dress, behave, and talk similarly, but wear different colored clothes, one in brown, the other in blue or gray. These Doppelgänger figures announce that once again Peter Shaffer has utilized the imagery of twinship to further his dramatic display.

But the prime pair in *Amadeus* are the antagonists, Salieri and Mozart. Salieri at thirty-two is Court Composer to Joseph II, Emperor of Austria; Mozart, the former child prodigy, now twenty-five and newly arrived at court, is a threat to the musical establishment. When Salieri recognizes Mozart's genius compared to his own mediocrity, he berates God in an impassioned speech. Salieri says he had made a pact with God, that he had agreed to be virtuous in return for God's blessing him with musical ability and success (p. 8). God in fact had rewarded the Court Composer with fame and financial success despite his second-rate music, but the appearance of Mozart underlines Salieri's mediocrity and outrages him. It is unfair that Mozart, a socially inept, sniveling, childlike creature, be beloved of God and blessed with genius. For this inequity, Salieri plans revenge on God, and Mozart will be its chief vehicle. He would like to kill his rival, but instead determines to sabotage his career, prevent him from earning a living, keep his compositions from being widely played, and thus drive him to a pauper's grave. He will also seek vengeance by seducing Mozart's wife, Constanze, and by renouncing his own virtuous behavior. "From this time," he shouts at God, "we are enemies. . . . To my last breath I will *block* You on earth as far as I am able" (p. 47). Salieri, doomed to appreciate Mozart's music, envies him his ability to write masterpieces. He pretends to side with and guide Mozart as he proceeds to destroy him, but sometimes finds himself feeling affection and pity for the young man, and guilt over his own vengeful acts.

Mozart is in fact an infantile genius. His speech abounds with anal remarks and playful redundancies ("Paws-claws—paws-claws—paws-claws," on p. 16, for instance). He calls Salieri's latest opera "dog shit. Dried dog shit" (p. 32). He playfully beats his wife and loves to have her hit him, preferably on the buttocks. He is also a womanizer who seduces his pupils—as well as Salieri's star student, Katherina, a beautiful girl whom the Court Composer wishes to seduce himself but, because of his moral scruples, cannot. Mozart characterizes Salieri's music as that of a man who "can't get it up" (p. 37).

As part of his revenge, Salieri takes on Mozart's immorality. First he tries to seduce Constanze, but is shy and inept. (Here he is like Mozart in his lack of social graces.) Finding the sexual act with Constanze repulsive, he does not consummate it. But after failing with Frau Mozart, he succeeds with Katherina and she becomes his mistress.

The revenge continues. Salieri keeps Mozart from obtaining the students he needs to sustain himself financially. Salieri tries unsuccessfully to deter the first production of the *Marriage of Figaro*, but is successful in preventing the repeated performance it deserves. Mozart, for his part, had a love-hate relationship with his father and depended on him for guidance. When his father dies, Mozart turns to Salieri as a replacement (as twins turn to their siblings for comfort and love). Salieri rewards him with bad advice by agreeing with Mozart to reveal the secrets of the Freemasons in "The Magic Flute." As a result, he loses their economic and moral support.

Mozart is in despair. He is ill, he takes to drink, he cannot support himself and his wife. In his unheated apartment, he composes a final Requiem Mass commemorating his own death. Salieri appears masked, dressed both as a man who has requisitioned the Mass and as a messenger of death who examines Mozart's composition.

> [*He tears off a corner of the music paper, elevates it in the manner of the Communion Service, places it on his tongue and eats it.*]
> [*In pain*] I eat what God gives me. Dose after dose. For all of life. His poison. We are both poisoned, Amadeus. I with you; you with me. [p. 88]

As Mozart removes Salieri's mask, the elder musician identifies himself. "*Ecco mi.* Antonio Salieri. Ten years of my hate have poisoned you to death" (p. 88). Having thus revealed his identification with Mozart—both men are figuratively poisoned—and his wish to be rid of him, Salieri watches Mozart as the latter plays with him as if Salieri were his father. Mozart says: "Papa . . . Papa . . . Take me, Papa. Take me. Put down your arms and I'll hop into them. Just as we used to do it! . . . Let's sing our little kissing song together . . ." (p. 89).

Although Shaffer makes it clear that Salieri, consumed with guilt for his "murder" and pity for his victim, attempted suicide many years later, in 1823, his attempt in the play follows quickly on the heels of Mozart's death. This is reminiscent of the announcement of Pizarro's death in *The Royal Hunt of the Sun*, shortly after Atahualpa dies, even though in actuality the Spaniard died years later.

In addition to the appearance of the Venticelli as secondary but prominent twinlike figures, the interaction between the protagonists, Salieri and Mozart, suggests that once again Peter Shaffer has utilized his personal twin experience in the production of a compelling drama.

The two men are similar. Both are musicians. Both have difficulty in sustaining an adult genitality in the psychoanalytic sense. Derivatives of orality, anality, and a playful sadomasochism pervade Mozart's character, while Salieri is seen as a gluttonous, orally fixated man enthralled by delicacies of taste and tongue. He loves Veronese biscuits, Milanese macaroons, and snow dumplings with pistachio sauce (p. 7). Although Mozart is a womanizer and seducer, his phallic sexuality suggests immaturity. He says that Salieri writes like a man who "can't get it up" (p. 37), but one suspects that without pregenital aids he too would face difficulties of penile performance. Aside from his musical sublimation, which is beyond suspicion, Mozart's behavior is now maladaptive. He is maladroit socially, offends people, loses friends, can't achieve an adequate income or control expenditures. He looks to his father for guidance and strength, but cannot abide by his advice and hates his beloved parents; his mother does not appear as a potent person in the play.

Salieri, by contrast, is the practical, achieving man. But he too has his social deficiencies. As revealed in the scene with Constanze, he is shy, clumsy, and unoriginal in his lovemaking as well as in his music. Salieri's characterization of himself as "clumsy" (p. 43), a word that can easily apply to his opponent, is a key adjective. The contrasts between the two men override their similarities. Mozart is much more inept socially and financially, but overwhelmingly superior musically.

Like twins each envies the other, but Salieri's envy dominates the play. Mozart recognizes his own genius, but feels it unjust that Salieri has pupils and position. Like a twin, Salieri rails against his Creator for the unfair division of abilities. Instead of accusing his parents, he accuses God the Father of causing the inequity. He hates both his rival, Mozart, and God, against whom he seeks revenge through his rival. His hatred for Mozart is thinly disguised: Salieri claims that Mozart is simply the vehicle for his attack on God.

Twinlike hatred for his antagonist comes in conflict with his love, admiration, and pity. He identifies with Mozart. Both, he says, are poisoned by God. His desired union with Mozart is a bit more disguised than is Alan Strang's desire for union with Equus and Dr. Dysart's desire to possess Alan's traits. Salieri ingests the pages of Mozart's Requiem as if it were a communion wafer representing God. He attempts by suicide (albeit failed) to reproduce Mozart's fate in himself, murdering himself as he had killed Mozart. And earlier in the play he had taken on certain of Mozart's less desirable traits, giving up morality and becoming a womanizer of sorts.

Not that all is twinship, however. Mozart's oedipal involvement with

Salieri is apparent. The younger man wishes to possess the powers of the older man, and does indeed seduce the woman Salieri loves. After Mozart's father dies, he turns to Salieri as a substitute parent and advisor. In the end he imagines himself playing infantile games with Salieri as Papa. Mozart, as noted, turns to Salieri as a bereft or deprived twin turns to his sibling for comfort, love, and nurture.

The protagonists' oedipal involvement is suspect in that what we see primarily is the older man's envy and jealousy of the younger, a reverse oedipal configuration more typical of the rivalry of an older sibling with a newly arrived younger one. The oedipal wishes thus bear the mark of twinship.

The Salieri and Mozart of *Amadeus*, then, display many of the traits of twins: an increasing similarity as the play progresses; mutual identification; complementary characteristics; mutual envy with associated rage at the "twin" and parent (or surrogate) held responsible for inequities; guilt over the aggressive intent to the alter ego and confusion of self- and object-representation. The preoccupation with halves and doubles is manifest for the most part not in the protagonists but in the repeated appearance of the Venticelli. At one point, however, Mozart does say to Constanze: "I will bite you in half with my fangs-wangs! My little Stanzerl-wanzerl-banzerl" (p. 16). (Perhaps Mozart's rhyming penchant also connotes an interest in doubles.) At another point, Salieri sets the stage by saying, "The Place is Vienna. The year—to begin with—1871. The age still that of the Enlightenment: that clear time before the guillotine fell in France and *cut all our lives in half*" (p. 9; italics added).

There are other manifestations of twinship in Peter Shaffer's plays in addition to the personalities of the protagonists, the interaction of the characters, and the author's preoccupation with doubles and halves. That Peter Shaffer wrote two "double bills"—*White Lies* and *Black Comedy; The Private Ear* and *The Public Eye*—suggests yet another variant of the twin theme. And in *Black Comedy*, a fascinating reversal occurs. Whenever it is supposed to be dark, as when the lamps are off, the stage is bright; when the audience understands that it is light, the stage is pitch black. As if they understood that this reversal signifies the complementary wishes of twins, the publishers have printed BLACK COMEDY twice on the cover of the paperback edition: a white mirror image as well as a proper red rendition of the title (see Glenn, 1974b.)

Every author uses his own personal experience to make his philosophical statements come alive and move the audience or to enhance the entertainment he intends (Baudry, 1979; Greenacre, 1957; Glenn, 1974c;

Meyer, 1972). But how specifically does the existence of disguised twins in these plays stir the viewers and arouse their emotions?

We know of the tremendous appeal of twins to most of us. We are fascinated by them and often harbor a conscious or unconscious wish to be a twin. Through being a twin, one imagines he can possess the added power of double strength or the ability to trick adversaries. Twins as a team, we imagine, are more impervious to harm; if one is destroyed another identical being survives. Fantasied twinship also appeals to our narcissism in that the double, the mirror image, unconsciously represents the mother of our infancy, with whom we felt fused (Brody, 1952). The twin in disguise may be unconsciously identified not as a twin, but simply as a double. In either case, the appearance of hidden twins stirs unconscious resonances of persisting childhood wishes and related defensive maneuvers.

The emotions aroused may also reflect the intensity of the author's feeling about certain issues, such as his sibling and oedipal rivalry. Further, the presence of disguised twins can provide for the audience a fresh defensive stance. The audience may be more capable of tolerating the strength of oedipal feelings, for instance, when they are softened and concealed within the twinship theme.

An essential ingredient of creativity is the author's capacity to regress as he works (Kris, 1952) and to facilitate a complementary regression in his audience. Many twins, having undergone unusual gratification intermixed with frustration in childhood, find themselves easily capable of regression followed by "snapping back" to more mature functioning (Glenn, 1966, 1974c).

Members of an audience do not react identically, of course. In many good dramas, the author appeals to a broad spectrum of human emotions and fantasies. For some people a large variety of unconscious emotions reverberate. For others a narrow range, perhaps consisting only of oedipal feelings or sadomasochistic propensities, is engaged. The plays discussed succeed in evoking narcissistic concerns, desires for power, feelings of rivalry with siblings and parents, heterosexual and homosexual wishes, and oedipal and sadomasochistic urges. As Aristotle has observed, the audience purges itself of pity and terror. The author also offers means of mastery and new solutions (Barchillon, 1971), not only through the primitive unconscious core that is stirred, but also through the author's conscious philosophical intent. The audience perceives its own defensive and adaptive mechanisms, and appreciates those of the author and his creations, without necessarily being aware of what moves it.

REFERENCES

Abraham, H.C. (1953), Twin relationship and womb fantasy in a case of anxiety hysteria. *Internat. J. Psycho-Anal.*, 45:219–227.

Arlow, J.A. (1960), Fantasy systems in twins. *Psychoanal. Quart.*, 29:175–199.

Barchillon, J. (1971), A study of Camus' mythopoetic tale, *The Fall*, with some comments about the origin of esthetic feelings. *J. Amer. Psychoanal. Assn.*, 19:193–240.

Baudry, F.D. (1979), On the problems of inference in applied analysis: Flaubert's *Madame Bovary*. *The Psychoanalytic Study of Society*, 8:331–358, eds. W. Muensterberger & L.B. Boyer. New Haven: Yale University Press.

Brody, M.W. (1952), The symbolic significance of twins in dreams. *Psychoanal. Quart.*, 21:172–180.

Burlingham, D.T. (1952), *Twins: A Study of Three Pairs of Identical Twins*. New York: International Universities Press.

Cronin, H.J. (1933), An analysis of neurosis of identical twins. *Psychoanal. Rev.*, 20:375–387.

Demarest, E.W., & Winestine, M.C. (1955), The initial phase of concomitant treatment of twins. *The Psychoanalytic Study of the Child*, 10:336–352. New York: International Universities Press.

Gardner, G.E., & Rexford, E.N. (1952), Retardation of ego development on a pair of identical twins. *Quart. J. Child Behavior*, 4:367–381.

Gifford, S., et al. (1966), Differences in individual development within a pair of identical twins. *Internat. J. Psycho-Anal.*, 47:261–268.

Glenn, J. (1966), Opposite sex twins. *J. Amer. Psychoanal. Assn.*, 14:736–759.

——— (1974a), Twins in disguise: a psychoanalytic essay on *Sleuth* and *The Royal Hunt of the Sun*. *Psychoanal. Quart.*, 43:288–302.

——— (1974b), Twins in disguise, II: content, form and style in plays by Anthony and Peter Shaffer. *Internat. Rev. Psycho-Anal.*, 1:373–381.

——— (1974c), Anthony and Peter Shaffer's plays: the influence of twinship on creativity. *American Imago*, 51:270–292.

——— (1976), Alan Strang as an adolescent: a discussion of Peter Shaffer's *Equus*. *Internat. J. Psychoanal. Psychotherapy*, 5:473–489.

——— & Glenn, S. (1968), The psychology of twins. In: *Supplement to Dynamics in Psychiatry*, ed. S.A. Karger. Athens, Greece.

Greenacre, P. (1957), The childhood of the artist. *The Psychoanalytic Study of the Child*, 12:47–72. New York: International Universities Press.

Hartmann, H. (1934–1935), Psychiatric studies of twins. In: *Essays on Ego Psychology*. New York: International Universities Press, 1964.

Herbert, I., ed. (1977), *Who's Who in the Theatre*. 16th ed. London: Pitman.

Joseph, E.D. (1959), An unusual fantasy in a twin with an inquiry into the nature of fantasy. *Psychoanal. Quart.*, 28:189–206.

——— (1961), Report on panel: the psychology of twins. *J. Amer. Psychoanal. Assn.*, 9:158–166.

——— (1975), Psychoanalysis—science and research: twin studies as a paradigm. *J. Amer. Psychoanal. Assn.*, 23:3–31.

——— & Tabor, J.H. (1961), The simultaneous analysis of a pair of identical twins and the twinning reaction. *The Psychoanalytic Study of the Child*, 16:275–299. New York: International Universities Press.

Karpman, B. (1953), Psychodynamics in a fraternal twinship relation. *Psychoanal. Rev.*, 40:243–267.

Klein, D.A. (1979), *Peter Shaffer*. Boston: Twayne.

Kris, E. (1952), *Psychoanalytic Explorations in Art*. New York: International Universities Press.

Lacombe, P. (1959), The problem of the identical twin as reflected in a masochistic compulsion to cheat. *Internat. J. Psycho-Anal.*, 40:6–12.

Leonard, M.R. (1961), Problems in identification and ego development in twins. *The Psychoanalytic Study of the Child*, 16:300–320. New York: International Universities Press.

Lidz, T., et al. (1962), Ego differentiation and schizophrenic symptom formation in identical twins. *J. Amer. Psychoanal. Assn.*, 10:74–90.

Maenchen, A. (1968), Object cathexis in a borderline twin. *The Psychoanalytic Study of the Child*, 23:438–456. New York: International Universities Press.

Mesnikoff, A.M., et al. (1963), Intrafamilial determinants of divergent sexual behavior in twins. *American Journal of Psychiatry*, 119:732–738.

Meyer, B.C. (1972), Some reflections on the contribution of psychoanalysis to biography. *Psychoanalysis and Contemporary Science*, 1:373–391.

Myers, P. (1976), *Notable Names in the American Theatre*. Clifton, N.J.: White.

Orr, D.W. (1941), A psychoanalytic study of a fraternal twin. *Psychoanal. Quart.*, 10:284–296.

Peto, A. (1946), Analysis of identical twins. *Internat. J. Psycho-Anal.*, 27:126–129.

Rank, O. (1925), *The Double*. Chapel Hill, N.C.: University of North Carolina Press, 1971.

Reilly, J.M., ed. (1980), *Twentieth Century Crime and Mystery Writers*. New York: St. Martin's Press.

Schoenberg, H. (1980), Mozart's world: from London to Broadway. *New York Times*, Section 2, pp. 1, 35 (Dec. 14).

Schwartz, A.U. (1973), Personal communication.

Shaffer, A. (1973), *Sleuth*. New York: Dodd, Mead.

——— (1979), *Murderer*. London/Boston: Marion Boyars.

Shaffer, P. (1973), *Equus*. New York: Avon Books (1975).

——— (1980), *Amadeus*. New York: Harper & Row.

Vinson, J., ed. (1977), *Contemporary Dramatists*. 2nd ed. London: St. James Press; New York: St. Martin's Press.

Wakeman, J., ed., (1975), *World Authors: 1950–1970*. New York: H.W. Wilson.

Wiedeman, G. (1973), Discussion of further observations on plays by twins, by J. Glenn at Psychoanalytic Association of New York, convention, March 1973.

... if you know whether a man is a decided monist or a decided pluralist, you perhaps know more about the rest of his opinions than if you give him any other name ending in *ist*. To believe in the one or in the many, that is the classification with the maximum number of consequences. . . . —*William James, 1907*

I will tell you the perfect truth, I have to fill a double place. I have to be my brother as well as myself.—*Henry James, 1875*

It is tempting in our individualistic culture to assume that we are all distinct psyches cut off irrevocably from each other by the unique constellation of qualities given us at birth. From this atomistic perspective, the skin forms the impenetrable boundary of person and the development of a unique personality is a given, a foreordained conclusion rather than an uncertain possibility. When we think of writers who are brothers, it seems natural to be drawn along by this idea. William James (1842–1910) was a psychologist and philosopher; Henry James (1843–1916), his next younger brother, was a novelist and playwright—both separate men of talent who happen to have been brothers. But to stop there obscures how tentative that admirable outcome was. If we do, we will fail to appreciate the immense difficulty the two brothers had establishing their psychological separateness from each other. Individuation, the process of differentiation from the general, collective

9

A Singular Life: Twinship in the Psychology of William and Henry James

HOWARD M. FEINSTEIN

psychology (in this case, a "twin" brother), was slow and painful. Both brothers nearly foundered in illness before taking separate directions and firming the boundaries between them. Indeed, for a time, they seemed like Siamese twins joined by their ailing backs and doomed to fused invalidism forever.

There were many elements in the James family atmosphere that discouraged psychological separateness. Henry James Sr. (1811–1882) was the "wild" son of a rich Albany merchant and banker. His rebellious youth had been a trial for his Calvinist father. His refusal to prepare for the law or some other lawful career, his radical theological ideas, and his alcoholism finally wore out the father's patience. He cut Henry off from his estate (estimated at three million dollars when he died in 1832) and consigned him, he thought, to work for the rest of his life to support his family. But Henry Sr. challenged his father yet one more time and broke the will. But the litigation took fourteen years, and before it was finished the seemingly invincible rebel broke down and became immobilized by anxiety, in 1844, at the age of thirty-three. He was cured by a Swedenborgian conversion, and describing and integrating that experience became the central preoccupation of the remainder of his leisured life. Raised in the shadow of these events, his son Henry would create a fictional oeuvre in which the threat of madness and the mystery surrounding inherited wealth were recurrent themes. As for William, the fear of inherited madness would both delay his marriage and shape his choice of career (Feinstein, 1977).

Henry Sr.'s eccentric ideology was by turns exceedingly liberal (anti-institutional, optimistic) and intensely conservative (emphasizing guilt over sin as the *sine qua non* of spiritual development). His confusing religious passions spun an immobilizing web around his sons even as he exhorted them toward salvation by following the God within (as he did). Mary James (1810–1882) supported her husband's ideas and dutifully moved the family from city to city and from country to country in search of an education for the children that would fulfill Henry Sr.'s utopian ideals. By 1860 (William was eighteen and Henry seventeen), the brothers had attended nine different schools in four different countries and had rarely stayed in one place for a full school year. Six years spent in Europe effectively cut them off from their American friends and forced them in upon each other. The three younger children (there were five in all, four sons and a daughter) tagged along to whichever destination seemed to meet William's educational needs and their father's whim. The other two boys, Garth and Robertson, were paired, as were William and Henry. They eventually fought in the Civil War, worked in the Midwest for the railroad, and married in tandem. Alice, like her brother Henry, never married and eventually made invalidism her career. Stimulating, privileged, yet erratic and unpredictable, the James family atmosphere subtly undermined independence.

As his father had feared, once he got his hands on his inheritance, Henry James Sr. never worked to support his family, though he wrote extensively as an amateur theologian and man of letters. In our culture, choosing a vocation can be an important step in establishing a separate identity. The James family undercut this individuating thrust between father and son and between brothers. When William came of age, he wanted to be a painter. William's talent for drawing was apparent from an early age. His brother Henry recalled, "As I catch W.J.'s image, from far back, at its most characteristic, he sits drawing and drawing, always drawing, . . . and not as with a plodding patience, which I think would less have affected me, but easily, freely, and, as who should say, infallibly . . ." (1913, p. 207). When William decided that the God within urged him toward painting, his father was deeply disappointed, urged science upon him instead, and after a heated exchange of letters reluctantly agreed to a trial of study with the painter William Morris Hunt in Newport, Rhode Island. The experiment was short-lived, barely six months in all. Henry Sr.'s fainting spells in Newport subtly threatened that should William persist it would kill him (Feinstein, 1977, pp. 226–233). William abruptly gave in to his father's wish and entered the Lawrence Scientific School at Harvard in 1861. Once he started preparing for a scientific career, William complained of vague illnesses that necessitated long breaks in his studies for rest and treatment as he inched toward an M.D. degree, which he finished in 1869.

Illness was to serve from then on as a lens that focused the family's conflicts over individuation. For William and Henry Jr., sickness would become both an expression of the psychological connectedness between them and a means of breaking free of that tie. Near the end of their lives it would serve once again to reaffirm their fraternal bond.

The brothers' ill health was nurtured by their parents, who were ambivalent about work and convinced of the value of leisure. There was never any doubt where their father stood on the matter. Typical is the following: "I am determined. . . ," he told his friend J.J. Garth Wilkinson in 1852, "to take holiday for the rest of my life [he was forty-one] and make all my work sabbatical, and expressive only of irrepressive inward health and impulsions" (Perry, 1935, vol. 1, p. 23). Though he applied himself steadfastly to his literary labors, he maintained a lifelong suspicion of the dangers of too much work. Mary James, following her husband's lead (as she did in most intellectual matters), shared this suspicion. When William was abroad and undertook to write some reviews for publication as a gesture of self-support, she lamented, "I fear he is working himself to death to meet his expenses . . ." (Mrs. Henry James Sr. to Alice James, Jan. 14, 1870, ms. [Harvard]). Of William's friend Oliver Wendell Holmes Jr., she remarked:

> His whole life, soul and body, is utterly absorbed in his *last* work upon his Kent. He carries about his manuscript in his green bag and never loses sight of it for a moment. . . . His pallid face and this fearful grip upon his work, makes him a melancholy sight. [Perry, 1935, vol. 1, p. 519]

A corollary to her belief in the dangers of overwork was Mrs. James's conviction that physical exertion should be avoided by her frail sons. Thus, to Henry, who was enjoying an exhilarating walking trip in the Alps, she cautioned: "you might easily over estimate your strength and sink down with sudden exhaustion . . ." (Mrs. Henry James Sr. to Henry James Jr., Aug. 8, 1869, ms. [Harvard]). Again to Henry, who was this time enjoying horseback riding in Rome and finding it salutary: "Do not run any risks darling Harry, by staying too long in Rome, and do not overdo the horseback exercise" (Mrs. Henry James Sr. to Henry James Jr., April 1, 1873, ms. [Harvard]).

The parents were convinced that human energy was scarce, had to be expended parsimoniously, and was easily exhausted. Scarcity rather than abundance, weakness instead of strength, ill health rather than health was their natural expectation. Their sons learned the lesson well.

William made the energy-supply problem explicit in a letter to a friend. "How I envy you your fund of energy. I have a little spoonful ready for each day and when that's out, as it usually is by 10 o'clock A.M., I'm good for nothing" (Perry, 1935, vol. 1, p. 373). Henry spoke in those terms too. In Europe, enjoying a vigorous grand tour in search of health, he feared that the hot Italian summer would deplete his energy. "I have laid in such a capital stock of strength and satisfaction in Switzerland," he wrote, "that I shall be sorry to be compelled to see it diminished and if I find it is melting away beneath the southern sun I shall not scruple . . . to cross over from Verona into southern Germany . . ." (Edel, 1953, p. 131). Both brothers obviously adhered to their parents' view of limited energy.

Mary James shared her husband's belief that work was dangerous to health and cultivated that attitude in her children. Yet she operated under different laws herself. An 1873 letter to William, for example, reads like a list of wounded from the front. She reported the current status of "our invalids"—Alice, "poor child," had one of her fainting attacks "from a little overexertion"; father had an attack of eczema of the face [apparently Herpes Zoster or "shingles"] and is "nervous and sleepless"; Aunt Kate "is progressing slowly" under Dr. Munro's care and "certainly bears well much more fatigue." But Mary, like a surviving heroine surveying the slain minions strewn about her, proclaimed, "The poor old mater wears well I am happy to say; strong in the back, strong in the nerves, and strong in the legs so far, and equal to her day" (Edel, 1953, p. 44).

Her strength and endurance were the more remarkable when repeatedly juxtaposed to the weaknesses of the boys. William reported that sickness did not keep *her* from her household tasks: "Mother is recovering from one of her indispositions, which she bears like an angel, doing any amount of work at the same time, putting up cornices and raking out the garret-room like a little buffalo" (1920, vol. 1, p. 80). Others were expected to be short of energy but Mary remained stalwart and ever ready to shoulder her caretaking tasks.

Though work was unappealing to the Jameses, pleasure was also suspect. Sabbatarian scruples over game playing or singing would have been unthinkable in Mr. James's liberal household. Yet they showed a subtle lack of hospitality for pleasure. This attitude also nurtured the brothers' illnesses. Work that is supposed to be sabbatical and leisure that is supposed to be uplifting both require money. No matter how extensive the resources of a family, if it shared a distrust of pleasure and leisure, money could not easily be spent on traveling for amusement. It was far simpler to justify travel for reasons of health. The elder Henry had been amply provided for by his inheritance (his income was about $10,000 a year), but numerous family trips abroad had cut into his capital. Furthermore, he had invested heavily in a Florida plantation which employed hired black labor and was run by his two younger sons. With its failure, although the family was still well off, there was no longer enough money to maintain parents and children in leisured extravagance. Between 1866 and 1873 sickness became a means by which William and Henry struggled for a lion's share of the family resources.

If both wanted to go abroad but there was only money enough for one, then surely the sicker of the two should go. If both were equally ill, then the one who had most recently had his turn at the cure should remain behind. When abroad, if he responded too quickly to the benefits of the cure, or seemed to be enjoying himself too much, then his travel might be cut short because it was using limited family resources for pleasure while others required "treatment." Both Henry and Mary James kept a sharp eye on the letters written by their traveling invalid children to monitor expenditures and healthful returns.

It is against this background of ambivalence about work, and political maneuvering for financial support for leisure, that we can appreciate William's excited announcement to his friend Tom Ward in September 1867 (he was then twenty-four and had fled from medical school to Europe for the cure). "I don't know whether you have heard or not that I found myself last November, *almost* without perceptible exciting cause, in possession of that delightful disease in my back, which has so long made Harry so interesting" (Perry, 1935, vol. 1, p. 244).[1] The announcement to Ward was intended to explain the reason for his 1867 flight to Europe. It was also a declaration by this ever self-aware young man that *his* illness was connected with Harry's illness in a puzzling manner. "It is evidently a family peculiarity," was all that he could make of it. He could not see, as we can more easily with the clarity that time provides, that his back problem was the latest in a long series of events confirming an especially close fraternal bond.

In later years, when he described William's illness in his autobiography, Henry James, the novelist, confirmed that tie by moving effortlessly and imperceptibly from "he" to "us." The reader was thereby invited to share in the belief that, save for grammatical usage, there was really no separation between them. He remembered "a sharp lapse of health on my brother's part which the tension of a year at the dissecting table seemed to have done much to determine; as well as the fond fact that Europe was again from that crisis forth to take its place *for us* as a standing remedy, a regular mitigation of all suffered, or at least of all wrong, stress" (1914, p. 444; italics added). In the immediacy of the event as well as in the recollections of old age, William and Henry saw illness as a confirmation of their brotherly attachment.

The fraternal bond was of long standing, having been fostered by closeness in age, shared aesthetic interests, and the constant deracination of their childhood. In play, in school, and in family life, William was followed by his admiring younger brother. Henry wanted to be with him and to be like him. But much to his chagrin, William was "always round the corner and out of sight" (1913, p. 9). This closeness was intensified by their shared fate as the earliest subjects for father's educational experiments. Henry characterized them himself as a mythological twinship. They were, he recalled, "a defeated Romulus, a prematurely sacrificed

---

[1] Though William identified his "interesting" disease of the back as a link between himself and Harry, he was not entirely accurate in naming him as the first to suffer with this "family peculiarity." In 1856, Mary James wrote to her mother-in-law about back trouble that had begun to plague the elder Henry. "The effort he has made in walking for so many years has occasioned a weakness in his back which at times gives him great trouble" (Mrs. Henry James Sr. to Catherine Barber James, August 25, 1856, ms. [Harvard]).

Remus," served up to their father's radical educational program (1913, p. 221). Where William went, Henry followed, albeit in the shadows. William's artistic talents declared themselves first; and here, as in so many other areas, Henry imitatively tried his hand. "The gratification nearest home was the imitative, the emulative—that is on my part," Henry recalled. "W.J. drew because he would, while I did so in the main only because he did . . ." (1913, p. 264). When William studied with Hunt, so did Henry. When William moved to Cambridge, Henry soon followed to attempt a Harvard degree as well.

In Europe with the family in the 1850s, they had mined the treasures of the museums together and learned to depend on each other for an attentive ear and an appreciative eye. Shared aesthetic sensibility deepened their sense of "we-ness." Again this is made clear in the younger brother's autobiographical recollections, which consistently link them as a pair. They liked Benjamin R. Haydon (English painter, 1786–1846) because he pointed to something that "*we* could do, or at least want to do. . . . *We* found in these works remarkable interest and beauty. . . . The very word Pre-Raphaelite . . . thrills *us* in its perfection. . . . *We* were not yet aware of style, though on the way to become so . . ." (1913, pp. 314, 315, 345; italics added). In old age, when the division between them had been effected, recognized by the world, and praised, it was easier to say that William was meant for science and Henry for art. But in the searching time of youth, they were aesthetic twins and it was unclear whether they would go on yoked in that twinship and become artists in tandem.[2]

As in so many other fields of fraternal endeavor up to that time, William was the first to fall ill. As indicated, his nervous symptoms began when he entered the Lawrence Scientific School in September 1861. Henry injured his back at the end of October, less than two months later. When the doctor found no organic cause for his back pain, Henry followed William to Cambridge and tried a year at Harvard Law School. Though unsuited to his talents, it justified leisured study. In their twenties, a subtle change took place in the balance of the fraternal relationship. While William reluctantly pursued science, Henry wrote fiction and succeeded in getting his works published. When their parents moved to Boston, both brothers lived with them, and there was ample opportunity for William to observe how efficiently Henry's back problem protected literate leisure. William's frail health justified intermittent withdrawal from

[2] Leon Edel has emphasized the rivalrous aspects of the twin theme. I am interested in a different psychological problem, individuation. See Edel (1953), pp. 240–252. For a modern instance of psychological fusion in identical twins see Wolfe (1975).

scientific study, but Henry's back made it possible to spend full time pursuing his art.

Henry wrote of his activities as an invalid variously to his correspondents as "eating of the lotus to repletion, . . . loafing and talking aesthetics all day," or the "pursuit of a dreary hygienic course of no work," depending upon his mood (1974, pp. 60, 68). But it was plain for all to see that illness secured a path for him that his brother's open rebellion of 1859 had failed to sustain. He didn't expose himself, as William had, to a direct confrontation with his father over art. Perhaps he had learned from his older brother's failure. Gradually the balance between them shifted and, as Henry gained strength and competence as an artist, he became the leader of the pair. It was William's turn to recede into the shadows.

William's back problem emphasized his kinship with Henry. It also afforded him an opportunity while abroad to revive the aesthetic interests they had once shared. On the surface, it appeared that he had put an ocean between them when he fled from Harvard Medical School in 1867, but his letters emphasized how much one brother was always in the other's consciousness. Harry was a wished-for or imagined witness to William's aesthetic revival. Delight in the Parisian theater prompted the exclamation, "Dear Brother, how much I would have given to have you by my side so that we might rejoice together" (Perry, 1935, vol. 1, p. 236). While enjoying the peaceful, cultivated landscape around Dresden he confided, "I have wished so often . . . that Harry might be here for an hour at a time just to refresh himself with a sight of something new . . ." (p. 241). Harry should "read Goethe's Faust—it is a good piece . . ."; Harry would want to read Balzac's *Modeste Mignon*; Harry would understand his feelings reading that "imperturbable old heathen Homer" (p. 268). Fresh from viewing Titian and Veronese he pined, "I'd give a good deal to import you and hear how some of the things strike you . . ." (p. 267). The older brother obviously missed the younger as he rattled the door to art which he had closed seven years earlier.

William was well aware that Harry wanted to be in Europe too. He had managed to acquire Harry's "interesting" infirmity, and was abroad because of it enjoying the aesthetic stimulation that Harry craved. Harry was miffed. Rather than acknowledging William's literary or artistic acumen, he irritatedly fastened on one of William's hortatory asides. "Don't try to make out that America and Germany are identical and that it is as good to be here as there. . . . Only let me go to Berlin and I will say as much." To underscore the point and prick the fraternal conscience, he added, "Life here in Cambridge—or in this house, at least—is about as lively as the inner sepulchre" (Perry, 1935, vol. 1, p. 251).

It was not his style to fight openly with his brother, but the very symptom that enabled William to get to Europe ahead of him provided the opportunity for Henry to strike back.

He knew William believed the illness they shared would follow the same course. Since Henry's back gave way first, it was assumed that changes in his back foreshadowed changes in William's, improvement or decline in one to be followed by improvement or decline in the other. So Henry spitefully minimized the improvement of his health (it had already been described to William by other family correspondents). "I am no worse but my health has ceased to increase so steadily, as it did during the summer. It is plain that I shall have a very long row to hoe before I am fit for anything—for either work or play." Ever mindful of what he was doing—and both of them were often penetratingly aware—he denied his intent. "I mention this not to discourage you—for you have no right to be discouraged, when I am not myself— . . ." (1974, p. 80).

Whether Harry saw William's back problem as imitation or shared fate is not clear. But he could not avoid noticing that this once admired older brother was trying to copy his early individuating success as a writer. And to make matters worse, William entreated him to provide editorial assistance and rescue him from idle diffusion. If Harry had drawn because William could, why shouldn't William write because Harry could? William announced the project in a letter: "The other day, as I was sitting alone with my deeply breached letter of credit, beweeping my outcast state, and wondering what I could possibly do for a living, it flashed across me that I might write a 'notice' of H. Grimm's novel which I had been reading." He felt inadequate compared with his younger brother, and complained that he had no facility as an author. After "sweating fearfully for three days, erasing, tearing my hair, copying, recopying, etc.; etc.," he passed his work on to Harry for judgment. "I want you to read it, and if, after correcting the style and thoughts . . . and rewriting it if possible, . . . send it to the *Nation* or the *Round Table*" (Perry, 1935, vol. 1, p. 245). The review was published, as were five others written during William's 1867–1868 stay in Europe. Henry dutifully proofread copy for him. It is emblematic of his vocational indecision that his first effort was not a scientific paper but an aesthetic review, edited and rewritten by his already accomplished literary brother. In his uncertainty, William scrambled to keep pace with Harry and to obscure the separation the younger brother had been patiently trying to effect.

The mutual sympathy represented by their shared symptomatology at times degenerated into name-calling. Each accused the other of feigning illness, of "imagining" himself to be physically ill. And when accused,

each insisted on his sincerity and the dismal state he endured. William
was the first to admit his suspicions. Full of the latest medical wisdom,
which he had crammed in preparing for his exams, he "reluctantly" prof-
ferred his considered opinion. "The condition of your back is totally incomprehensible to me. . . . My diagnosis of it now wd. be simply dorsal
insanity" (William James to Henry James Jr., June 12, 1869, ms. [Har-
vard]).

Henry's turn to accuse his "twin" of feigning would come four years
later. By then his separate course was clear. He was in good health and
no longer needed the symptoms that William held to so tenaciously. His
accusation can be inferred from William's pained retort. "I don't know
whether you still consider my ailments to be imagination and humbug
or not, but I know myself that they are as real as any one's ailments ever
were, and that with the exception of my eyes [he had had a weakness of
the eyes since 1865 that made it hard to read medicine though they
worked well enough for philosophy and literature] which can now be used
4 hours a day the improvement I have made in 12 months is very
slight . . ." (William James to Henry James Jr., May 25, 1873, ms. [Har-
vard]). Four years earlier, Henry had been far less secure.

When he first went abroad in 1869, Henry's back still ached and provided the necessary justification for dipping into his father's inheritance.
Henry was adept at his invalidism. When he seemed to be enjoying
himself too much in Europe, he had been criticized by his Cambridge-
bound parents. He wrote a defense to his father, whose side of the exchange can be inferred from the son's remarks.

> To have you think that I am extravagant with these truly sacred
> funds sickens me to the heart, and I hasten in so far as I may to
> reassure you. When I left Malvern, I found myself so exacerbated
> by immobility and confinement that I felt it to be absolutely due
> to myself to test the impression which had been maturing in my
> mind, that a certain amount of regular lively travel would do me
> more good than any further repose. As I came abroad to try and get
> better, it seemed inexcusable to neglect a course which I believed
> for various reasons to have so much in its favor. . . . [1974, p. 115]

Having made show of concern for limited funds and the evils of idle
pleasure, Henry deftly concluded that what he needed for *really* good
health was *more* pleasurable travel. "I have now an impression amounting
almost to a conviction that if I were to travel steadily for a year I would
be a good part of a well man" (p. 115).

Seven weeks later, he replied to a remonstrance against extravagance from his mother's pen. Here too he balanced carefully between accepting parental injunctions against pleasure and insisting upon his need, as one weak in body, to cater to the pleasures of the spirit. He wisely commended the plan for its utility in increasing his capacity to work:

> I duly noted your injunction to spend the summer quietly and economically. I hope to do both—or that is, to circulate in so far as I do, by the inexpensive vehicle of my own legs. When you speak of your own increased expenses, etc., I feel very guilty and selfish in entertaining any projects which look in the least like extravagance. My beloved mother, if you but knew the purity of my motives! Reflection assures me, as it will assure you, that the only economy for me is to get thoroughly well and into such a state as that I can work. For this consummation, I will accept everything—even the appearance of mere pleasure-seeking. [1974, p. 124]

That Henry had learned well the puritanical judgment of selfishness and mere pleasure-seeking was clear. He had also learned that illness and the need for treatment made divine what might otherwise have been labeled diabolical, even in his parents' liberal household. Energy and capital flowed freely for healing, while the sluices shut decisively against pleasure and idleness. Henry wrote,

> When I think that a winter in Italy is not as you call it a winter of "recreation" but an occasion not only of physical regeneration, but of serious culture too (culture of the kind which alone I have now at twenty-six any time left for) I find the courage to maintain my proposition even in the face of your allusions to the need of economy at home. It takes a very honest conviction thus to plead the cause of apparently gross idleness against such grave and touching facts. I have trifled so long with my trouble that I feel as if I could afford now to be a little brutal. My lovely mother, if ever I am restored to you sound and serviceable you will find that you have not cast the pearls of your charity before a senseless beast, but before a creature with a soul to be grateful and a will to act. [1974, pp. 124–125]

A month later his mother reassured Henry that he could do what he wished. He was so successful at the politics of invalidism that he got her to apologize for having questioned his motives. The coffers were wide open, with Mary James urging Henry to let your "prudent old mother" take care of everything. She added:

> If you were only here for an hour, and we could talk over this subject

of expense, I could I know exorcise all these demons of anxiety and conscientiousness that possess you, and leave [you] free as air, to enjoy to the full all that surrounds you, and drink in health of body and of mind in following out your own safe and innocent attractions.

The only promise that she wished to extract was that henceforth he would "throw away prudence and think only of your own comfort and pleasure, for our sakes as well as your own" (Mrs. Henry James Sr. to Henry James Jr., July 24, 1869, ms. [Harvard]).

Henry's letters from Europe during 1869 also showed he was pulling against his ties to William. Soon after the crossing he wrote, "Has Willie felt my absence in any poignant—or rather any practical degree; if so—if he misses me round the room he mustn't scruple to send for me to return" (1974, p. 96). The offer could hardly have been serious, as he had barely arrived and was thoroughly enjoying himself in London. As his health improved, he generously extolled the fact, knowing that William would consider it a good omen. But there is a distinct sign of relief joined with a fraternal shove of "good riddance" in his query: "I am of course especially anxious to hear from Willy—as I hope he has by this time understood. Who in the world does his share and runs his errands and me over here? It's terrible to think" (1974, p. 105). When William announced a new program of rest from the study of science, Harry, as an expert on the back, gave his blessing: "I heartily applaud your resolution to lie at your length and abolish study. As one who has sounded the *replis* of the human back, I apprise that with such a course you cannot fail to amend" (1974, p. 113).

He served willingly as an observer for the pair, as William had done for him. He knew where William's heart was, and magnanimously met the need. "What you will care most to hear about is the painters . . . ," and he described them in lavish detail. Giotto's Chapel in Padua made him "long for the penetrating judgment and genial sympathy of my accomplished William" (1974, p. 146).

As much as he longed for William's presence, Henry was not about to rush back. He was determined to exploit illness-protected leisure to the hilt. "When you tell me of the noble working life that certain of our friends are leading, in that clear American air, I hanker woefully to wind up these straggling threads of loafing and lounging and drifting and to toss my ball with the rest." But, he resolved, "having waited so long I can wait a little longer" (1974, p. 186). Henry knew what he wanted to do far better than William. Although William's trip abroad served to forestall his scientific career, it failed to rescue his artist self. Henry, by contrast, pursued his development as an artist steadily. He alone would attain the goal that had once seemed a shared destiny. There was a sharp edge to his plea, "Envy me—if you can without hating!" (1974, p. 216). And there was a poignant note in the words that he would put in the mouth of Roderick Hudson in his first novel (1875). "I will tell you the perfect truth, I have to fill a double place. I have to be my brother as well as myself" (p. 47). In 1875, when that was written, the twins had been divided and Henry was the sole emergent artist of the pair.

But in 1869 conscience and illness did set limits on indulgence. In Italy for the first time, Henry found his body turning on him. Amid the sensual Italian feast, he became constipated to such a degree that intestinal obstruction was feared. Henry delicately alluded to the matter as "an old trouble." William seized upon the complaint and wrote graphically about it, sparing no details (William James to Henry James Jr., October 25, 1869, ms. [Harvard]). The affliction gave his Cambridge-bound brother a chance to confirm their bond once again.

Having himself the same complaint, he entered into Henry's bowel difficulties with the enthusiasm of a neophyte physician and the compassion of a fellow sufferer. And when he wrote, there were moments when he slipped imperceptibly from "I" to "you," the same sort of pronominal indifference seen in Henry's letters and so suggestive of the brothers' psychological fusion. "If it continues 3 months longer in spite of what Doctors can do for *you* in Italy *I* would post for Malverne again and see what England can do for *me*" (William James to Henry James Jr., November 1, 1869, ms. [Harvard]; italics added). The brothers traded remedies, but Henry never showed as intense an involvement with the subject as his psychological twin, who at times reached rhapsodic heights: "You can with difficulty conceive of the joy with which I received . . . the news of the temporary end of your moving intestinal drama. If I could believe it to be the beginning of *the* end the happiness wd. be almost *too* great. . . ." He evidently caught himself overdoing and stepped back with the remark, "I dare say you'll thank me at last for dropping the subject . . ." (William James to Henry James Jr., December 5, 1869, ms. [Harvard]).[3] The issue symbolized by stasis of the bowel was one of dis-

[3] It will be no surprise to those who have followed the logic of Erik Erikson's epigenetic scheme, which correlates organic modes with normal psychological crises, that this pair of talented young men who were so close, and yet who needed to become uniquely themselves, suffered from constipation. Concurrent with gaining sphincter control—the organically patterned task of the toddler—a child's developing ego will further separate him from a pre-

cipline vs. desire. William confirmed this in a characteristically hortatory exclamation to his brother: *"Never resist a motion to stool* no matter at what hour you may feel it. That is a *hauptsache* in the discipline of the gut" (William James to Henry James Jr., June 1, 1869, ms. [Harvard]). We can easily hear the psychologist of "Habit" in that brotherly advice. William had so thoroughly habituated himself to stifling his own desires out of filial obligation that he no longer was sure of the difference. If the division of the two brothers was to proceed, it was essential that desire be properly recognized and distinguished from self-deforming discipline if each was to become himself. Henry knew the difference. He wanted to be a writer and accepted the discipline of that craft. And the early stories that he wrote during this difficult period show how acutely aware he was of the pull of this psychological twinship and the need to disengage from it.

William could see the risk too, at least where *others* were concerned. In one of his brilliant epistolary vignettes written from Germany in 1860 he described two old ladies as a fused pair who

> have been so shut out from the world and have been melting to-
> gether so long by the kitchen fire that the minds of both have
> become confounded into one, and they seem to constitute a sort of
> two-bodied individual. I never saw anything more curious than the
> way in which they sit mumbling together at the end of the table,
> each using simultaneously the same exclamation if anything said at
> our end strikes their ear. . . . they always speak together, using the
> same words or else one beginning a phrase, the other ending it. It
> is a singular life. [Perry, 1935, vol. 1, p. 197]

But it is in the fiction of Henry James where one finds the twin rela-
tionship most thoroughly delineated and explored. The short stories are particularly revealing, because their brevity makes the author's intentions nakedly clear. Three will illustrate the point: "De Grey: A Romance" (1868), "The Romance of Certain Old Clothes" (1868), and "A Light Man"

viously imagined unity with his parent. The issue of autonomy, of dividing from significant others, meets its earliest heightened challenge coincident with and through control of the bowels.

As Erikson has pointed out, psychological issues recur in later stages of the life cycle. Earlier crises are constantly reopened and earlier solutions perpetually reworked. In young adulthood, which Erikson has labeled a time of identity formation, following one's will becomes a paramount issue once more. In a family context that has made separation difficult, it may have to be fought out symbolically, once again through controlling one's own stool. (See Erikson, 1968, pp. 107–114.)

(1869). They were written when the pull of the brothers' attachment was intense yet on the verge of being severed, as William opted reluctantly for science and Henry succeeded with art. An analysis of these tales reveals the younger brother's understanding of the bonds that tied him to the older and shows how urgently he wanted to break away from "the singular life."

Henry built the De Grey romance with familiar Jamesian elements: a family that "enjoyed great material prosperity," a father who acted in such a manner "as to incur the suspicion of insanity," and a family curse that casts a "shadow of mystery" over the household (H. James, 1973, pp. 277–278). Henry represents William through the character of Paul, George De Grey's son and heir, and characterizes himself as Margaret, a young woman living as a companion to Mrs. De Grey. (Though not consanguineous, the two stand functionally in a sibling relationship by having the same maternal protector.) Henry was brutally frank in his evaluation of George De Grey, the father of this family. His insane temperament and idleness made him "not to be wished . . . as an example" (p. 278). Paul, his son, was urged instead to select a career since "in America, in any walk of life, idleness was indecent . . ." (p. 279). Paul goes abroad and spends his time, like William, "roaming about Europe, in a vague, restless search for his future . . ." (p. 293). On his return, he and Margaret fall in love and activate the De Grey curse. For generations, the first passionate lover of a De Grey son has inexplicably fallen ill and died.

This story expresses an obvious fear of sexual passion, but even more important is the portrait of the sibling bond in the relationship between Paul and Margaret. Though they inhabit separate bodies, the boundary between them is vague. When Margaret cries out in terror, Paul hears her though miles away. When one is hurt, the other feels the pain. When Margaret is told of the curse, she courageously refuses to be separated from her brother/lover. But her challenge leads to disaster. Instead of preventing the curse she redirects it. Paul falls ill. "As she bloomed and prospered, he drooped and languished" (p. 306). At the end, Paul dies in spite of Margaret's brave attempt to save him. But she does not escape. She becomes insane. In concluding, James underlined this twin–shared body connection: "The sense had left her mind as completely as his body, and it was likely to come back to one as little as to the other."

Henry was obviously weighing the cost of his intense attachment to William. In "De Grey," he imaginatively posed the troublesome question, could he survive and still remain one with his brother? If he attempted to rescue his ailing twin, did it mean that both would fall prey to the curse of illness and insanity? Writing this story was a decisive step along his own literary path, yet in the tale he expressed his worry that he might condemn himself to paired invalidism with William's submerged artist self. If work output was any measure, Henry "bloomed and prospered" while William "drooped and languished" in the spas. Yet even though an ocean separated them, he winced when his twin cried out.

In "The Romance of Certain Old Clothes" (1973, pp. 210–226), Henry presents another view of their "singular life." With William abroad, thanks to Henry's back pain, writing tepid critical letters about Henry's writing, and imitatively composing reviews that he expected him to edit (not without complaint—"My *schriftstellersiches Selbstgefühl* [writer's sense of self] was naturally rather mangled by the mutilations you had inflicted on my keen article about Feydeau . . ." [Perry, 1935, vol. 1, p. 263]), Henry was furious. The pages of this romance bristle with barely concealed rage at an older sibling who wastes his opportunities in Europe or who usurps the life of the younger. William first appears in this tale as Bernard, a devalued older brother who was not very "clever," "the wit of the family" having been "apportioned chiefly to his [two younger] sisters" (1973, p. 210). While in Europe to study, Bernard accomplished very little ("without great honor") but did have "a vast deal of pleasure" (p. 211). Henry's portraits are so thinly disguised it is remarkable that the only comment William made on the story was to criticize its "trifling" quality (Perry, 1935, vol. 1, p. 264). The main action centers on the pair of sisters, Viola and Perdita. Though "dissimilar in appearance and character," they had "but one bed" and one objective—to marry the same man (1973, p. 213). Arthur Lloyd, a friend Bernard brought back from England (the family lives in Massachusetts like the Jameses), was a novel attraction that threatened to split the twins. Arthur chooses Perdita, the younger, and makes Viola bitterly jealous. She is chided by the triumphant Perdita, who declares, "Come, sister, . . . he couldn't marry both of us" (p. 216).

But as Henry crafted the story, that is exactly what happens. The singular life continues to the marriage bed, serially rather than coincidentally, but no matter. It is with the same husband. James also used the wearing of another's clothes as an emblem for usurping the other's life. He acknowledged that the older sister was more artistic and therefore more suited to the clothes (and the life) that in fact await the younger. He wrote that Viola had "the very best taste in the world," and when the cloth for the wedding gown arrived it matched her coloring better than the bride's. The bride-to-be admitted as much with a blend of cunning and innocence. "Blue's your colour, sister, more than mine. . . . It's a pity it's not for you. You'd know what to do with it" (p. 217). Indeed she did know what to do with it. Immediately after the wedding, Perdita is horrified to discover Viola wearing her wedding clothes. Following Perdita's death after childbirth, Viola takes her sister's place as Arthur's wife. But this undifferentiated twinship, like the love of Margaret and Paul in "De Grey," is destined for a violent end. Perdita's dying wish is to preserve some separateness for herself by preventing her rapacious older sister from wearing her clothes. She makes her husband promise that he will preserve them as a legacy for her daughter. Once again a legacy is a curse. When Viola forces her husband to give her the key and opens the chest, Perdita's avenging spirit murders her. Henry was unusually graphic and gothic in describing the corpse of the vanquished older sibling. "Her lips were parted in entreaty, in dismay, in agony; and on her bloodless brow and cheeks there glowed the marks of ten hideous wounds from two vengeful ghostly hands" (p. 226). Significantly, soon after the story was written, Henry ordered a suit made of the same cloth used by William's tailor before he went abroad (Edel, 1953, pp. 249–250).

"The Romance of Certain Old Clothes" can be read as an allegory of Henry's struggle to individuate from William. William may have had more artistic ability (better taste in clothes) and may have been intended for the artistic career they both desired (the cloth for the wedding gown was more Viola's color), but Henry was furious at William's attempt to usurp his place, to rob him of his triumph by becoming a successful writer (wearing the wedding clothes). As far as Henry was concerned, it was high time they stopped sharing the same bed! Or was it?

On the question of sexual identity, the romances are ambiguous in the extreme. What is to be made of the fact that Henry represents himself as a young woman in both? Or that he makes Viola resemble Shakespeare's heroine? (In *As You Like It*, Viola is a woman dressed as a man.) Or that the lover in "Old Clothes" is merely a pretext for displaying the attachment between two siblings of the same sex? It can be suggested that Henry James's early stories be read as the creation of a young artist who had become painfully aware of himself as a female consciousness masquerading in the body of a man. It is not surprising that the brothers' "singular life" blurred sexual distinctions between them. And it should come as no shock that in Henry's fictive world there is a strong homosexual strand in his bond to his brother William.[4]

---

[4] Richard Hall (1979) has called Leon Edel to task for leaving a "peculiar timidity" at the center of his monumental biography of Henry James. Hall quite rightly points to a tendency to "wash out the sexual content" of his analysis (particularly in the early volumes), in favor of the rivalrous theme and to thus obscure the fraternal incestuous strivings (whether acted upon or not) that were central to Henry's psychology. Following Edel, Hall believes that

In "A Light Man," Henry wrote a story that is so transparently homosexual (at times even pornographic) that it is a wonder it has escaped
wider critical notice. Where else in Henry James's works do we read of
one man saying of another, "How I should like to give him for once, a
real sensation!" (1973, p. 359)? And where else in the entire Jamesian
corpus do we watch as the orgasmic sensation is masterfully delivered,
man to man?

> The remainder of this extraordinary scene I have no power to de-
> scribe: . . . how I, prompted by the irresistible spirit of my desire
> to leap astride of his weakness, and ride it hard into the goal of my
> dreams, cunningly contrived to keep his spirit at the fever point,
> so that strength, and reason, and resistance should burn themselves
> out. I shall probably never again have such a sensation as I enjoyed
> to-night—actually feel a heated human heart throbbing, and turn-
> ing, and struggling in my grasp; know its pants, its spasms, its
> convulsions, and its final senseless quiescence. [p. 367]

The frank orgiastic eroticism is embedded in this story published in
1869, while Henry was abroad and deftly manipulating his parents to
keep the money flowing from his father's inheritance to support his traveling cure. The tale is built on James family history (a symbiotic sibship,
a weak father-figure) even as it augurs the shape of Henry's future erotic
life. From the outset gender is in question. The story's title plays on that
of the Robert Browning poem "A Light Woman," which alludes to a figure
who (like Shakespeare's Viola) is something other than she appears to her
lover.[5] The triangle in James's version, however, is all of one sex—male.
Also, as in the previous two stories, an inheritance plays an important
role. In fact, the orgiastic scene quoted was intended not to describe
homosexual intercourse but rather the effort of a ruthless young man
(Maximus) to force his aged benefactor (Frederick Sloane) to put him in
his will. (The letters squeezing money from his father's inheritance were
written by Henry in May 1869, and "A Light Man" was published in
July.)
      Maximus and his friend Theodore blend qualities we have already noted
in William and Henry. Maximus is at loose ends, plagued by the eternal

William's marriage in 1878 caused a shift in Henry's novels from male to female heroines.
This change seems less striking when placed in the context of his early stories, which
typically represent a female consciousness. From the very outset of his career in his twenties,
Henry James's psychological core was ambivalently feminine and fused with his older, more
masculine "twin."
      [5] "And I,—what I seem to my friend, you see: / What I soon shall seem to his love, you
guess: / What I seem to myself, do you ask of me? / No hero, I confess" (R. Browning, 1855).

questions of youth: "What am I? What do I wish? Whither do I tend?"
(p. 346). He is also frankly opportunistic, "scanning the horizon for a
friendly sail, or waiting for a high tide" to set him "afloat" (p. 347).
Theodore rescues him with an invitation to stay at the home of his "eccentric" employer. Like William, Theodore has returned from studying
science in Germany with the determination to pursue his vocation. But
"the inner voice failed him" (p. 353). He is at work, instead, helping
Sloane to write his memoirs.

James places Sloane in a fatherly relation to the two young men by
age—he is seventy-two—and as a former friend of Maximus's mother and
Theodore's father. In short, the two are brothers imaginatively set in
place by James to battle for favor and money from their father, just as
William and Henry were doing when the tale was written. Maximus
accepts the invitation, declaring unashamedly that at least he will "obtain
food and lodging" while he "invokes the fates" (p. 348).

Theodore's sex is ambiguous. He greets Maximus with "formidable
blushes" as his friend "strides into his arms—or at all events into his
hands." The richly homoerotic tone of the meeting is projected onto the
landscape as the two walk arm in arm from the town past a lake "lapping
and gurgling in the darkness" as it offers "its broad white bosom to the
embrace of the dark fraternal hills" (pp. 348–349).

Sloane has qualities reminiscent of Henry James Sr. Besides being old,
he is rich, in ill health, and "fancies himself as a philosopher" (p. 359).
Henry has a harsh judgment to pass on this side of his life. In his view,
"his mind is haunted by a hundred dingy . . . theological phantasms."
What is worse, "He has never loved anyone but himself . . ." (p. 359).[6]

Sloane is ambiguously feminine. His library is "a sort of female study."
He is also "depraved," "unclean," and "immoral," but not in the fashion
of "a *viveur*" because "he's of a feminine turn . . ." (p. 357). Retired to
his country house, he has for the past ten years entertained "an unbroken
series of favourites, *protégés*, and heirs presumptive," but each has made
"some fatally false movement" and now the field is clear for Theodore
and Maximus (p. 358). Once again, Henry constructed a plot with siblings
as blushing lovers who fight to get into the same bed. This time the
homosexual intention is blatant. Sloane plays his sadomasochistic part to
perfection. When the new arrival fills in for Theodore, who has fallen ill,
and reads and gossips with Sloane, the old man gives him "a venerable

---

[6] Henry James Sr.'s entire speculative life stood in judgment here. By 1869 he had
published all but one of his major theological works, declaring that redemption depended
upon transcending selfishness. From his son's perspective (sharper here because veiled in
fiction), Henry Sr., though he urged the abandonment of self in theory, never loved anyone
but himself, and distorted his sons' lives chasing after his theological phantasms.

grin" and declares, "Max,—you must let me call you Max—you're the most delightful man I ever knew" (p. 361). This time it is Max who blushes. Sloane pleads with his new beloved—"I wish very much that I could get you to love me as well as you do poor Theodore" (p. 362)—and places in his hand the weapon that will ultimately be used to assault and then kill him—the threat of departure. He wheedles and moans: "You'll not get tired of me and want to go away?" (p. 362). Sloane then turns on Theodore, his former favorite, and treats him with "brutality" (p. 363). Maximus senses that Sloane enjoys being treated the same way, so he makes sure that he is "beaten" and "bullied" and "contradicted." The old widower is "vastly thankful" (p. 363).

When Maximus concludes that his money troubles would be over if he married, he exclaims, "My only complaint of Mr. Sloane is, that instead of an old widower, he's not an old widow (or I a young maid), so that I might marry him . . ." (p. 356). The story reaches a climax when Max threatens to desert Sloane unless the widower wills him all of his money. But the document gets destroyed and Sloane dies before he can execute another. Neither brother wins. Rather than destroying each other (as in "Old Clothes"), in this denouement the brothers declare their love. Theodore admits, "I loved you, even as my rival" (p. 371). Despite all the sadomasochistic byplay and blushing affection that has taken place, Maximus replies, "I don't understand the feeling between men" (p. 372). His tone is unconvincing, and he most certainly was not speaking authentically, either for himself or for the author. Henry James imaginatively understood homosexual love all too well.

In 1873 William began to teach part-time at Harvard. He found the work satisfying and his health and spirits improved. But when President Eliot offered him a full-time position, all of his old doubts about science and work resurfaced. He became ill and fled to Europe to be with Henry. From Florence, where he was living in a hotel with Henry, he wrote, "At present Harry is my spouse" (Perry, 1935, vol. 1, p. 351). But the two had gotten out of tune with each other. William had so successfully submerged his artistic inclinations that he was poor company. Whereas earlier his response to European art centers was fresh and vital, he now spoke in conventional, moralistic terms that grated on Henry. He found Florence offensive because of its "swarming and reeking blackness" (Perry, 1935, vol. 1, p. 351). Rome seemed to him "the incarnation of Satan" (p. 162). Not only was he aesthetically dull, he did not grasp Henry's individuated intentions. He kept writing of Henry's future as if it were indistinguishable from his own. He wanted him to return to

America (as *he* had to). He wanted him to choose "a position of literary drudgery" (as *he* accepted the drudgery of teaching) (p. 351). He was convinced that writing was abnormal and bad for Henry's "mental hygiene," and compared it unfavorably with a "mechanical, routine occupation" (as *he* had decided that philosophy was morbid and the physiology laboratory was better for *his* health) (p. 356).

What William did not understand was that Henry might have been willing to offer him sympathy when he cried out in distress, as Paul De Grey had run to Margaret's side, but that he had decided once and for all that he would not share the same destructive fate. William returned to Cambridge sooner than he had planned. In *The Principles of Psychology* (1890), his first major book, William's comments on the psychology of habit hearkened back to that somber parting. "Habit is thus the enormous fly-wheel of society, its most precious conservative agent. . . . It dooms us all to fight out the battle of life upon the lines of our nurture or our early choice, and to make the best of a pursuit that disagrees, because there is no other for which we are fitted, and it is too late to begin again . . ." (vol. 1, p. 121). He had made an early choice to train for science and that was to be the line of battle for him whether it disagreed or not.

He was eventually able to evolve within science and carve a niche for himself as an interpreter of science to philosophers and of philosophy to scientists. His artist self would find expression in the grace of his prose. But in 1873 William was uncertain of his future as he left Europe and his aesthetic twin behind.

William had joked about Harry being his "spouse." In 1878 it was Henry's turn to use the same figure on the occasion of his brother's marriage. Though intended as a humorous acknowledgement of the delay of his letter of congratulations (written five days after the wedding), it referred painfully and awkwardly to yet one more decisive wrench from their twinship. William had decided to marry Alice Gibbens and Henry wrote: "As I was *divorced* from you by an untimely fate on this unique occasion, let me at least *repair the injury* by giving you, in the most earnest words that my clumsy pen can shape, a tender bridal benediction" (1975, p. 177; italics added). Would a fate ever be "timely" that cut such a fraternal tie in favor of another? Henry's imagery is ambiguous, covering as it does both the minor fault of having missed the date and the more serious "injury" that cannot be "repaired" with earnest words, the choice of another lover.

A week later he wrote again, and this time Henry imagined himself Viola-like in his sibling's place. "I wrote you briefly the other day, in first hearing that your marriage was coming off immediately—so that you know my sentiments about it. I can best repeat them by saying that I rejoice in it as *if it were my own.*" But then he drew back, "or rather much more" (1975, p. 178; italics added). Like the Viola he had created ten years earlier, he had not been chosen; the wedding clothes were not for him.

As Edel has noted, William's marriage provoked a change in Henry's inner life that was reflected in his fiction. The tendency toward feminine identification, evident in his early stories, became dominant. He now made heroines the main characters in his longer works. Edel credits this to Henry's identification with the second-class status of younger siblings, but Hall's reading is more to the point. It is also a matter of "sexual intrigue" between the brothers. In *Confidence*, the short novel Henry wrote in the weeks following William's marriage, the heroine is named Angela (Henry's pet name in the family was "Angel"), and the plot revolves around a woman who cannot marry the man she loves (Hall, 1979, part 1, p. 31). Henry might imagine what it would be like to be such a woman, but fate had given him a different body and decreed that he could never marry the brother who had for so long been his psychological twin.

Henry James was not content to restrict formal literary control to his fictional world. He also attempted to shape his own biography. He set traps for future scholars, left false clues, and destroyed letters. He tried in every way within his means (as he warned his nephew and literary executor) to "frustrate as utterly as possible the post mortem exploiter— . . ." (Edel, 1972, p. 142). In his view, the literary vision was privileged. Art had priority over life as lived. Yet Henry knew that in spite of his wish to "discredit and dishonour such [biographical] enterprises" one "can't prevent them." What he may have been less aware of was how accurately some of his early fiction reads as a blueprint of his future. We have already seen how the difficulties of separating from William and the homoerotic tension of that fused fraternity were described in fiction that "predicted" the "injury" done by William's marriage. "A Light Man" peered thirty years into the future of Henry's private life with uncanny clarity. He was to become a Frederick Sloane, retired to his country house to write. He would die at the age of seventy-two, after a series of homoerotic love affairs. And the lovers of his old age were incarnations of his youthful fiction.

Hendrik Anderson was twenty-seven and James fifty-six when they met and James fell in love. There were many connections that bridged the gap between Anderson and James's early rendering of his psychological twinship. Anderson was a sculptor (like Roderick Hudson), his older brother was a painter (like young William), and they had both been raised in Newport, the scene of William's artistic experiment. He was a man of ordinary gifts who like Maximus was looking for "aid in the hard climb to fame and fortune" (Edel, 1969, p. 307). Henry invited him to his country house, where his protestations of affection and fears of abandonment echo the dialogue between Maximus and Sloane thirty years earlier. "I wish I could . . . put my hands on you (oh, how lovingly I should lay them!) . . ." (p. 313). "I was absurdly sorry to loose you . . ." (p. 311). "Don't 'chuck' me this year, dearest boy . . ." (p. 314). When Anderson's older brother died, Henry's expression of love and sympathy pointed to his earliest relationship with his brother William and the homoerotic link between them: "lean on me as on a *brother* and a *lover*" (p. 313; italics added). The two were together on half a dozen occasions at most, and whether they were actually lovers is unknown; the fraternal and fictional resonance, however, is unmistakably evident.

Hugh Walpole was by contrast a *literary* young man on the make (he was twenty-four). Wangling an invitation from Henry, he declared his desire "within my compass of the safely combustible, to feed your flame" (Edel, 1972, p. 398). Walpole was "a nice boy, full of anxiety and good feeling" like Theodore of "A Light Man," but he was not inhibited by any of that young man's puritanism (p. 397). He had access to the underworld of Victorian sexuality and fed Henry's imagination with reports of "immorality on stone floors" (a liaison between a priest and a professed homosexual writer)—reports that were never quite detailed enough to satisfy Henry. "When you refer to their 'immorality on stone floors,' and with prayer books in their hands, so long as the exigencies of the situation permit of the manual retention of the sacred volumes, I do so want the picture developed and the proceedings authenticated" (p. 408). It was Hugh Walpole who undertook, like Maximus, to give his aged patron a "real sensation." From the youth's first visit to Lamb House, James gushed erotic affection verbally. "I shall be here, at your carriage door with open arms. . . . Bring a love-scene . . . and read it to yours . . ." (pp. 399–400). But when life threatened to intrude on art, when the imagined act craved expression in action, James protested to the inviting young lover, "I can't, I can't" (p. 407).

Here too the blueprint was provided thirty years earlier by his youthful imagination. In "A Light Man" Maximus chides his elderly patron for living in his imagination rather than daring to experience life. Sloane deceives himself by thinking that "he has drained the cup of life to the dregs; that he has known in its bitterest intensity, every emotion of which the human spirit is capable; that he has loved, struggled, and suffered. Stuff and nonsense, all of it. He has never touched with the end of his lips the vulgar bowl from which the mass of mankind quaffs its great floods of joy and sorrow" (H. James, 1973, p. 359). The very evaluation that unsympathetic critics would make of James's style at the height of his career, he had already made of Frederick Sloane's character in 1869. H. G. Wells merely echoed this self-fulfilled prophecy when he poked fun at Henry for splitting "his infinitives" and filling "them up with adverbial stuffing . . . for tales of nothingness. . . ." He was like a "hippopotamus . . . picking up a pea . . ." (Edel, 1972, p. 535).

Not the least of these Maximus-like echoes came from William. He saw his brother (now, in 1899, quite separated from him) as "limited," a "queer boy" who "had taken an oath not to let himself out to more than half his humanhood in order to keep the other half from suffering . . ." (Hall, 1979, part 2, p. 26). William reserved his most impatient barbs for Henry's late style. His own more masculine way was "to say a thing in one sentence as straight and explicit as it can be made. . . ." Henry by contrast chose "to avoid naming it straight, but by dint of breathing and sighing all round and round" to create "the illusion of a solid object." William pleaded for an interlude when Henry would write according to "accepted canons" (1920, vol 2, p. 278). By the 1890s both were literary, yet the twinship of their youth had been largely dissolved. Still the older brother could see, as only a perceptive psychologist and former fused twin could, that something was missing, some vital part that made Henry seem there only by half. And in their last years, the symbolism of illness would reconfirm their "singular life."

One streaming moonlit night in July 1898, while camping in the Adirondacks after a strenuous day of climbing, William James had a mystical experience. He later described it to his wife as a "Walpurgis Nacht" in which memory and sensation all "whirled inexplicably together" to create "one of the happiest lonesome nights" of his life (1920, vol. 2, p. 76). His early ideas on the psychology of religion, being worked up for the Gifford Lectures—*The Varieties of Religious Experience* (1902)—gave shape to it all. To the fifty-six-year-old James it felt as if "the Gods of all the nature mythologies were holding an indescribable meeting" in his breast "with the moral Gods of the inner life." The sensation in his chest may also have been an ominous harbinger of disease, as afterward he began to complain of constant pain in the region of his heart. He soon informed a friend that his "heart has been kicking about terribly of late, stopping, and hurrying and aching . . ." (vol. 2, p. 78). Unfortunately, William did not distinguish this early sign of the illness that would eventually kill him from the neurasthenic symptoms that had plagued him all his adult life.

His initial reaction was to hide it from his family and to refuse to "give up to it too much." He really needed rest but was fearful of stalling his life as he had thirty years before. Once again he headed to Europe for two years of cure.

Henry had been feeling vaguely depressed and the news of William's illness was unsettling. He heard the physiological details from Dr. Baldwin, a friend who while at Bad Nauheim for the cure had examined the ailing William. Henry's note to the doctor shows how vulnerable he was even in late middle age to the belief that he and his brother were one. He told Dr. Baldwin that the details of William's heart disease made *him* "feel sick and sore," as if *he* had the illness, and he nervously informed his medical friend that he had begun to restrict his own activities to take care of *his* heart. "I am coddling my organ at such a rate that I no longer bicycle up anything less level than a billiard table" (Edel, 1969, pp. 317–318). William, by contrast, chaffed at the "moral repulsiveness" of the invalid life at the baths. "Everybody fairly revelling in disease, and abandoning themselves to it with a sort of gusto. 'Heart,' 'heart,' 'heart,' the sole topic of attention and conversation" (1920, vol. 2, p. 95). He had spent his entire adult life fighting his own tendency to abuse illness and found the stance hard to give up. Yet he realized that his mountain-climbing days were over. He wrote to a former climbing companion the sad truth. "I fear we shall ascend no more acclivities together. 'Bent is the tree that should have grown straight!' " (vol. 2, p. 95). At Bad Nauheim, his health improved briefly but then the angina returned. After consulting yet one more heart specialist in London, William finally "consented," in Henry's words, "to be really ill" (Edel, 1969, p. 323). He postponed the Gifford Lectureship and extended his leave from Harvard, suspecting that the *Varieties* would be his "own last will and testament" (1920, vol. 2, p. 112). He was wrong. His major philosophical works, *Pragmatism* (1907), *The Meaning of Truth* (1909a), and *A Pluralistic Universe* (1909b), were yet in front of him.

When he returned to Cambridge in 1902 he confessed to a friend that he had "a bad conscience" about leaving Henry to his loneliness at Lamb House and summarized his appreciation of the temperamental differences that separated them so radically in their old age. "He and I are so utterly different in all our observances and springs of action, that we can't rightly judge each other" (1920, vol. 2, pp. 168–169). True, the differences were dramatic, but the language of bodily symptoms continued to point to the links that had bound them from boyhood to a shared existence. Henry continued to believe that *he* had heart disease. In a Christmas letter in 1908 William acknowledged their common symptom and commiserated with his ailing twin. "The accursed 'thoracic symptom' is a killer of enterprise with me, and I dare say that it is little better with you" (vol. 2, p. 317). He had absconded with Henry's back pain in 1867 and now he and Henry would share the same cardiac sickbed for the last decade of William's life.

Once again the troublesome psychosomatic question—was there an organic basis for the heartache?—became central to their lives. William had in fact injured a valve in his heart but as for Henry, the doctors could find no organic disease. He was despondent about the poor reception of his New York edition (his first royalty check was for $211), complained of palpitations and shortness of breath, and wrote to the same Dr. William Osler who had treated his brother (Edel, 1972, pp. 434–435). Osler referred him to a London specialist, Sir James Mackenzie, who finding no signs of heart disease shrewdly interpreted this to Henry in terms of the literary style of "The Turn of the Screw." Henry admitted that he had used ambiguity in that story to invite the reader to fill in "all sorts of horrors" with his imagination. The doctor "tapped Henry on the chest and said: 'It is the same with you, it is the mystery that is making you ill' " (Edel, 1972, pp. 435–436). Mackenzie later published the case as an example of his method of treating a cardiac neurosis. He reported that his patient had been "greatly cheered" by his therapy. But he had spoken more wisely than he realized. It was the mystery of psychological fusion that was making Henry ill and that would *not* be cured by simple reassurance. Henry continued to speak of having had a "cardiac crisis" (Edel, 1972, p. 436).

In "De Grey," written forty years earlier, Margaret had cried out when Paul was hurt, just as Paul had run to Margaret, hearing her cry of pain though miles away. Now William heard the frantic cry across the ocean and sailed to be with his ailing twin. He had been kept informed of Henry's condition and once again Dr. James diagnosed an ailment of his brother's as a nervous breakdown (Edel, 1972, p. 441). At first Henry protested that his "illness had no more to do with a 'nervous breakdown' than with Halley's Comet: I had no nervous breakdown whatever—and no reason to have one" (Allen, 1967, p. 475). But the weight of medical opinion could not be ignored and he reluctantly confessed to Edmund Gosse that he was the victim of "a sort of nervous breakdown" (Edel, 1972, p. 441).

William's wife Alice now found herself in the difficult position of having to minister to the two invalid brothers, much as Mary James, their mother, had done in the 1860s. Henry found her presence comforting and his spirits began to lift. Then William needed attention as his strength ebbed.

She was not as sure as Mary James had been that she was "equal to her day." "If I can only do my part!" was the uncertain wish she confided to her diary (Allen, 1967, p. 484). And that part was trying indeed as first one brother and then the other clutched at his heart and at hers. William wanted to go to Bad Nauheim but Alice was afraid that Henry would relapse so she let him leave Lamb House alone. Then she gathered Henry up and headed for Nauheim after reading William's wretched letters of relapse. The three were together on William and Alice's wedding anniversary, but William was too ill to get out of bed. Then they returned to Rye. On the trip William regained his strength and Alice recorded in her diary that "Henry [was] suffering again" (Allen, 1967, p. 488). The three decided not to stay at Rye but to return to America instead. Alice James tried to take encouragement from the doctor's observation that William's heart had gotten "*much* better." According to Allen, the fluctuations in William's condition were probably due to his going in and out of heart failure from aortic insufficiency. She buoyed herself with the hopeful thought, "We have a right to expect improvement now all along the line." How unhappily that patient quest for "improvement" had dominated their mother's life fifty years before! That they were paired in Alice's mind is clear from her diary. In June she had written, "William cannot walk and Henry cannot smile" (Edel, 1972, p. 442). And on the eve of her return to America, she wrote to her mother that "in our perplexities, our journeyings, our decisions . . . these two men have been always full of consideration for me—a good record for two nervous invalids . . ." (Allen, 1967, p. 489).

But the doctor's encouragement was illusory. They returned to Chocorua, the family summer home, where William died in Alice's arms. Before the end came, he asked Alice to "go to Henry when his time comes" (Allen, 1967, p. 491). In a letter to Grace Norton Henry confessed his "blackest fears at the prospect of losing my wonderful beloved brother out of the world in which, from as far back as in dimmest childhood, I have so yearningly always counted on him . . ." (Edel, 1972, p. 446). After William's death, Henry resumed the unfinished letter and for one final, grief-stricken time spoke of himself as if he were a pair. "Think of us, dear Grace,—think of us!" (p. 447). The loss felt like an amputation. He confided to Edith Wharton: "My beloved brother's death has cut into me, deep down, even as an absolute mutilation . . ." (p. 448). Now, it was his turn to "fill a double place."

When Henry's time came in 1916, Alice was there as she had promised. He lay dying of a stroke and murmured, "I should so like to have William with me" (Edel, 1972, p. 559). On the twenty-third of February, he asked her, in his confusion, to tell William he would be leaving in two days. He lost consciousness on the twenty-fifth and died two days later. Their singular life had finally ended.

REFERENCES

Allen, G.W. (1967), *William James: A Biography*. New York: Viking Press.
Browning, R. (1855), A light woman. In: *Men and Women*. London: Chapman and Hall.
Edel, L. (1953), *Henry James: The Untried Years (1843–1870)*. New York: Lippincott.
——— (1969), *Henry James: The Treacherous Years (1895–1901)*. New York: Lippincott.
——— (1972), *Henry James: The Master (1901–1916)*. New York: Lippincott.
Erikson, E.H. (1968), *Identity, Youth and Crisis*. New York: Norton.
Feinstein, H.M. (1977), *Fathers and Sons: Work and the Inner World of William James—An Intergenerational Inquiry*. Unpublished doctoral dissertation. Cornell University, Ithaca, N.Y.
Hall, R. (1979), An obscure hurt: the sexuality of Henry James. *New Republic*, 180(17):25–31, 180(18):25–29.
James, H. (1875), *Roderick Hudson*. New York: Harper, 1961.
——— (1913), *A Small Boy and Others*. New York: Scribner.
——— (1914), *Notes of a Son and a Brother*. New York: Scribner.
——— (1973), *The Tales of Henry James (1864–1869)*, ed. M. Aziz. Oxford: Clarendon Press.
——— (1974), *Henry James: Letters (1843–1875)*, ed. L. Edel. Cambridge: Harvard University Press.
——— (1975), *Henry James: Letters (1875–1883)*, ed. L. Edel. Cambridge: Harvard University Press.
James, W. (1890), *The Principles of Psychology*. 2 vols. New York: Holt.
——— (1902), *The Varieties of Religious Experience: A Study in Human Nature*. New York: Longmans, Green.
——— (1907), *Pragmatism: A New Name for Some Old Ways of Thinking*. New York: Longmans, Green.
——— (1909a), *The Meaning of Truth: A Sequel to "Pragmatism."* New York: Longmans, Green.
——— (1909b), *A Pluralistic Universe*. New York: Longmans, Green.
——— (1920), *The Letters of William James*, ed. H. James. 2 vols. Boston: Little, Brown.
Perry, R. (1935), *The Thought and Character of William James*. 2 vols. Boston: Little, Brown.
Putt, S. (1966), *Henry James: A Reader's Guide*. Ithaca: Cornell University Press.
Strouse, J. (1980), *Alice James: A Biography*. Boston: Houghton Mifflin.
Wolfe, L. (1975), The strange death of the twin gynecologists. *New York*, 8(36):43–47.

Lytton Strachey is accorded wide recognition for his contributions to biography; James Strachey is acknowledged as the peerless translator and editor of Freud. Lytton (1880–1932) and James (1887–1967) were brothers, close in their relationship to each other and both related significantly to Bloomsbury and its sociocultural ambience. To what extent did this sibling relationship influence the work each produced, and how is this shown? What intimacies and battles of spirit do their lives portray?

Lytton Strachey's reputation has undergone many shifts among literary critics, but he has remained widely read by the general public. James is barely known outside the psychoanalytic community, although recently his relationship to Rupert Brooke has stimulated interest in his own personal life (Lehmann, 1980; Partridge, 1981). Both brothers led lives that were strikingly parallel up to a certain point, after which they diverged in their careers although maintaining close personal ties.

The approach taken here is psychoanalytic. The life and work of each man is explored in terms of the major events in his life, the primary emotional and sexual relationships each formed, and of course the unconscious forces, meanings,

10

Lytton and James Strachey: Biography and Psychoanalysis

MURRAY H. SHERMAN

My sincere thanks and appreciation go to Dr. Roy Huss and Dr. Phyllis Meadow, whose thoughtful comments and criticism have been incorporated in this essay.

329

and intentions that lay beneath these outward occurrences.

The personal details of the Stracheys' lives are dealt with extensively, since it is here that basic character is most clearly pictured. The lifework of Lytton and James is briefly presented and some psychoanalytic implications cited. The different patterns of sexual development of the two brothers are then examined, especially the unconscious meanings of these differences. Some comments regarding the specifics of how Lytton and James both became literary people are also offered.

This study has been made a great deal more feasible and meaningful by the publication of Holroyd's biography (1967, 1968) of Lytton Strachey. Holroyd was the first writer to describe Lytton's homosexuality. He portrayed the details of his most significant relationships and treated them as normal events in the life of a gifted, intricate man. His minute and personalized descriptions of many people and events aroused renewed interest in the Bloomsbury circle and in itself appreciably increased the acceptance of homosexuality as a normal disposition.

Since 1968 many biographies, journals, and letters have revealed more about the Bloomsbury group and made these lives increasingly meaningful to us. Most recently the correspondence of James Strachey and Rupert Brooke[1] has become available, which in turn makes it feasible to explore James's homosexuality.

Sexuality has always held a central position in psychoanalytic theory, although some theorists believe Freud exaggerated its significance. The Bloomsbury group rebelled against the sexual mores of their time and led unconventional lives in many ways. Although a few members were consistently heterosexual in their behavior, the predominant pattern was homosexual and the leader in this regard was Lytton Strachey. He was completely open in expressing his desires and in fact offended certain homosexuals who would have preferred discretion. This openness has in recent years become increasingly characteristic of homosexuals in our own culture.

The Brothers: Their Lives

Lytton and James were born into a family highly distinguished in its lineage. Their father, Sir Richard Strachey, traced his family to 1547 and their mother, Lady Jane Grant Strachey, could trace her ancestry to 1539.

---

[1] I am deeply indebted to the curators of the Henry W. and Albert A. Berg Collection in the New York Public Library, whose full cooperation made the James Strachey–Rupert Brooke correspondence available to me.

Many of the Stracheys had been distinguished in public life and in literature. One of the earliest Strachey ancestors had embarked for Virginia, been wrecked off the coast, and had then helped build ships that took the survivors back across the Atlantic to England. His account of this adventure is believed to have furnished material for Shakespeare's *The Tempest* (Holroyd, 1967, p. 4).

Other Stracheys were equally known for adventurous careers, public achievements, and friendships with key figures in political life and in literature. Among the noted figures with whom the Strachey family formed close relationships were John Locke, Lord Clive of India, Robert Southey, Walter Savage Landor, James Mill, and Thomas Carlyle. The Stracheys were men of action who also expressed themselves in vivid, effective writing.

Lytton and James were the two youngest sons in a family of ten surviving children. Their father was seventy years old when James was born, although their mother was twenty-three years younger than her husband. Sir Richard had a distinguished career as a military engineer decorated for active service in India, and later became a top administrator in organizing India's public works and transportation. He also made scientific discoveries in botany and in meteorology, for which he was awarded a medal by the Royal Meteorological Society. He was knighted in 1897.

Richard Strachey had married Jane Maria Grant in 1859. They did not seem well matched either physically or emotionally. He was quite short in stature and of a meticulous, abrupt temperament. She was tall, commanding in appearance, and volatile in behavior. Lady Strachey was vigorous, unconventional in habit, and determined that both she and her family be literary and artistic. She was acquainted with many men and women of eminence, among them Galton, Huxley, Carlyle, Tennyson, and George Eliot.

Neither parent seemed suited to raise the large family they brought into the world. By the time Lytton and James were born, both parents had acquired a rigidity that exaggerated their eccentricities. Sir Richard would spend most of the day engrossed in novels that he read by the dozen. Lady Strachey often devoted her energies to instilling literary tastes in her children but did so in a way that was insensitive and alienating. She would read aloud from literary classics, often addressing children who were squirming in discomfort. Frequently she read romantic or bawdy novels that were far above their comprehension. Both parents were conspicuously preoccupied or absent-minded—Sir Richard absorbed in his novels and unaware of anything happening in the room, Lady Jane often coming into the room and suddenly forgetting why she was there (L. Woolf, 1960, p. 188).

There were hordes of visiting relatives who invaded the household. They provided a liveliness and hubbub that was keen but shattering. A continuous din of conversation and argument often pervaded the atmosphere. At one point a visitor, Leonard Woolf, noted three Strachey relatives arguing on the front lawn while at each of eighteen windows a Strachey face stared in attentive interest. Woolf (1960) remarked that the Stracheys were "the most remarkable family I've ever known, an extinct social phenomenon" (pp. 187, 191).

Another visitor, Bertrand Russell (1967), described an occasion when it seemed to him that each of the Strachey children looked and acted just like the others. As a result the evening seemed to Russell to consist of the same individual entering and leaving and interacting with himself or herself over and over again, until he began to doubt his sanity (p. 103).

The Strachey habits seemed strange and otherworldly. There was the famous Strachey voice that often consisted of squeaks, odd tonalities, and atypical registers that one writer (Sanders, 1953, p. 83) traces to the eighteenth century. Another writer, David Garnett (1955), was "struck by the rigidity of the Strachey outlook. We had to conform to Strachey habits: the Stracheys would not even pretend to adapt themselves to manners or customs which were not their own" (p. 18).

The age discrepancy between Lytton and James Strachey and their parents produced an emotional gap that was painful and distancing. Their older brothers had moved out of the house and the family life was dominated by Lady Strachey and her daughters. The dominance by women certainly influenced the sexual orientation of both brothers. There was also a sense of being tied to an ancient history in which the Strachey family had played and was still playing a vital role, especially a literary one. Sir Richard and his own family of origin were so advanced in years that at dinner "someone might casually say something which implied that he remembered George IV (which he might) or even Voltaire" (Holroyd, 1967, p. 27). It is not surprising that a literary sense seemed actually inbred in Lytton and James.

From his earliest years Lytton impressed even his unconventional family as being strange and eccentric. At the age of three he would march back and forth "chanting what was apparently an epic poem full of high-sounding phrases" that were interspersed by what his mother called "Dickey Songs." These songs had heroes whose names were made-up nonsense titles. Lytton would also conjure up unlikely tales that he then enacted in dramatic fashion. He told his mother, "Yesterday in the streets I saw a cow eating the birds," and then dramatized a dreadful conflict in which he killed the cow with a broom and exclaimed, "Go to be dead!

Now the cow is dead" (Holroyd, 1967, p. 17). Lady Strachey remarked that Lytton never stopped talking, that he was "the most ridiculous boy I ever saw." When James Strachey was five years old, he commented upon one of his brother's letters, "I know that's from Lytton, he's always so absurd. . . . He's a funny little creature" (Holroyd, 1967, p. 48).

Holroyd believes that the "prevailing atmosphere of femininity in which he grew up produced a definite retrograde effect upon Lytton's emotional development" (1967, p. 43). He was often dressed in girls' clothes and in family plays was given the female roles. Although intellectually advanced, he became very shy. His physical health seemed impaired from the earliest years. His mother and sisters continually insisted that he was too weak and fragile to join his older brother playing cricket or to indulge in any strenuous play. Throughout his lifetime Lytton was plagued by a variety of physical ills. He was expected to eat a plate of porridge at each meal, was dosed with glasses of port wine, and at one period was fed almost exclusively on raw meat. When he was in his teens he would be sent with one of his older sisters to a health resort and treated like a patient recovering from surgery. There would be "convalescent teas in the hotel lounge followed by slow, hypochondriac parades along the front to examine the sea" (Holroyd, 1967, pp. 112–113). When he was in his twenties he suffered from "indigestion attacks, palpitations of the heart, high fever and piles" (Holroyd, 1967, p. 294). There were few periods in his entire life when he felt fully well.

Lady Strachey took full charge of Lytton's education, which was conscientiously directed at developing his literary gifts and compensating for his frail physical frame. Unfortunately her judgment was poor and Lytton came under the influence of brutalizing boys' schools that intimidated him and further impaired his health. One headmaster was determined to restructure the total world in which his charges lived. He went so far as to do away with water closets and had the boys use outdoor latrines. Cold baths, hard physical labor, and flogging were intended to strengthen character but sent Lytton into fever, dizziness, and unconsciousness.

When he was fourteen Lytton was sent to another school where he was subjected to the kind of bullying that was rather typical of the English boys' school. The first year was extremely trying for Lytton and he wrote complainingly to his father, perhaps the only time in his life when he did so. Sir Richard responded with a rather formally worded but supportive and sympathetic letter in which he encouraged Lytton to resist "any absolute acts or attempts at indecency such as is well known are not unheard of at schools" (Holroyd, 1967, p. 66). At this Lytton braced up and decided to brave the storm. The bullying decreased and he did succeed in finding an acceptable social niche for himself. His academic achievements were impressive, especially in mathematics, English, and French. He also began developing crushes on older boys who were physically strong and of impressive physique.

The only consistently positive educational influence Lytton experienced before his college years was that of Marie Souvestre, a Frenchwoman of striking carriage and culture who ran a school for young women (Eleanor Roosevelt was one of her pupils). Lady Strachey sent her younger daughters there and formed a close attachment to this woman, whom she greatly admired. Marie Souvestre in turn influenced the Strachey family and Lytton spent periods of time informally at the school from his earliest years through the 1890s. He had started to learn French at the age of seven, but Marie Souvestre inspired him to a true passion for the French language and literature.

At nineteen Lytton emerged as a highly gifted youth with outstanding talent for literary expression, but someone with almost no direct channel for self-expression and little means of relating socially to others. He was oppressed by a whole realm of physical ills, detrimentally dominated by his mother and sisters, and unable to develop his abilities in any positive direction.

A dramatic change occurred in 1899 when Lytton went up to Cambridge. There he formed a close circle of friends with whom he remained on truly loving terms for the rest of his life. His painful loneliness and feeling of isolation subsided and he began to relate to the world around him. At Cambridge he developed his literary tastes and talents and was soon acknowledged by fellow students as a leader in serious discussion. The friendships formed became the nucleus of what was to be the Bloomsbury circle. He was highly successful academically and was awarded a Chancellor's Medal for the best poem in heroic verse. As a result of further examination he was made a scholar at Trinity College, Cambridge, which made his mother ecstatic and elicited a letter from his father in which he said he was making Lytton a gift of a "portrait of your mother to whom so much of your literary training is in truth due" (Holroyd, 1967, p. 151).

In 1902, Lytton was elected to the Apostles, a secret fraternal society that had been in existence for nearly a century. In the world of the Apostles Lytton came to full bloom. Together with his fellow member Maynard Keynes he exerted an enormous influence in the Society. Keynes was also homosexual and together they succeeded in making homosexuality the predominant tone of the Apostles. Strachey was stridently antireligious and was successful in making these opinions dominant ones, although his caustic outspokenness offended certain students who could not bear to be in the same room with him. While at Cambridge Lytton was won over by the ethical philosophy of G.E. Moore, whose concept of the "good" and its desirability was conceived by Lytton to be an endorsement of homosexuality.

Unfortunately, despite Lytton's high achievements at Cambridge, he was not appointed to the faculty. His mother, severely disappointed, then planned for Lytton to become eligible for a civil service position or to become a Fellow of the university, but he also fell short of these goals. When he came down from Cambridge, Lytton felt very much as if he were closed out from a world of warmth and fellowship. He began to write numerous literary pieces for the *Spectator* and other publications, but for a long while felt very much shunted about and at odds with the world. His Cambridge friends were settled and getting their careers under way, but Lytton, still supported by his mother, felt lost and aimless. Lethargy, illness, and disenchantment engulfed him. He became absorbed in a continuing series of affairs with men, which at first enthralled him but invariably moved on to scorn and disillusionment. Perhaps the most significant of these relationships was a deep love for his cousin Duncan Grant, who at first returned Lytton's adoration and filled him with unbelieving joy. Before long, however, Duncan turned to Keynes, which created one of the most painful episodes in Lytton's life. Grant later became one of England's outstanding artists, and at his death in 1978 at the age of ninety-three was the last survivor of the original Bloomsbury circle.

Although Lytton Strachey was successful in his literary criticism that appeared in the *Spectator*, he was deeply dissatisfied with his lack of status and independence. His cousin St. Loe Strachey was editor of the *Spectator* and their relationship, although superficially cordial, was a strained one. Lytton could easily feel that he was being accommodated for family reasons. By 1910, however, he had achieved a certain literary reputation and was commissioned by the Home University Library to write a critical survey of the entire corpus of French literature, later entitled *Landmarks in French Literature* (1912). The book was well received and established Lytton as an acknowledged authority. His literary career and social life gained momentum.

In 1915, Lytton met Dora Carrington and at this very first encounter impulsively embraced and kissed her. Her first reaction was to complain about "that horrid old man with a beard [who] kissed me!" (Holroyd, 1968, p. 184). Almost immediately, however, Carrington (who never used her first name) fell totally and passionately in love with Lytton, a love so

profound that any separation at all from him made Carrington feel that
her world was cold and in shadow. Although there were some efforts
directed to a sexual union, Lytton's antipathy toward female sexuality
prevented it. Carrington's own sexual orientation was bisexual.

The lack of sexual intimacy did not impair the strength or tenderness
of the bond that was to hold this couple together for the rest of their lives.
Initially, Lytton felt self-conscious about his lack of sexual attraction to
Carrington and when she proposed their sharing a house, he demurred,
as she recorded in her diary (Carrington, 1970):

> (L) But it's too incongruous. I'm so old and diseased. I wish I was
>   more able.
> (C) That doesn't matter.
> (L) What do you mean? What do you think we had better do about
>   the physical?
> (C) Oh I don't mind about that.
> (L) That's rather bad. You should. I thought you did care. What
>   about those boys when you were young?
> (C) Oh that was just being young. Nothing.
> (L) But do you mind me being rather physically attracted [to boys]?
> (C) I don't think you are really. . . . I knew it long ago and went
>   into it deliberately. [p. 64]

It was with Carrington's help that Lytton was able to break away from
his mother's home and establish his own together with her. His shyness
and timidity were such that he was literally unable to ask a maid to get
him a cup of tea or to prepare meals. Carrington's devotion was so total
that to some of her friends she appeared to be Lytton's slave. She was
not domestically inclined but learned to run a household that harmonized
with Lytton's needs and compensated for his timidities. She learned to
serve acceptable meals, although visitors were always careful about what
they ate. On one occasion she was on the verge of serving Lytton a half
cup of undiluted iodine when interrupted by an observant friend. This
absent-mindedness is remindful of Lytton's mother.

The life that developed between Carrington and Lytton was interde-
pendent and involved. Each carried on affairs very much as they had
before they started living together. In 1918 they met Ralph Partridge,
who had been a wartime friend of Carrington's brother in the army. Ralph
fell in love with Carrington and Lytton fell in love with Ralph. Although
Ralph had not been homosexual, he was able to return Lytton's affections.
For a few years a stable and reciprocally affectionate *menage à trois*

existed, the primary basis for which was the passion between Carrington and Ralph, approved and supported by Lytton. Carrington, who at first was highly insecure with Lytton, began to feel more certain of her place with him. Lytton basked both in Carrington's relationship with Ralph and in his own deep passion for him. In a letter to Ralph, Lytton wrote, "I send my fond love and all the kisses and etceteras that I didn't dare to send you by Carrington for fear of their being intercepted en route" (Holroyd, 1968, p. 377). In another letter Lytton wrote to Ralph, whom he addressed as "my angel," "I hug you a hundred times and bite your ears. Don't you realize what I feel for you? how profoundly I love you? . . . I am always your own Lytton" (Holroyd, 1968, p. 460).

After a while this harmony became disturbed by Ralph's jealousies over Carrington's flirtations, and he began to press her to marry him. Although Carrington had profound misgivings, she eventually gave way and became Ralph's wife in 1921. However, she immediately started an affair with Gerald Brennan, a writer, who had been Ralph's best friend in the army. She continually deceived Ralph about the affair, but he discovered her lies and suffered acutely.

Ralph eventually tired of Carrington's infidelity and deceitfulness, and left her for Frances Marshall. Carrington became attracted to Ralph once again, shunning Gerald. She could not alter her mode of life but was candid about her sexual conflicts. Carrington (1970) wrote to Gerald:

> I pray to God you will never have the misfortune to get involved with such a hopeless character as me again. . . . You know I have always hated being a woman. . . . I am continually depressed by my effeminacy. It is true . . . I have a female inside which is proved by [my having sex relations] but afterward a sort of rage fills me because of that very pleasure. . . . All this became clear really last summer with H[enrietta]. Really I had more ecstasy with her and no feeling of shame afterwards. . . . Probably if one was completely S[apphic] it would be much easier. Somehow it is always easier if I am treated negatively, a little as if I was *not* a female. . . . [pp. 324–325]

Ralph finally moved away to be with Frances, although he continued to visit Lytton and Carrington. Gerald[2] passed out of the picture and Carrington turned more to homosexual relationships and to heterosexual affairs that were demeaning to her.

Lytton continued his own love life, but this became increasingly ec-

---

[2] For Brennan's own account of his affair with Carrington, see Brennan, 1975.

centric. Even at Cambridge he had appeared strange and different from
others. He spoke in oddly accented and inconsistent registers and adopted
odd mannerisms and poses. As he grew older the eccentricities became
more deeply accented and conspicuous. He dressed in theatrical garb
that startled most people.

> He was by this time sporting a conspicuous, bright yellow coat worn
> over a beautiful new suit of 'mouse-coloured corduroys' and an or-
> ange waistcoat; and his outlandish, heavily-haversacked figure
> caused some stir among the local populace as he stepped out gaily
> along the roads and fields, especially since he was also wearing
> golden earrings. These he told [his brother] James, were a great
> solace to him, though outraging the good citizens. . . . 'They eyed
> me with the greatest severity but I bearded them'. [Holroyd, 1968,
> p. 61]

The affairs in which Lytton engaged became characterized by various
artifices. His lagging passions were stimulated by an increasing fetish for
men's ears, and with his partners Lytton roleplayed various master-slave
parts. "For the evening's entertainment, he would sometimes produce
one-act farcical playlets for his guests to perform, in which all the men
were women and the women men, and ingenious plots hurried the actors
into a bewildering, hermaphroditic confusion" (Holroyd, 1968, pp.
480–481).

Lytton's literary productivity grew increasingly successful. Beginning
with *Eminent Victorians* in 1918 his work found wide acceptance and
popularity with the public and with critics. His later biographies, *Queen
Victoria* (1921) and *Elizabeth and Essex* (1928), were enormously popular.
He achieved financial and social security and found the fame and acclaim
for which he had always hungered. Carrington's emotional and sexual
tribulations brought concern and sometimes grief, but their relationship
remained the rock to which the security of each was anchored. Nevertheless, Lytton's physical ailments continued to assail him. He developed
an undiagnosed cancer of the bowel and died in 1932 at the age of fifty-
one.

Carrington knew no way to continue her own life without Lytton. She
wrote in her diary (1970):

> It was only [because] I knew he disliked me to be dependent that
> I forced myself to make other attachments. Everything was enjoyed
> to be [only because I was] with him. He was, and this is why he
> was everything to me, the only person to whom I never needed to

lie, because he never expected me to be anything different to what I was. [p. 491]

To a friend she wrote, "You see that my weakness is that I only led, or tried to lead, a 'good' life to please Lytton, left to myself I lapse (secretly) into superstition and mooning about" (1970, p. 498). Six months prior to Lytton's death and in response to a literary contest, Carrington had written an excellent biographical caricature of him in parody of his own style. The piece playfully ended with his accidental death at age ninety-nine. The entry easily won first prize. After Lytton died, Carrington guiltily reproached herself for having anticipated his death without preventing it (Holroyd, 1968, pp. 671–672). Two months after Lytton's cremation Carrington committed suicide with a shotgun. She was thirty-nine years old.

Data about James Strachey are much less available to us than facts about Lytton. However, he has often been mentioned and described by writers in the Bloomsbury circle, of which he was a peripheral in the Bloomsbury circle, of which he was a peripheral Holroyd's biography also provides significant details.

As the last child in a large family, James was uncle to a number of his siblings' children who were older than he. As a child he was often called "Uncle Baby." Lytton, seven years older than James, was the only brother consistently at home; there were three sisters—five, twenty-one, and twenty-five years older than he. James adored and idealized Lytton. Because of the age discrepancy between the brothers the effects of feminine dominance and emotionally distant parents would seem to apply even more keenly to James than to Lytton but, as shall be seen, the results were not comparable.

Some of the earliest description available about James comes from an account of when he first met Rupert Brooke in preparatory school at age ten (Hassall, 1964, pp. 29–30). Brooke was to become the most significant figure in James's later adolescence and young manhood. When they met, both children wore their hair down over their forehead, most unusual for boys at that time. A teacher encountering them roared, "Back to the changing room, both of you. You look like a couple of *girls.*" Rupert and James often studied together and competed for grades. Rupert looked up to James for his excellence in school subjects, whereas James admired Rupert for outstanding skill at cricket, a game at which James was, in his own words, "quite hopeless."

The writer David Garnett met James at a costume ball given by the latter and a sister in 1910. He caught his first sight of the two Stracheys as they danced a pas de deux down the full length of the center aisle. The costume James wore was conspicuously bizarre. He was

> chiefly greasepaint from the hips upward, but wore full Turkish trousers of blue gauze or butter-muslin, cut low enough at the waist to reveal his navel. On his head was a black astrakhan wig, and round his neck a big gold or silvergilt necklace in the form of a cobra with jewelled eyes. [Garnett, 1953, p. 207]

David and James became good friends. In 1913 they went picnicking with three sisters, one of whom, Noel Olivier, was important to James and, as will be seen, to Rupert Brooke. At this picnic James is pictured as having just been ill. Garnett recalled that James "immediately transformed our party," in that his four companions catered totally to his

> concern for . . . health and comfort. . . . Between every meal a glass of ovaltine was prepared and administered to James as though it were a sacrificial rite. . . . I was immediately struck in him by what I later discovered was a very marked characteristic of the whole family; an astonishing inelasticity of values, a rigid adherence to certain limitations which they have imposed upon themselves. . . . To know the Stracheys well, one has to be ready to accept the atmosphere in which they live. [Garnett, 1953, pp. 257–258]

In 1905 James went up to Cambridge and took over the same room that Lytton had occupied. Because of his resemblance to Lytton he soon became known as Little Strachey, and Lytton the Great Strachey. Lytton asked his friends, especially Maynard Keynes, to look after his brother. James became part of Lytton's circle of Cambridge friends and he too was elected to the Apostles, the Society that figured so prominently in the lives of both brothers. James and Lytton also shared certain love interests and confided in each other regarding their affairs. The brothers introduced friends to each other who, they felt, would be attractive partners.

Much of James's social life centered upon the Apostles. The predominant tone of the Society remained homosexual, continuing the influence exerted by Lytton and Keynes. One observer, Rees (1968), states that the major sexual emphasis both at Cambridge and Oxford was homosexual up until World War II, and that this emphasis exerted a significant influence upon all of British society in that period.

James's personality while at Cambridge is described by Holroyd (1967) as so lethargic as to be inert. When Lytton went to visit, he was appalled at the half-eaten breakfast. Eggshells and tea stains covered the table and the room was freezing cold. James was sunk in appalling gloom and radiat[ed] an atmosphere of apathy and oppression that ate into one's very bones. His fundamental disease, in Lytton's estimation, was that he could rouse himself to take no interest in anything but the few people he admired or was in love with. . . . The poor creature seemed quite unable to think, or read or work at all. Instead he spent all his time dreaming over a solitary fire, which eventually went out because he was too dilatory to put on more coal. . . . The very contemplation of anything difficult was poison to his system and brought on a complete collapse. Already at twenty, he didn't appear to have adequate stamina for the slightest exertion, and made no positive use—even as an analgesic—of his mind. [p. 307]

It was while he was at university that Lytton induced James to study German, saying it might be useful to him at some future time (Letter of James Strachey to Rupert Brooke, June 28, 1909).

When James was about to go up to Cambridge he wrote to Rupert Brooke, who had tried several times, fruitlessly, to initiate a correspondence with him. Brooke responded and the two men continued to be close friends for many years. Brooke in fact was the grand passion of James's life, and his lasting influence upon James can be traced in detail through their correspondence.

James's initial letter in July of 1905 conveys a decidedly subservient tone as he begs forgiveness for having ignored Brooke's prior efforts to be in touch and begs to be excused for his inadequate ability to express himself. By the end of the next year James was openly adoring Brooke's beauty, as in fact did many other men. Brooke possessed a rare combination of strong but delicate features, an unusually clear, translucent complexion, and a stalwart body (Hassall, 1964, p. 26).

At this time the two young men shared an anti-Victorian stance that stressed freedom of sexual impulses and revolt against all religious restrictions. Brooke was dominated by a strong and intimidating mother, and he retained a strict puritan streak in his nature that later proved disastrous. His published poetry brought fame at the age of twenty-four, and he was immortalized by the following lines written just before World War I: *If I should die, think only this of me; / That there's some corner of a foreign field / That is for ever England.* He was one of the first English soldiers to die in that war.

The love between James and Rupert was continual pursuit by James and ever-tantalizing retreat by Brooke. James wrote: "what must you think of me in order to treat me as you have? . . . I'm frightened of this part of the letter, and everything depends on it. Be kind. . . . [Michael] seemed to think the physical side of love less ugly than you did. . . . they are good feelings" (Letter of April 2, 1907). James pleaded for Brooke's sexual acceptance, was allowed superficial favors, but was never permitted the full intimacy he sought. This specific structure of the relationship continued on James's part for as long as the two men knew each other.

For his own part, Brooke experienced comparable pursuit by other men and also women, almost all of whom he kept at bay. Although James and Brooke met frequently, it was never enough for James. He complained: "you didn't give me a word or even a look which should belong to me. . . . I suppose all my tears have been unreasonable" (Letter of March 21, 1909). He begged simply to be allowed to be in Brooke's mere presence, to sit and be treated as a dog or cat or piece of furniture (Letter of July 1, 1909). He would be good and not offend Brooke by sexual impositions. On the few occasions that Brooke seemed ready to accept a visit, James would suddenly become timid, wonder if he were truly welcome, and offer to stay away if this was his friend's preference.

Despite these conflicts James and Brooke remained essentially the good and close friends they had been at the age of ten. Brooke admired James for his scholarly mind; James worshiped Brooke's physical presence and everything else about him. "Sometimes I remember that it's You and my love that make the universe magical. . . . And isn't it splendid to be the only person in the world who loves you? You don't pretend that the others do? They may *say* but I *know* that the curve of your nostril is beautiful, and that you're cleverer than I am, and that you're the greatest poet in the world" (Letter of August 16, 1909).

The relationship continued unchanged for as long as James was at Cambridge. Brooke also went to Cambridge and was considered for membership in the Apostles. As a former leader and guiding light in this secret society Lytton Strachey was a major person whose approval was necessary for Brooke's acceptance. As a kind of entrance examination several written questions were posed to Brooke and his responses passed upon. One of the questions was, "Are you in favour of war at any price?" In view of Brooke's death in the not so distant future, his response seems tragically ironic: "Certainly I approve of war. . . . It kills off the unnecessary" (Hassall, 1964, p. 68).

Lytton had never taken to Brooke, and a rather strained relationship existed between them. He questioned Brooke's depth of intellect and feeling (Hassall, 1964, pp. 70–71) but, perhaps because of James's feelings, approved the membership. But the strained feeling between the men persisted. Later on, when at a Cambridge lecture Brooke expressed admiration for H.G. Wells, Lytton "lost his temper and delivered a violent personal attack" (Harrod, 1951, p. 147). The reasons for Lytton's ill feelings toward Brooke are obscure but may have been compounded of envy for his good looks and attractiveness to men plus misgivings over James's infatuation with him.

When James graduated from Cambridge, his family influenced their cousin St. Loe Strachey to hire him as his private secretary at the *Spectator*. James remained with the publication for six years and although he disliked many aspects of his work, he recognized that it brought him out into the world. In addition to chores like correspondence, James wrote book reviews and popular articles. The nature of the latter may be surmised from some of the titles: "The Limitations of Logic," "Thinking and Reading," "The Meaning of Individuality." There were also such articles as "The Poetry of Swift," "Oliver Goldsmith," and "The Duke of Wellington" (Sanders, 1953, pp. 319–320). The Strachey family had been making contributions to the *Spectator* since 1875, and once again James was following in Lytton's footsteps.

Beginning in 1911 and following Brooke's lead, James began to develop a sexual interest in women (Letters of June 7, July 17, and December 7, 1911). One of these women so resembled Rupert that a friend of James approached the young woman and jokingly inquired whether her name were Miss Brooke (Letter of March 13, 1911). Most remarkably, in 1911 Brooke wrote to James and asked him to explain how to use contraceptives because he was contemplating intercourse with a young woman he was seeing. Both men were then twenty-four. James replied not only with details of various methods but also drawings of condoms and syringes. He advised Brooke, perhaps partly with tongue in cheek: "isn't it all too incredibly filthy? Won't it perhaps make you sick of it?—Come quietly to bed with me instead" (Letter of April 10, 1911).

For several years prior to this incident Brooke had been secretly in love with Noel Olivier, who was only fifteen when he first declared his passion for her. Noel was the same young woman with whom James later went on the picnic in 1913. Some time in 1911 Brooke became acquainted with Katharine Cox, known to her friends as Ka. Much of the interchange between James and Brooke from 1911 on centered on the relationship of the two men with Noel and Ka. Both young women were primarily attracted to Brooke, but his interests waxed and waned. At one point James felt he was in love with Ka (Letter of July 17, 1911). Ka in turn seemed at various times attracted to James, then to Brooke, but in December of 1911 an event occurred that dramatically changed all their lives (Hassall, 1964; Lehmann, 1980).

A group of friends gathered for a reading party at Lulworth. Ka induced

Lytton to invite his friend Henry Lamb because of her interest in him, and at one point Ka and Lamb went off together. Ka had previously been kept at a certain distance by Brooke. She now told him that she was in love with Lamb, whereupon Rupert promptly proposed marriage but was refused (Hassall, 1964, pp. 296–297). Ka became fixed upon marrying Lamb (Holroyd, 1968, pp. 25–29). Brooke suddenly developed a consuming hatred for Lytton that surpassed reason and in fact evolved into a full paranoid rage that centered on Lytton but led eventually to his estrangement from all his Bloomsbury friends. Simultaneously, Brooke also fell under the spell of a passionate love for Ka, who agreed to continue their relationship. It was too much for Brooke to handle; it became obvious that he was severely disturbed emotionally. Feelings of rage, disgust, jealousy, and self-loathing overwhelmed him. He lost fourteen pounds and was persuaded to consult a "nerve specialist" (Hassall, 1964, pp. 297–298). His mother sent him to Cannes and to Munich so that he could rest and recover. Ka joined Brooke, and they became lovers and agreed to marry, but Brooke was afraid to face his mother. Eventually Ka and Rupert decided marriage was not feasible. Their close relationship, however, lasted to the very end of Brooke's life, and in his will he left Ka his papers and her choice of his manuscripts (Hassall, 1964, p. 517).

What the correspondence between James and Brooke reveals is that even after Brooke's partial break with reality and his virulent hatred of Lytton, the friendship between them continued for some time. The correspondence indicates that Brooke encouraged James to be with Ka and with Noel, and that James was initially more successful sexually with these young women than was Brooke. Both men were in acute conflict. James, it would seem, kept company with Ka and with Noel partly out of compliance with Brooke's urging, but he was continually afraid of overstepping the bounds of what Brooke desired (Letters of May ?, 1911; August 7, 1912). At one point James wrote of how sorry he felt for Ka, whom he was treating so badly (Letter of July 10, 1912). Although Brooke indicated a wish for James to see Ka and Noel, he became severely disturbed when James did so.

In August 1912, when James visited Brooke at his home, Brooke was so enraged at Lytton and in fact at all of Bloomsbury that James was forced to leave abruptly (Lehmann, 1980, p. 17). Even after this event, deeply traumatic to both men, they continued to correspond. However, where Brooke previously had been distressed but not directly hostile to James, he now became grossly abusive in a manifestly deranged way: "to be a Strachey is to be blind . . . to have undescended spiritual testicles; to be a mere bugger. . . . Buggery still hangs about you" (Letter of August 6, 1912).

Brooke also lashed out at James for his "thin, dirty little feelings for Ka. . . . I have loved Ka. . . . I know what she's like—that she's incredibly brave, incredibly honest & a woman. You find her useful as a sleeping draught" (Letter of August 8–9, 1912).

Brooke indicated suicidal thoughts; he wished James would stab him to death. Even after these disturbed and inflammatory letters—and to the very end of their correspondence—James sorrowed for the loss of Brooke, expressed love for him, and continued to invite visits. Peculiarly, he seems not to have recognized how severely disturbed Brooke had become. One of the very last letters from James, written from Moscow in 1914, offered to share a London flat with Brooke. At this time, World War I was fast approaching and Brooke was appalled at James's pacifist beliefs. His last letter in 1914 impugned James's manhood as well as his intelligence.

When war came both Lytton and James declared themselves conscientious objectors. James did work for the Quakers during the war, developed an interest in the subject of love, and also felt drawn to Fabian socialism. He was dismissed from the *Spectator* because of his pacifist views, but the Stracheys induced John Middleton Murry to hire James as a drama critic for the *Athenaeum* (V. Woolf, 1976, p. 341).

James came to a study of psychoanalysis through his interest in psychical research and the writings of Frederic Myers (1893), who was the first author in England to cite Freud (pp. 50–52). In 1918 James spoke to friends about earning a living in the field of psychoanalysis and he gave a club lecture on onanism (V. Woolf, 1977b, p. 221). He also started medical school, as this was Ernest Jones's recommendation to all analytic candidates, but dropped out after several weeks.

During these years James was keeping company with Noel Olivier. In 1916 he also began to date Alix Sargant-Florence, whom he had mentioned in a letter to Brooke in 1912. Alix was one of a small circle of young women, including Carrington, whom Virginia Woolf characterized as "cropheads." These young women attended various social functions with the Bloomsbury people. Alix was Carrington's oldest friend and had been on intimate terms with her for many years.[3] Alix began a determined pursuit to win James away from Noel and was characterized by Carrington (1970) as his "second wife," Noel being the first (p. 138).

Alix was then a recent college graduate. She was hired by the Woolfs

---

[3] The details of the early relationship between Carrington and Alix are not available. When Garnett was editing Carrington's correspondence (1970), her letters to Alix were the only ones whose original texts were not given him. James instead supplied typescripts of these letters (p. 15).

as their first assistant at the Hogarth Press, but the work so bored her
that she resigned after only one day. At the time Alix was subject to
serious depressions. Carrington (1970) described in her diary how she
went to see Alix and "found her in a sad plight . . . sitting fully dressed
in outdoor clothes on a bed, with a gas fire roaring in a tiny room, remains
of 12 days' meals, for she hadn't left the room for that number of days!
Her face was pale grey with deep red rims round her eyes" (p. 59).

Noel Olivier was also courted by Virginia Woolf's brother Adrian. For
James Strachey she was, in Woolf's words (1978), "the unattainable romance" (p. 136). Later she became a physician and married a fellow doctor
in 1921. When Woolf met Noel for lunch two years later, Noel spoke of
how she cried when rereading Rupert Brooke's love letters to her (V.
Woolf, 1978, pp. 229–230).

Alix's pursuit of James was a stormy one. Her steely determination
made Virginia Woolf's "blood run cold" (Woolf, 1977b, p. 237). At one
point James came to a mutual friend

> in an appalling state of fright. He said that Alix was on the point of
> killing herself. [She and James] had quarreled over something quite
> unimportant. Alix had lost her temper . . . and dismissed him for
> ever. [Her friend] found her sitting on the edge of her bed, which
> had not been made, in a room strewn with old food and litter,
> sobbing. She was completely broken down. . . . Carrington was
> sent for. Just before Carrington arrived, James made his way in;
> there was a reconciliation scene. . . . [James] won't admit he's in
> love. . . . [V. Woolf, 1976, pp. 369–370]

Alix then took rooms at 41 Gordon Square in London and James went to
live with her there. In 1920 they married, on Alix's twenty-eighth birthday.

James had written to Freud inquiring about psychoanalysis and in response was invited to come to Vienna for study and analysis. The following
month the couple went there to live and both were analyzed by Freud,
perhaps the first case of psychoanalytic conjoint marital therapy. After
only several weeks of analysis, Freud asked James and Alix to make a
translation of "A Child Is Being Beaten" (J. Strachey, 1966, p. xxi). In
1921 James wrote his mother that he and Alix were translating Freud's
clinical essays (eventually to become Volume III of the Collected Papers):

> [Freud] thought of the plan on purpose to be of help to us in two
> different ways. First of all, it'll give us a specially intimate knowledge
> of his methods, as we are able to talk over with him any difficulties

that occur to us in the course of the translation; and we now go on Sunday afternoons specially to discuss whatever problems we want to. In the second place, our appearance as official translators of his work into English will give us a great advertisement in psychological circles in England. [Holroyd, 1968, p. 442n]

James and Alix returned to London in 1922, reestablished themselves at 41 Gordon Square, which became both a rooming house for various members of Bloomsbury and their own offices for analytic practice. They remained at this location until 1953, when they retired to devote themselves fully to the editing and translating of the Standard Edition of Freud's work.

Upon their return from Vienna for a holiday, Virginia Woolf (1978) recorded her observations: "Freud has certainly brought out the lines in Alix. Even physically, her bones are more prominent. . . . James . . . is the least ambitious of men—not ambitious even of being a character—low, muted, gentle, modest . . . not at all possessive, masculine or dominating" (pp. 135–136). Earlier she had characterized James as "soft as moss, lethargic as an earthworm" (1977b, p. 221). Allowance should be made, in Woolf's comments, for her preference for Alix, and perhaps for jealousy toward the young couple.

Both James and Alix went on to enjoy successful careers as psychoanalysts and analytic writers. In 1924, at James's suggestion to Leonard Woolf, the Hogarth Press took over the International Psychoanalytic Library, which eventually included all of Freud's writing (V. Woolf, 1977a, p. 119n).

Of the Stracheys' later life together little is available. A recent volume by Partridge (1981) describes a party given by Alix in 1930:

> About a hundred people stood close together in a stuffy basement, shouting, bellowing rather, into each other's open mouths, and sometimes twining their arms vaguely about one or two necks at once. The atmosphere was choking, the food and drink good. Almost all were homosexuals—young man after young man pushed his pretty face round the door, and a crowd of truculent Lesbians stood by the fireplace, occasionally trying their biceps or carrying each other round the room. [p. 175]

One of James Strachey's analysands, the well-known object relations theorist D.W. Winnicott, wrote an obituary article (1969) when James died of a heart attack in 1967. Winnicott mentions the shy and unaggressive nature of James's personality, but emphasizes his vast erudition, cultural sophistication in literature, music, and ballet and, above all, his "unassailable intellectual honesty." Winnicott states that his ten-year analysis with Strachey gave him a keen appreciation for the fact "that a process develops in the patient, and that what transpires cannot be produced but it can be made use of. . . . my experience of analysis at the hand of Strachey . . . has made me suspicious of descriptions of interpretative work in analysis which seem to give credit to the interpretations for all that happens . . ." (p. 130).

Anna Freud's obituary (1969) emphasizes the many difficulties inherent in translation and Strachey's determination not only to translate but also to clarify through editorial exposition: "The founder of psychoanalysis is considered fortunate to have found a translator of this stature. It may be said that James Strachey, too, was fortunate to find an author and a subject matter worthy of his efforts" (p. 132).

Alix Strachey died in 1973. Her obituary was written by the analyst M. Masud R. Khan (1973), who cited Virginia Woolf's description of the young Alix as "tall and grave . . . austere and melancholy." In his own contacts with Alix, Khan found her "gracious, hospitable, courteous and resolutely distant." He was also impressed by the very large contribution she made to the Standard Edition and "the extraordinary range of her own scholarship" (p. 130). Alix's obituary in the *Times of London* read: "Strikingly good-looking when young, her personal distinction, exquisite manners, gentleness and lucid calm remained to the end of her life; and these, with frequent flashes of wild gaiety and originality, and her clear speculative mind, always made a conversation with her the most stimulating and enjoyable of experiences" (May 7, 1973).

A more realistic picture of James and Alix Strachey is given by Holroyd in his description of how James and he worked together as he wrote his biography of Lytton. Holroyd paints a vivid portrait of the Stracheys as he visited with them in their final years. Alix Strachey had been described to him as "a once brilliant cricket player and avid dancer at the night clubs and now an authority on cowboys" (Holroyd, 1971, p. 12). The first time Holroyd met James was for an "interview" regarding his fitness as Lytton's biographer. Holroyd was dismayed by Strachey's extensive silences. In between them, he learned that James had suffered from retinal detachment, had undergone a series of eye operations, and walked with an unsteady gait. Holroyd also discovered that he was an authority on classical music. Alix "came in, austere and intellectual, very thin, with deeply-lined parchment face and large deeply expressive eyes" (Holroyd, 1971, p. 13). She told how she was beginning to study physics. As she and James went on, Holroyd became oppressed by the stultifying overheating of the rooms and by their meager fare.

> Lunch was a spartan affair. Though extremely generous in spirit, my hosts were by temperament ascetic, and lived very frugally. We ate spam, a cold potato each, and lettuce leaves. In our glasses there showed a faint blush of red wine . . . but I was the only one who so much as sipped any. . . . Everything, spam, potato, lettuce, cheese and biscuits, was, like the windows, swathed in protective cellophane. [p. 13]

Holroyd was engaged in a continuing battle with Strachey in order to write the kind of biography he wanted. It was a struggle, for James metamorphosed into the strictest guardian of every bit of Lytton's letters and papers. He expressed frequent peevish dissatisfactions about the way his cherished brother was being portrayed. The final product pleased the general public and the critical audience more than it did the surviving brother.

The Brothers: Their Work

It is not the intent of this chapter to summarize or critically evaluate the whole of Lytton Strachey's contribution to literature. His three major biographical volumes (omitting the journalistic essays) will be described and the response of some critics to his writings will be indicated. Certain stylistic features will be noted and their psychoanalytic implications explored.

Eminent Victorians (1918) consists of biographical essays on Cardinal Manning, Florence Nightingale, Dr. Thomas Arnold (headmaster at Rugby and father of Matthew Arnold), and General Charles G. ("Chinese") Gordon. The essays are not intended to be definitive. Rather they are pen portraits, selectively constructed to convey Strachey's own distinctive viewpoint of these four lives. He presents the meaning that the individual might convey to a critical rather than admiring writer. He was suspicious of popular acclaim and aimed at examining the underpinnings of outward events.

Strachey took public figures, widely admired, and described them in light of their less flattering attributes. Cardinal Manning was painted as inhumanly cold and relentlessly ambitious. Florence Nightingale was shown more as a ruthless administrator than as a lover of humanity. The public, reacting to its disillusionment over public figures who had led them into war, greeted *Eminent Victorians* with enthusiastic endorsement. They delighted to see idols with feet of clay fall down before their eyes. The book continues to attract audiences today. Its lucid, readable style, pungent insights into human frailties, and urbane wit consistently inform and entertain.

Nevertheless, from a critical point of view *Eminent Victorians* is acknowledged less for its intrinsic worth as biography than for its landmark status as setting a new style in English biography. Before the book appeared, most biographies consisted of eulogistic recitals of formal events and public records that chronologically detailed a life history. Lytton Strachey wrote a three-page Preface to *Eminent Victorians* that has come to be regarded as a kind of manifesto of freedom for biographers, and this preface is perhaps more often quoted in the critical literature than the book itself. The parts most often cited are the famous sentence, "it is perhaps as difficult to write a good life as to live one," and Strachey's denigration of the traditional "two fat volumes . . . with their ill-digested masses of material, their slipshod style, their tone of tedious panegyric . . ." (1918, p. viii). He is explicit in extolling brevity and incisive fact passed through the sieve of the writer's own subjective comprehension.

To a psychoanalyst, the paragraph that strikes a particular chord of recognition is the following:

> It is not by the direct method of a scrupulous narration that the explorer of the past can hope to depict that singular epoch. If he is wise, he will adopt a subtler strategy. He will attack his subject in unexpected places; he will fall upon the flank, or the rear; he will shoot a sudden, revealing searchlight into obscure recesses, hitherto undivined. He will row over that great ocean of material, and lower down into it, here and there, a little bucket, which will bring up to light of day some characteristic specimen, from those far depths, to be examined with a careful curiosity. [p. vii]

These words, besides suggesting an unconscious image of sodomy, call to mind Freud's concept of the free-floating attention with which a psychoanalyst listens to the free associations of the supine patient. Via this method, a plumb line is dropped into one's own depth of feeling and inner associations, and often emerges with an obscure particle of striking relevance.

The extent to which this Preface, and in fact *Eminent Victorians* generally, was influenced by Freud is a matter of some importance. Kallich, who has addressed the issue at length, was informed in direct correspondence with James Strachey (Kallich, 1958) that Lytton was in no way influenced by Freud in *Eminent Victorians*, and apparently James was so apprised by Lytton himself. Nevertheless, Kallich (1962) believes that "there is a good deal of Freudian influence on Lytton Strachey's published works [of biography], the shorter studies of personality as well as the longer ones. The fact is that Lytton Strachey lends himself to this [Freudian] approach because of his interest in two types of motivation—the sexual and the unconscious" (p. 34). Kallich (1961) in fact believes that the Freudian zeitgeist had already penetrated British thinking before 1914 (p. 9).

There is much to support Kallich's thesis, despite James Strachey's disclaimer and despite Holroyd's conviction (1968) that Freud had no influence on either *Eminent Victorians* or *Queen Victoria* (p. 586). In James's letter he said that it was only after he and Alix discussed Freud with Lytton that he used Freudian ideas. Such use occurred particularly in *Elizabeth and Essex* (1928), which was attributed by James to the influence of Alix. The book was dedicated to both of them.

Nevertheless, in addition to the general tenor of the passage quoted above from the Preface, there is other evidence of the very early influence of Freud upon Lytton Strachey. The word "unconscious" occurs in a specifically Freudian sense in *Eminent Victorians*, where he writes: "The Christian Religion was still preserved intact by the English priesthood, but it was preserved, as it were, unconsciously . . ." (1918, p. 19). In *Queen Victoria* (1921), the queen is described as having been "induced . . . to give, unconsciously no doubt, false reasons to explain away her conduct" (p. 112). Both of these usages of "unconscious," in the sense of latent but active, conform quite specifically to Freud's own formulation; in *The Psychopathology of Everyday Life* (1901), for example, he speaks of "the influence of thoughts which have become active but have at the same time remained entirely unconscious" (p. 273).

In more recent years, additional information has come to light. A book of Strachey's previously unpublished works (1973) includes a piece entitled "According to Freud," in which there occurs a direct allusion to *The Psychopathology of Everyday Life*, which appeared in English in 1914. The editor of the volume states that "the date of the piece must be 1914. . . ," and Freud's influence is directly evident in Lytton's article, which mentions "the impossibility of [psychic] accidents, and the unconscious self, and the sexual symbolism of fountain pens" (pp. 113–114).

It thus appears that Lytton Strachey was informed about the Freudian unconscious before he wrote *Eminent Victorians*. The extent to which this awareness influenced his writing is uncertain. The piece "According to Freud" presents a comic parody of Freud, and reflects a skeptical if not scornful attitude toward psychoanalysis. James might have had ample ground for saying his brother was uninfluenced by Freud, since he may well have heard Lytton speak of psychoanalysis in a negative vein.

Under the tutelage of James and Alix, Lytton did come to an acceptance of Freud. By the time of *Elizabeth and Essex* (1928) he quoted precisely the same two lines of Virgil that Freud had used as the motto for the *Interpretation of Dreams: Flectere si nequeo superos, Acheronta movebo*—"If I cannot bend the beings in Heaven, I will stir the shades below" (p. 96). The use of Virgil seems to have occurred in cryptomnesic fashion, and it is possible that this was the mode of Freud's influence also on *Eminent Victorians*.

The stylistic feature of *Eminent Victorians* to which all critics (e.g., Iyengar, 1939) allude is that of the acid irony that permeates the volume. Strachey's method is to present a presumably laudable trait or feature of the individual in such a way that it is shown to be a vice. This irony is most conspicuous in the chapter on Cardinal Manning, where Strachey's antireligious convictions are clearly manifest. Psychoanalysts have had little to say about irony. Freud (1905) did make some passing comments in his book on wit, where he noted that the technique of irony (stating the opposite of the sense intended) is similar to that of jokes, in that both are rooted in unconscious attitudes (p. 174). Reik (1952) believed that irony is effective because the reader experiences an unconscious affinity to the actual, explicit statement in its obvious rather than ironic sense. He describes how this is true also for the writer of irony, and this would imply that Strachey in his own unconscious maintained a deep longing for religious convictions. Lytton unconsciously may have felt that religion could have helped him deal more effectively with his homosexuality. His irony then expressed deep disappointment, disillusionment, and aggression directed against religion. From a psychoanalytic perspective, religion may have been the scapegoat for Lytton's parents.

The total corpus of Strachey's biographical volumes is not large. In addition to *Eminent Victorians*, there are two further works—*Queen Victoria* and *Elizabeth and Essex*. In *Queen Victoria* the acid irony that characterized *Eminent Victorians* is softened, especially in regard to the Queen herself. The reading public gave *Queen Victoria* an even more enthusiastic reception than *Eminent Victorians*. Its sale made Strachey wealthy. He was able to pay off old debts and to purchase and modernize the home in which he and Carrington lived until the end of their lives. Readers of the book were both relieved and delighted to discover that Strachey had not turned his acidity upon its royal principal. The volume has the further distinction of being one of the first biographies to deal with a regal figure from the viewpoint of human character rather than political or historical events. Strachey's public eminence increased to where he himself became a notable figure, conspicuous wherever he went and welcomed with respect in Britain's leading houses.

Elizabeth and Essex is less of a biography than either of Strachey's previous works. Rather, it is a kind of dramatic tapestry on which he paints vivid scenes of Queen Elizabeth as she deals with scheming courtiers, outguesses wily councilors, and simultaneously engages in a sort of playacting romance with handsome and virile young suitors, of whom Essex was a tragic instance.

A rather lurid theme of traumatic sexuality runs through *Elizabeth and Essex*, often reducing it to melodrama. Strachey dwells upon suspicions of sexual abuse in Elizabeth's youth, shows her as a woman with hysterical infatuations and frustrations, and supplies details of mutilation and castration in the legal punishments of that day. Although the main characterization is that of Elizabeth's resolute genius in guiding England to her destined preeminence among nations, the tenor of action at times approaches farce and lacks majesty or magnificence.

Strachey's writings have always elicited a wide range of responses from literary critics. Certain of these were ad hominem reactions to his public image or to actual encounters with him. However, it was immediately evident that Strachey had initiated a new mode of biography in Britain, although the French had for some time produced comparable biographical writing that had influenced Strachey's own stylistic stance. Ever since *Eminent Victorians* he has been credited with the debunking mode of biography that undercuts and deflates people in high places. His intimate characterization, incisive brevity, and emphasis upon psychology rather than history have had many imitators. Among those who have followed in his footsteps are André Maurois, Harold Nicolson, and Emil Ludwig. Of these, Maurois (1929) has been most direct in his frank admiration and admission of debt:

> Read a page of a Victorian biography and then read a page of Mr. Strachey. . . . a book by [him] is above all a work of art. Undoubtedly Mr. Strachey is at the same time an exact historian; but he has the power of presenting his material in a perfect art form. . . . a biographer, such as Mr. Strachey, . . . has the power to diffuse through his record of facts the poetic idea of Destiny, of the passage of Time, of the fragility of human fortune . . . and brings us in fact a secret comfort. [pp. 9, 142]

Strachey was greatly admired by Max Beerbohm, who delivered a Rede lecture in 1943 that praised his mastery of narrative and style (Beerbohm, 1943). Edmund Wilson (1952) believed that Strachey's major contribution was his deflating of Victorian smugness. However, he also stated that Strachey's "irony [in *Eminent Victorians*] was so acid that it partly dehumanized his subjects" (p. 551). Wilson added an interesting observation: "It is sometimes the case with first-rate people that their lives seem to come to an end—sometimes very suddenly—just when they have finished performing their function" (p. 551).

Strachey is credited also with having influenced other literary trends and events. Edel (1957) believes that Virginia Woolf's *Orlando* (1928) was written in part as a kind of parody of Strachey's biographical style. Harrod (1951), the biographer of Maynard Keynes, believes that the economist's attack on Woodrow Wilson after World War I was influenced by his friend Strachey's biographical style (p. 115).

Strachey has often been attacked because he slanted facts, introduced events that never occurred, or even misquoted public speeches in order to convey the impression he desired (Johnson, 1937, pp. 511–512). His introduction of interior monologues, most notably Queen Victoria's death scene, has drawn criticism, and he has been accused of excessive use of clichés and writing "purple prose" (Farrelly, 1950). Muir (1940) wrote of the death scene that it is "one of the worst falsetto purple patches that he ever wrote."

Some attacks on Strachey's work convey so virulent and oppressive a feeling that it must be surmised that they were motivated by his personality, affectations, or homosexuality. Crutwell (1968), for example, states that Strachey was "immature" because his homosexuality prevented the "normal responsibilities of family and parenthood" (p. 732). He goes on to say that in Strachey's later life "he was much more prosperous and . . . the ambisexual circus which surrounded him became more numerous, more frenzied, and more complex in its anatomical gyrations" (p. 736).

But Strachey's most venomous critic was Frank Swinnerton, a noted British writer. His enmity toward Strachey and his distaste for *Eminent Victorians* is puzzling because it was Swinnerton's own enthusiasm and endorsement of the book when it was still in manuscript form that made its publication possible. Swinnerton wrote that once the manuscript was in his hands he could not put it down (Holroyd, 1968, p. 250). Apparently, later encounters with Lytton, together with his reaction to the book's success, produced abhorrence, for Swinnerton (1951) later wrote:

> Sick and sorry [Strachey] may have been, but he had a sportive mind. If one could have seen behind that disguising beard, one might possibly have found that he was smiling. Certainly he was amused by anybody dead; he may have been amused by one yet alive. . . . He shrank from the loud and efficient, the smug and successful. He did not like them, and could not crush them; but he could think of all sorts of amusing things to say which discredit

them. . . . All his work was taken from books, and not from men. He was a bookworm and a talker with bookworms, a male blue-stocking. [pp. 283–286]

An endorsement of *Elizabeth and Essex* came from Freud himself, who wrote its author a qualified letter of approval. Freud noted the difficulties in discerning the motives of others, even those with whom we are in close touch, and he compared the interpretation of historical figures to the analysis of dreams to which we have no associations. "And, with reservations such as these, you have approached one of the most remarkable figures in your country's history. . . . you have touched upon her most hidden motives with . . . boldness and discretion, and it is very possible that you have succeeded in making a correct reconstruction of what actually occurred" (quoted in Holroyd, 1968, p. 616).

James Strachey, of course, is known primarily as the incomparable editor and translator of Freud's Standard Edition, for which he won the Schlegel-Tieck prize for translation in 1966—a measure of the universal acclaim accorded him. Perhaps the most gratifying tribute is the fact that his commentaries have been translated for the German version of the twenty-four volumes of the Standard Edition. He also wrote several psychoanalytic articles, including "Some Unconscious Factors in Reading" (1930) and a piece on the pharoah Akhenaten (1939). In 1934 he published a major contribution to the theory of psychoanalytic technique entitled "The Nature of the Therapeutic Action of Psychoanalysis." This incisive and profound essay has since its first appearance been considered of primary theoretical and clinical significance. A recent authoritative anthology on analytic technique (Bergmann and Hartman, 1976) includes the paper as a milestone in the theory of psychoanalytic treatment. Half a century later, Strachey's views on transference interpretation are so compelling that the editors consider him "the foremost advocate of this point of view" (p. 27).

The article itself centers on Strachey's introduction of the concept of a "mutative interpretation," a term that has remained current and tied to his name. Strachey emphasized the significance of the punitive superego in the impaired functioning of neurotic patients. Once a transference has started, the patient begins to develop a more benign superego but still experiences impulses to regard the analyst as punitive. With the help of the analyst's transference interpretations he becomes able to question and mitigate his own self-punitive tendencies, and such interpretations are therefore termed mutative. Strachey believed that only transference interpretations are capable of creating significant change in the analysand, and it is this extreme view of transference that Bergmann and Hartman feel Strachey best represents.

One theoretical frame that Strachey employs is Kleinian, centered upon the interlocking processes of introjection and projection, although the primary references in the article are to Freud's own views on analytic therapy and their development in the technical literature. Within British analytic circles Strachey was noted for his early and continued espousal of Melanie Klein's views.

The Brothers: Their Sexualities

In his adult years Lytton recalled and described a significant episode from his childhood. He remembered that his sister Dorothy, fourteen years older than he,

> evening after evening . . . kissed me a hundred times, in a rapture of laughter and affection, counting her kisses, when I was six. . . . in that same room, perhaps twenty years later, sitting on a sofa with [my nephew] Andrew, I suddenly kissed *him*, much to his surprise and indignation—"My dear man! Really! One doesn't do those things!" . . . It was on Sunday afternoons, when my mother was invariably at home, that the family atmosphere . . . reached its intensest and its oddest pitch. [1971, p. 22]

This passage illustrates a probable channel for Lytton's homosexual development. The sensual feelings inappropriately and perhaps seductively directed at Lytton by his sister were later associated with the oppressive atmosphere engendered by his mother. Feelings intended by mother and sister to be expressions of affection were experienced by him as overpowering intrusions—partly stimulating but mainly beyond his capacity for response or mastery. What Lytton in childhood experienced as helpless passivity was later to turn into an active expression of feelings of affection and sexuality. Identifying with his mother and sisters, he chose a younger male who represented himself as a child.

The influence of Lady Jane Strachey upon both Lytton and James was of course critical to their later choice of sexual partners. In Carrington, Lytton found someone who watched over him, took care of the household and other personal needs that his mother had met, and who provided continuing emotional security. Lytton turned to men to meet basic physical needs that his mother had been unable to satisfy.

In Rupert Brooke, James found a relationship that reproduced his mother's distance and inaccessibility on the one hand, and her limited physical accommodation on the other. Lytton too was a parental figure for James, who modeled much of his behavior on his idealized brother.

Later on, Freud became a determining parental figure for him, and it is likely that Melanie Klein filled a similar role. Primarily it was the brothers' identification with their mother that decreed a passive and unaggressive stance that was a basic component in their homosexuality.

The theme of Lady Strachey's determining influence upon both brothers is one that could be developed in considerable detail. However, the relationship of Lytton and James to each other is the focus here, and in particular the sexual differences between them rather than their common parental heritage. Rupert Brooke was an epochal figure to James; he became a derivative imago combining both parental love and deprivation. Although Brooke's figure reproduced Lady Strachey's in significant ways, the direct and specific details of his influence upon James determined the direction taken.

The relationship of James and Lytton to each other was conspicuously noncompetitive. Based on personal observation, Leonard Woolf (1969) said of James:

> All his life he was to some extent overshadowed by the greater brilliance, achievements, and fame of Lytton. In similar fraternal cases—not uncommon—more often than not the less successful brother is embittered and, consciously or unconsciously, bears a grudge against his more distinguished brother in particular, and even against the world in general. I never saw the slightest trace of this in James. He was devoted to Lytton and delighted in his success. He confronted the world with a facade of gentle, rather cold, aloofness and reserve, but behind this was a combination of great sense and sensibility. [pp. 119–120]

James maintained this adoring, totally noncritical attitude toward Lytton to the very end. When Holroyd was writing Lytton's biography, James was ludicrously oversensitive to anything that might be construed as criticism of his brother. James's written comments are retained in the biography in the form of footnotes. When Holroyd noted that Lytton at one time sported "a small rather dismal moustache," quoting from a Bloomsbury writer who knew and admired him, James responded with characteristic testiness: "What do you think you mean by this? What can you mean? . . . you might see from photographs [it was] a thick one, not in the least straggly. . . . This is a good example of your unceasing desire to run Lytton down . . . in this case to make people think he was impotent—which, believe me, he wasn't" (Holroyd, 1967, p. 129n).

When Holroyd (1968) described some of Lytton's youthful poetry as "expressions of hopeful, melancholy lust . . . [with] a truly phenomenal amount of copulation," James retorted:

> I have been positively staggered by some of your ethical judgements on the subject of sex and religion. Your remarks about Lytton's poems astound me. . . . the impression you give of holding up your hands in shocked horror at their fearful obscenity makes me wonder whether you've ever come across a young human being. . . . When I read these passages I wonder why on earth you ever set out to write this book—and I feel inclined to want the whole thing thrown out the window. The whole of Lytton's life was entirely directed to stopping critical attitudes of the sort you seem to be expressing. [p. 138n]

James's obloquy is inappropriate and reveals a defensive overidentification with his older brother.

A number of parallels in the lives of Lytton and James are striking. Physically, both were tall (6'1") and slender, with delicate constitutions that required careful diets, although Lytton was much more extreme in his constant ill health. They were remarkably intelligent, of a decidedly rational, intellectual bent and devoted to literary study. Temperamentally, both were socially shy and lacking in forthright aggressiveness. Although the brothers were eccentric, as all the Stracheys are said to have been, Lytton was an absolute model of eccentricity.

James closely followed Lytton in his career up to a point. He chose the same university and the very same room that Lytton had occupied, and he also set out on an identical writing career, producing similar articles for the same literary publications. Both were conscientious objectors in World War I and both moved in the same Bloomsbury circle. Lytton was an exemplar, or ego ideal, that James sought to emulate in place of the father who was emotionally remote from both of them.

These fraternal parallels carried over into the sexual realm. James was Lytton's confidant for many of his homosexual affairs, and to some extent they shared partners. However, in the course of James's infatuation with Rupert Brooke he followed Brooke in initiating heterosexual activity, and here he began to diverge from Lytton, who continued his homosexual activities all his life. Up to the time James met his future wife Alix, he chose women who were approved by Brooke. The one female who was not known to Brooke bore a striking resemblance to him. However, after Brooke died, James's choice of Alix seems to have been influenced by her close intimacy with Lytton's Carrington. The bond between James and Lytton was reinforced by the tie between Alix and Carrington. The relationship between James and Carrington was warm and affectionate but that between Lytton and Alix is not clear in the material now available, and in fact this uncertainty may be significant. Knowledge of how Lytton and Alix felt toward each other would clarify the psychodynamics of the foursome.

A key event in James's life that led to divergence from Lytton was his analysis with Freud. Certainly the analysis enabled James to enter upon an active, productive profession, something that up to then he had been conspicuously unable to do. His acute premarital conflicts presumably entered analytic discussion, and here too the resolution was sufficient to enable the couple thereafter to share a productive life together.

A significant psychoanalytic issue emerges at this point. Is it possible to determine what it was that enabled James to move toward a hetero-sexual object choice, while Lytton remained fixed on homosexuality? According to analytic theory, James, seven years younger than Lytton and even less assertive than his brother, might more likely be expected to remain fully homosexual. Actually, of course, the extent to which James moved toward heterosexuality cannot be gauged from the record of events now available. It is sometimes difficult even in a directly clinical situation to make this judgment. The pursuit of this question is therefore prob-lematical, but the exploration may prove worthwhile.

James was eighteen when he initiated the correspondence with Rupert Brooke. His attraction at that time was both physical and emotional. Brooke was a poetically expressive youth, mannered in his behavior and prone to dramatic posing. These qualities were highly appealing to James, who was languorous and neurasthenic. Preoccupied with physical ail-ments, he was self-absorbed and conspicuously lacking in goal orientation. But Brooke never permitted consummation of James's sexual feelings for him, and this is a key to James's further development. James could not help pursuing Brooke as an unattainable object; he needed Brooke as someone who remained forever unreachable. If Brooke ever expressed some direct availability, James would withdraw (Letters of February 24, 1910; November 7, 1910). In his distancing behavior Brooke reproduced the continuing physical presence and emotional unavailability of James's mother and father.

James adored Rupert and envied him. Brooke attracted people by a kind of magnetic aura. Despite a decided sexual ambiguity, or perhaps because of it, he drew admirers of both sexes. James tried to please Brooke in all things. He wanted Brooke to allow his unrequited love to continue eternally. In the most poignant passages in the correspondence, James pleads abjectly to be allowed to remain in Brooke's presence, if only to be treated as an object.

Brooke not unexpectedly developed contempt for James. In a letter to a friend he referred to James as a "dead twig" (Brooke, 1968, p. 202). After their relationship declined, Brooke (1968) wrote to Virginia Stephen (later Woolf), "God! how I hate the healthy unimaginative hard shelled dilettanti, like James and Ka" (p. 364). Later to Ka he wrote, "James is . . . so defenceless that it is not sport kicking him, after a bit" (p. 422). But no matter how disturbed Brooke became or how their relationship deteriorated, James could not help pursuing Brooke. Brooke reviled Lytton and grossly insulted James, but he could not drive James away.

The self-abasing bond that chained James to Brooke was predicated upon intense but repressed aggression that could not be expressed overtly but was instead turned against himself. Aggression was deeply buried in both Lytton and James, but with James there was the additional factor of his relation to Brooke. Since James was bound to fulfill all of Brooke's desires, he accommodated Brooke's wish that he relate sexually to women and thus turned sensual feelings toward both Noel and Ka. He diverted and fulfilled sexual wishes for Brooke and showed his love for him by displacing some of these feelings to young women chosen by Brooke. He sensed Rupert's unconscious wish that sex be consummated with Ka and did as he felt Brooke wanted. This was the hammer that broke their relationship.

Brooke could not tolerate the fact that James, whom he considered emotionally inferior, succeeded where he could not. Brooke also recognized that James was acting in accord with his own unconscious needs. He needed James to open a pathway for him to Ka, but this was an intolerable idea. The resulting conflict was so intense that Brooke could not remain rational. On the one hand, Brooke could not bear the idea of being sexually inferior to James; on the other, James had only done as unconsciously bidden by Brooke, but by doing so he had created a deeper and more intense homosexual bond that Brooke could not abide either.

Brooke's later abandonment of James released some of the latter's buried aggression and this enabled him to move on to marriage and a career in psychoanalysis. It also might be speculated that Brooke's emotional collapse somehow corresponded to James's unconscious hostility toward him. By fulfilling Brooke's unconscious wish that he possess Ka, he not only proved his love but also his destructive impulses. These were in fact realized in Brooke's paranoid torment.

In Lytton's life there was no one comparable to Brooke. His homosexual relations were consistently consummated and were regularly followed by disillusion and a train of equally disappointing relationships. The masochistic nature of these experiences, which has been described by Roy (1972), could apply as well to James's relation to Brooke. Both brothers turned their primitive aggression inward in continual self-abasing behavior.

Lehmann's biography of Brooke (1980) centers upon his breakdown following the events at Lulworth, but does not clarify just why he developed a paranoid hatred of Lytton in particular. Brooke's choice of Lytton was irrational, but it had a valid root in his unconscious. James Strachey for a long while, as shown in the correspondence, did not react to Brooke's collapse. He seems in his letters either to have overlooked it or actually not to have noticed Brooke's aberrant condition. Brooke was obsessed with the belief that Lytton had conspired with Ka that she and Henry Lamb betray him sexually, but he was not in the least angry with either Ka or Lamb. In fact, as noted, Brooke's passion for Ka suddenly caught fire and endured throughout his emotional disturbance. During this time he was in a paranoid rage centered upon Lytton. Brooke's accusations of Lytton can be viewed as a displacement from James, who had in fact betrayed Brooke, even if at his own bidding.

From the time of Lulworth in December 1911 until the middle of 1912 the relation of James and Brooke remained relatively cordial, although signs of stress were present. During this interval Brooke required the relationship with James even more than James did. It was a dramatic reversal of roles in this friendship bond. The relationship fulfilled both Brooke's unconscious but pressing homosexual tie to James and simultaneously permitted his heterosexual feeling for Ka. Thus Brooke was unable to express hatred for James's betrayal because it would have interfered with both repression of homosexuality and expression of sexuality with Ka. Brooke's precipitant paranoid hatred of Lytton and feeling of betrayal by him at Lulworth had been psychologically feasible because the delusion was a substitute for James's actual betrayal of him with Ka as well as with Noel. Other factors that supported Brooke's delusional formation were his prior unpleasant relationship with Lytton, as well as the many physical and emotional resemblances between the brothers. Brooke needed the emotional fuel of betrayal in order to mount an aggressive passion for Ka.

James's insistent sexual overtures to Brooke had served to keep Brooke's own homosexual impulses in check, since they enabled him to view James as the one with such passions. However, there is documentation of a single full homosexual episode of Brooke's that is dramatic both in its detail and its singularity. In a letter of July 10, 1912, Brooke described vividly and completely his own homosexual intercourse with a fellow student at Cambridge in 1909 (Lehmann, 1980, p. 7). Brooke wrote that he had been jealous of the homosexual sex that James, Lytton Strachey, and Maynard Keynes had been having and at that time he wanted no longer to remain a virgin. Immediately following this admission, Brooke's letters to James become manifestly more disturbed. There is one strikingly pathetic letter (July 12, 1912) in which he describes his inability to sleep because he visualized (hallucinated?) thousands of lice crawling across the ceiling and dropping disgustingly right upon him as he lay in bed (Hassall, 1964, p. 349). In the same letter he writes: "Am I wrong in thinking it feeble and unmanly not to wish to kill any man who dreams of the same cunt as you? . . . James, James, shall I have to turn to you to find my Brutus?"

Brooke was in terrible conflict over needing to share Ka sexually with James but simultaneously unable to tolerate his own homosexual emotions and castration feelings. Even after Brooke's accusations of buggery, even after he wrote, "Perhaps some day you'll grow up" (Letter of March 25, 1913), James remained apologetic in tone, although he responded that it was "a pity that your sorrows should have turned you into a Prig" (Letter of March 27, 1913). James bore the abuse and insisted upon his continuing love for Brooke until his letters were no longer answered.

The writing careers of Lytton and James Strachey evolved from a matrix of family tradition, the influence of parental and sibling relations, and the emotional support of human love. Lytton's career as a biographer blossomed after he met Carrington, and her love softened his ironical writing style. James's career as a psychoanalyst, writer, and editor developed from his loss of Rupert Brooke, the challenge of heterosexuality, and its resolution in relation to Alix and analysis with Freud.

There are also factors of cognitive skill and sublimation but these are most difficult to specify. Both brothers, possibly, were blocked in their early emotional development and especially in the expression of aggression and heterosexuality. Perhaps cognition took over realms more frequently allotted to emotional expression.

The Stracheys' sexuality developed along a common homosexual channel and later diverged. This divergence influenced the distinction between Lytton's biographical writing and James's career in psychoanalysis. Lytton retained a fluidity of sexual expression that perhaps permitted a literary type of writing, whereas James inhibited this fluidity and became increasingly detached from sexual feeling, which may have fostered his career in psychoanalytic practice, writing, and editing. Where biography provided Lytton a path to literary innovation, psychoanalysis gave James a way of helping others and of conceptualizing this work in written form. Both brothers were writers of distinction.

REFERENCES

Beerbohm, M. (1943), *Lytton Strachey (The Rede Lecture)*. Cambridge: Cambridge University Press.

Bergmann, M.S., & Hartman, F.R., eds. (1976), *The Evolution of Psychoanalytic Technique*. New York: Basic Books.

Brennan, G. (1975), *Personal Record (1920–1972)*. New York: Knopf.

Brooke, R. (1968), *The Letters of Rupert Brooke*, ed. G. Keynes. London: Faber & Faber.

Carrington, D. (1970), *Carrington: Letters and Extracts from Her Diaries*, ed. D. Garnett. New York: Holt, Rinehart & Winston.

Crutwell, P. (1968), Eminent Edwardians. *Hudson Review*, 21:726–736.

Edel, L. (1957), *Literary Biography*. Bloomington: Indiana University Press, 1973.

Farrelly, J. (1950), Lucky eminence. *New Republic*, 122:25–26.

Freud, A. (1969), James Strachey. *Internat. J. Psycho-Anal.*, 50:131–132.

Freud, S. (1901), The Psychopathology of Everyday Life. *Standard Edition*, 6. London: Hogarth Press, 1960.

———— (1905), Jokes and Their Relation to the Unconscious. *Standard Edition*, 8. London: Hogarth Press, 1960.

Garnett, D. (1953), *The Golden Echo*. London: Chatto & Windus.

———— (1955), *The Flowers of the Forest*. London: Chatto & Windus.

Harrod, R.A. (1951), *The Life of John Maynard Keynes*. New York: A.M. Kelley, 1969.

Hassall, C. (1964), *Rupert Brooke: A Biography*. New York: Harcourt, Brace & World.

Holroyd, M. (1967), *Lytton Strachey, Vol. 1: The Unknown Years (1880–1910)*. New York: Holt, Rinehart & Winston.

———— (1968), *Lytton Strachey, Vol. 2: The Years of Achievement (1910–1932)*. New York: Holt, Rinehart & Winston.

———— (1971), *Lytton Strachey: A Biography*. rev. ed. New York: Holt, Rinehart & Winston.

Iyengar, K.R. Srinivasa (1939), *Lytton Strachey: A Critical Study*. Port Washington, N.Y.: Kennikat Press, 1967.

Johnson, E. (1937), *One Mighty Torrent*. New York: Macmillan, 1955.

Kallich, M. (1958), Psychoanalysis, sexuality, and Lytton Strachey's theory of biography. *American Imago*, 15:331–370.

———— (1961), *The Psychological Milieu of Lytton Strachey*. New Haven, Conn.: College & University Press.

———— (1962), Lytton Strachey: an annotated bibliography of writings about him. *English Fiction in Transition (1880–1920)*, 5(3):1–77.

Khan, M. Masud R. (1973), Mrs. Alix Strachey. *Internat. J. Psycho-Anal.*, 54:370.

Lehmann, J. (1980), *The Strange Destiny of Rupert Brooke*. New York: Holt, Rinehart & Winston.

Maurois, A. (1929), *Aspects of Biography*. New York: Ungar, 1966.

Muir, E. (1940), *The Present Age from 1914*. New York: McBride.

Myers, F.W.H. (1893), *Proceedings of the Society for Psychical Research*, June 1893.

Partridge, F. (1981), *Love in Bloomsbury: Memories*. Boston: Little, Brown.

Rees, G. (1968), A case for treatment: the world of Lytton Strachey. *Encounter*, 30:71–83.

Reik, T. (1952), Saint Irony. *The Secret Self*. New York: Farrar, Straus & Young, 1953.

Roy, D. (1972), Lytton Strachey and the masochistic basis of homosexuality. *Psychoanal. Rev.*, 59:579–584.

Russell, B. (1967), *The Autobiography of Bertrand Russell*. Boston: Little, Brown.

Sanders, C.R. (1953), *The Strachey Family: 1588–1932*. New York: Greenwood Press, 1968.

Strachey, J. (1930), Some unconscious factors in reading. *Internat. J. Psycho-Anal.*, 11:322–331.

———— (1934), The nature of the therapeutic action of psychoanalysis. *Internat. J. Psycho-Anal.*, 15:127–159.

———— (1939), Preliminary notes upon the problem of Akhenaten. *Internat. J. Psycho-Anal.*, 20:33–42.

———— (1966), General Preface to the *Standard Edition*, Vol. 1. London: Hogarth Press.

Strachey, L. (1912), *Landmarks in French Literature*. London: Williams & Norgate.

———— (1918), *Eminent Victorians*. New York: Modern Library, n.d.

———— (1921), *Queen Victoria*. New York: Harcourt, Brace, 1949.

———— (1928), *Elizabeth and Essex*. New York: Harcourt, Brace, 1956.

———— (1971), *Lytton Strachey by Himself*, ed. M. Holroyd. New York: Holt, Rinehart & Winston.

———— (1973), According to Freud. In: *The Really Interesting Question*, ed. P. Levy. New York: Coward, McCann & Geoghegan, pp. 111–120.

Swinnerton, F. (1951), *The Georgian Literary Scene, 1910–1935: A Panorama*. New York: Farrar, Straus, 1951.

Wilson, E. (1952), *The Shores of Light: A Literary Chronicle of the Twenties and Thirties*. London: W.H. Allen.

Winnicott, D.W. (1969), James Strachey: 1887–1967. *Internat. J. Psycho-Anal.*, 50:129–131.

Woolf, L. (1960), *Sowing: An Autobiography of the Years 1880 to 1904*. New York: Harcourt Brace Jovanovich.

———— (1969), *The Journey Not the Arrival Matters: An Autobiography of the Years 1939 to 1969*. New York: Harcourt Brace Jovanovich.

Woolf, V. (1976), *The Letters of Virginia Woolf: 1912–1922*, Vol. 2, ed. N. Nicolson & J. Trautmann. New York: Harcourt Brace Jovanovich.

———— (1977a), *The Letters of Virginia Woolf: 1923–1928*, Vol. 3, ed. N. Nicolson & J. Trautman. New York: Harcourt Brace Jovanovich.

———— (1977b), *The Diary of Virginia Woolf: 1915–1919*, Vol. 1, ed. A.O. Bell. New York: Harcourt Brace Jovanovich.

———— (1978), *The Diary of Virginia Woolf: 1920–1924*, Vol. 2, ed. A.O. Bell. New York: Harcourt Brace Jovanovich.

During the past two centuries, Jewish life has developed from a self-enclosed, static, medieval world to one that is modern, open, and mobile; from a world in which all concerns were related to religion to one that is increasingly secular. The intellectual movement that rationalized this transition, that espoused and urged this modernization of Jewish life, was the Haskalah, the Jewish expression of the Western Enlightenment. Indeed, the impact of the Haskalah on Jewish life and thought is incalculable. There is scarcely an aspect of either that has not been affected, influenced, or stirred by it.

Modern Yiddish literature was not merely influenced by the Haskalah; it is no exaggeration to state that it would have been impossible without it. Its faith in human reason, rejection of Jewish medievalism and pietism, passion for the modernization of Jewish life—"Be a Jew at home and a man in the street!"—made possible a modern culture in Hebrew as well as in Yiddish and secular careers in Jewish learning and literature, thereby breaking the monopoly over the Jewish mind that had hitherto been held by Yeshiva and Torah. But the concept could succeed only in proportion to the breakdown of the self-contained, intellectually self-sufficient enclave of the world of Jewish piety. In a very real sense, modern Yiddish literature became possible only with the breakup of

11

The Brothers Singer: Faith and Doubt

JOSEPH C. LANDIS

that enclave; it became viable only as a successor to that world. What the Haskalah had urged, life effected. The movement of Yiddish and its culture during the century that followed the publication of *Dos Kleyne Mentshele* in 1864 by Mendele Mokher Sforim—a date arbitrarily accepted as the "beginning" of modern Yiddish literature—was toward a modern cultural entity, that was secular, rationalist, libertarian, and meliorist.

Within less than a century, that literature with its culture had completed a cycle. Having witnessed and experienced Western barbarism, it recoiled from its faith in the Enlightenment and the golden promises of Western culture. But it never returned to the faith of its pious ancestors, never longed for their faith. When the poet Yankev Glatshteyn thundered, in the thirties, "Good night, you great big stinking world. I return to the ghetto because I wish to," he was not urging the need for a return to traditional piety. Rather, his gall-dipped words were proclaiming the moral superiority of "backward" traditional Jewish life and Jewish morality over the bestial immorality of the modern Western world. Like his colleagues and readers he was too much the modern, too much committed to modern life for a return to ghetto piety. In like manner, the regrets and the tears, the *kaddish* of the mourner's prayer for the lost shtetl that is heard in contemporary Yiddish writing are an expression of regret for the loss of a Jewish world, not hunger for Jewish religious faith. Indeed, secular Yiddish culture has been little troubled by its departure from the faith of its forebears. It remains committed to the Enlightenment and to secularism. The need for faith, the plague of doubt—these are concepts that do not trouble it. But it is precisely this conflict, this confrontation that is illustrated in the two most famous brothers in Yiddish literature, Israel Joshua and Isaac Bashevis Singer, who represent an astonishing study in contrast in their attitudes to the world in which they were reared, in their resulting attitudes to God and man, and in the mainsprings of their work.

Both brothers have left us memoirs of their early years, which are wonderfully telling in illuminating their basic struggles to find a locus in a changing world and in elucidating their central fictional concerns. Indeed, to read these memoirs side by side is to perceive once again the paradoxical truism that siblings reared in the same home by the same parents are never reared in the same home by the same parents. To study these memoirs is to discover such contrasts in the brothers' perceptions of their world, in their reactions to it, and in their resulting weltanshauung as to suggest different places, different times. Indeed, as the times of their maturing were different, so were the places. These differences led Israel Joshua into the mainstream of modern Yiddish intellectual and literary life; they led Isaac to a lonely isolation from both the modern and the traditional world.

Israel Joshua, the older of the two by eleven years, followed the common road that led other contemporary Yiddish writers from the circumscribed world of piety to the open world and limitless horizons of modern culture. Like most, he found the shtetl enclave constricting and heeded the sirens' song beyond the invisible but very real walls of the shtetl.

The beginnings of that journey are recorded in a posthumously published memoir of his childhood, *Of a World That Is No More*, which appeared in Yiddish in 1946 and which, internal evidence suggests, was begun at least as early as 1935. Israel is quick to point an accusing finger at the oppressive piety of the world in which he was reared (his father a rabbi, his mother a rabbi's daughter, rabbinical forebears on both sides of the family), and the trauma of his experience with the heder, the religious school to which, like all other shtetl children, he was sent at the age of three. "I resisted the despised heder with all the determination of a three-year-old," he recalled. "In the end, I naturally gave in but I never grew to love the heder. At the same time, I formed a strong dislike for the Torah" (p. 25). Although he continued his religious studies—to do otherwise would have been unthinkable for a rabbi's young son—he had "nothing but unpleasant experiences with most of [his] teachers" (p. 25) and was thoroughly bored by the religious texts.

Equally negative was his reaction to the religious atmosphere at home.

> Our house was gloomy—one reason why, since childhood, I have preferred the street to the home.
> One cause of this gloom was the Torah, which filled every cranny of our house and weighed heavily on the spirits of those living there. Ours was more of a studyhouse than a home, a House of God rather than one of man. [p. 28]

The indictment continues.

> In our house everything was a sin. Calling my teacher, Reb Meyer, crazy was a sin. Catching flies on the Sabbath was a sin. Running was also a sin, since it did not befit Jews to run, only gentiles. No matter what one did or didn't do, chances were it was sinful. Doing absolutely nothing was certainly a sin. "Why are you wasting time?" Father would complain each time he caught me looking out the window. "A Jew must never be idle. He must study instead." [p. 34]

"The 'Jew' in question was a young child who spent ten hours a day in heder," he added with undisguised bitterness, "but apparently this wasn't enough. Every spare moment had to be devoted to the Torah" (p. 34).

The Sabbath was a day of rest in the shtetl, a day of inner peace, but not for Israel Joshua.

> Even on Sabbaths, there was no respite from the implacable Torah. In fact, Sabbath was to me an even greater torture than weekdays. True, there was no heder, for which I offered up lavish thanks. . . . [p. 35]

But Father always left late for synagogue and therefore returned late.

> When we finally came home, it would already be mid-day. The Sabbath meal . . . would be cold and tasteless. . . . The moment we finished eating, both Mother and Father settled down for the traditional Sabbath nap and my real period of torture began.
>
> "If you don't feel like napping, you can glance through the *Book of Morals*," Father would suggest. [pp. 35–36]

Yet Father was no tyrannical paterfamilias. Quite the contrary. But he was partner to a "mismatch" that intensified the dour atmosphere of the house.

> Another cause for . . . gloom was the mismatch between my mother and father. They would have been a well-mated couple if she had been the husband and he the wife. Even externally each seemed better suited for the other's role. . . .
>
> They were as different in spirit as they were in physique. Although Father was a devoted scholar and inspired researcher of fresh nuances in the Torah, it could not be said that he had an outstanding mind. He was more a creature of heart than of intellect, one who accepted life as it was and did not delve deeply into the way of things. . . . Nor was he plagued by uncertainty. He believed in people and, even more, in God. His absolute faith in God's Torah and in saints was boundless. He never questioned the ways of the Lord, he nursed no resentments, he suffered no doubts. For him it was enough that a thing had been written in the Torah to believe in it unquestioningly. [pp. 29–30]

Israel's mother, by contrast

> took after her father, the Bilgoraj rabbi. She was an accomplished

worrier, a fretter, a doubter; totally devoted to reason and logic; always thinking, probing, pondering, and foreseeing. She brooded about people, about the state of the world, about God and His mysterious ways. She was, in short, the complete intellectual. [p. 30]

At one point Father—"naive," a "helpless dreamer," in his wife's eyes, with an "absolute faith" in the Torah—became convinced that the Messiah was on his way. The year was 1905. The Russo-Japanese War could easily be the War of Gog and Magog that was to precede the coming. And there were passages in the Talmud that seemed to suggest 1905 as the year of redemption. The Messiah's failure to arrive, though it caused him some embarrassment and disappointment, did not diminish his faith one iota.

Not long thereafter, Father managed to let himself be fleeced out of a substantial inheritance from his mother and became the laughingstock of the town he served as rabbi. When the family found itself in desperate straits, Mother took out her last piece of jewelry for Father to pawn. He went to Warsaw, pawned the hat pin and returned, satisfied that his mission had been a success. However, "A thorough search of his pockets produced nothing":

> Father turned pale. "Woe is us, someone must have picked my pocket," he bleated. "What do we do now?"
> "Go wash up for dinner," Mother said. . . .
> But Father wouldn't eat; he opened a holy book instead. "The Almighty undoubtedly knows best," he mumbled, becoming engrossed in the text. [p. 246]

Israel's choice of the verb "bleated" seems characteristic of his perception of his father and indicates the scorn he felt for him.

Even the towering figure of his maternal grandfather, the rabbi of Bilgoraj, with whom Mother and the children spent summers, could not restore Israel Joshua's interest in religious studies. He did, however, "feel safe and secure and protected by his presence" (p. 84). If an undercurrent of contempt taints Israel's descriptions of his father, memories of his grandfather border on awe.

> Grandfather was tall, with dark piercing eyes, a refined but grim face, a gray beard and earlocks, and a rangy physique. He was sharp of speech, taciturn, dignified. For some reason I feared him immediately even as I loved him. I later found out that all the Jews in Bilgoraj shared these feelings, as did his own grown children. [p. 81]

He recalled that "a kind of implacable force seemed to emanate from
the tall, stern, imposing man who appeared to have been born for his
role as shepherd of a community. He ruled the city with wisdom and
justice, feared nothing and no one, did not let the smallest matter pass
unnoticed, and granted immunity to no one, no matter how rich, pious,
or powerful" (p. 131).

In contrast to so massive a figure, Israel's father inevitably shrivels.
"My Father was an ardent Hasid and the scion of generations of Hasidim"
(p. 17). Grandfather, on the other hand, belonged to the contemptuous
opponents of the pietistic Hasidim, "with all their mysticism, their singing, their dancing and gabble about miracles" (p. 17). Grandfather

> was a practical man with a deeply ingrained sense of duty. He
> contended that one should devote one's life to either the Torah or
> to . . . business. My father, on the other hand, was a visionary with
> a total dependence on God. He hated responsibility of any kind.
> His credo was: "With God's help, all will be well." . . . He was
> content with his Hasidim, his saints, and his Torah. In his spare
> time he wrote commentaries on the Gemara and innovations on the
> Torah. Grandfather thought little of his commentaries, his innova-
> tions, his court rabbis, and his banquets. [p. 17]

Indeed, "Grandfather saw that the young husband would amount to nothing and hinted to Mother that she should divorce him. But she adamantly
refused" (p. 18).

Not even Grandfather, however, could restore Israel's dissolving piety.
He continued to find the world of religious study dull. On the other hand,
the world of nature and the world of people were exhilarating. He had
a "passion for realism" (p. 13) and a passion for real life and real people,
a passion for the outside world which lay beyond the indoor realm of
religious study and the mystical, impractical, otherworldly atmosphere
that his father established in the house. These contrasting, opposing
moods seemed symbolized in his mind by the contrasting personalities
of his parents.

> I'd glance through the Book of Morals and follow its fanatic rant-
> ings about the vanity of vanities that consumed the world and I
> would grow deeply resentful. I longed for the outdoors—for the
> fields, the sun, the wind, the water, and the company of friends.
> The world was no pit of iniquity totally riddled with the vanity of
> vanities but an incredibly beautiful place abounding in indescribable
> joys. Every tree, every grazing horse, every foal, haystack, stork,

goose, and gosling called out to me and filled me with happiness and an appreciation of life. I waited for my parents to close their eyes, then fled like a thief from the prison of the Torah, the awe of God and of Jewishness.

I dashed out into the open, sun-drenched world. . . . The boys in the meadow welcomed me as one of their own. [p. 37]

Again and again he recorded his passion for life. "My friends were never the decent and respectable boys from good Hasidic families, but the sons of teamsters, artisans, and other common folk with whom I, the rabbi's son, had no business consorting" (p. 38). In the house of prayer he would edge away from the eastern wall where the men of status prayed and talked, to join the boys near the exit; there they

talked about horses, cattle fairs, fights, fires, epidemics, highway-men, thieves, soldiers, gypsies, and other such fascinating subjects. There were also always gangs of beggars there, men who had roamed the world and could spin marvellous yarns. Occasionally a soldier would drop in, a porter, or a village peddler from out of town. There were also youths from Warsaw employed in Leoncin as journey-men. . . . They told wondrous stories about the capital city, where lamps burned without naphtha, and other such miraculous phenom-ena. [pp. 38–39]

In the end, neither Leoncin or Bilgoraj could contain Israel: he began to quarrel with God. The first incident he recounts concerns a madcap teacher who, tipsy from celebrating the rejoicing customary on Purim, imagined he could fly and dived through the closed window of Father Singer's study. A sliver of glass pierced his left eye and destroyed it.

I looked down at my melamed lying so still on the green blanket with the yellow lions. He lay there without a sound as the blood kept trickling down his cheek. I felt deeply resentful against God for having permitted such an injustice, and on a holiday besides. [p. 68]

This was but the first of Israel's quarrels. On another occasion, he attended his grandfather's rabbinical court and was witness to the helpless exploitation of the poor by the rich. After one such lawsuit he "began to rage against God for allowing the poor to bear such suffering. 'Why doesn't God make everybody good, Grandfather?' I cried out." Even Grandfather could not effect a peace.

He tried to placate me with all kinds of explanations but I refused to be put off. Then he fixed his great piercing eyes on mine and said, "You are too young to understand such things. . . . Have faith in God and in the rightness of His deeds."

At the same time he looked up to the heavens, sighed deeply, and blurted out with feeling, "I believe, Lord of the Universe! I believe!"

From the way he seized his Gemara and resumed his studies, I knew that he wanted to rid himself of brooding thoughts and tormenting questions. [p. 131]

But it was the simultaneous death of his two younger sisters as a result of scarlet fever that brought about what seems to have been the definitive break. His distraught mother stretched her hands to heaven and cried:

"What have I done to deserve this, Father in heaven?"

The Father in heaven did not answer, but my father did. "Obviously it was meant to be," he said brokenly. "One dares not question the ways of the Lord . . . God is just . . . God is good."

"No, God is bad!" I shouted.

Father was aghast. "A Jew dares not say such a thing!" he said, shaking with fear. "God is righteous. . . ."

"He is evil! Evil!" I cried.

A God Who would hand over my little sisters to the Angel of Death could not be righteous—this didn't square with my concept of righteousness. Because of this resentment, I also quarreled with my tutor when we studied the Book of Job—I sided with Job, the victim and leper, instead of with Job's friends, who comforted him with words, or with God, Who justified His harsh punishment with boasts of His divine power and wondrous works. I raged against God so persistently that pious people stopped up their ears and warned me that I would pay for my arrogance. [p. 150]

Meanwhile, the world beyond both Leoncin and Bilgoraj was reaching young Israel. He met his much older cousin Fradel, who refused to marry a promising young rabbinic scholar and declared her intention of becoming a dentist. "The word 'dentist' filled me with such pride and awe that I could hardly breathe. I would only keep staring at this fantastic creature with the cigarette bobbing between her lips and wonder how she could be my blood relative" (p. 125).

His mother, still hoping that his father would learn Russian and pass the government examination which would give him a license to practice as a rabbi (he was rabbi of Leoncin illegally) and thereby gain a legitimate position in a larger community, bought a Russian grammar. His father steadfastly refused to study the "unclean" language, but Israel began to do so on his own. His mother encouraged him " 'so that when it's your turn to take the examination you'll breeze through it.' She hadn't the slightest doubt that I would grow up to be a rabbi" (p. 140). "The more Father sought to shield me from the outside world and bury me in holy books, the more I was drawn to life that penetrated even inside the Chamber of Justice, where I was supposedly immersed in the Torah. . . . for I was possessed of an insatiable curiosity about everything and everybody" (pp. 195, 199).

From the outside world one day came a group of young Jewish painters and decorators, hired by the Squire of Leoncin to refurbish his manor. Their free Warsaw ways antagonized the pious Jews, who rejoiced when a squad of police arrived in town to arrest them for seditious activities, but Israel "choked back bitter tears and for a long time gazed after the strangers"; they had, he wrote, "disturbed my life in such a way that I would forever after be restless" (p. 220).

And from the outside world came news one day that Theodore Herzl was dead, even then famous as the founder of modern Zionism, "the luxuriantly bearded man who wanted to lead the Jews to the land of Israel" (p. 217). His father had no idea who Herzl was. Another influence was a young student named Sheike, who was left with Father Singer to study the Gemara: "but the boy had a mind of his own. From him I learned about Zionism, socialism, about strikes and revolutions, about the assassination of policemen, officers, generals, and even emperors. . . . One day he taught me a seditious song . . ." (p. 221). When Sheike, who showed no fear of peasant dogs, went home, "he left me with a nagging urge for something better, bigger, and more exciting than I had" (p. 222).

Israel Joshua's memoir, which begins with his earliest recollections at the age of two, ends as he is approaching his thirteenth birthday and is beginning to feel the emotional impact of approaching adolescence. In 1908 the family moved for a short time to the heart of a Jewish orthodox neighborhood on Krochmalna Street in Warsaw. Israel continued his Talmudic studies until he was seventeen, but all the while he was secretly reading books in Yiddish and Hebrew and trying his hand at drawing, painting, and writing. At eighteen he left home, supporting himself at all kinds of jobs, studied Polish, Russian, German, and other secular subjects on his own. When the World War I broke out, he hid to avoid service and took his first steps toward a literary career in Yiddish.

Of a World That Is No More is in essence the story of Israel Joshua Singer's gradual estrangement from the quasi-medieval shtetl world of Jewish piety that was still very much alive at the beginning of the twentieth

century. It is a story of the gloom of that world, of his boredom with the
irrelevancy of Talmudic studies, of his ill-concealed disdain for his ineffectual and mystical father, of his admiration for the clear-minded prac-
ticality of his intellectual mother, of his increasing estrangement from
God, of his passionate fascination with nature and life. At his sudden
death in 1944 at the height of his literary fame, he was regarded as one
of the three greatest living Yiddish novelists (along with Sholem Asch and
Dovid Bergelson). A social realist, his fiction portrayed people with uncommon vivacity and color; but always he had remained the
skeptic—skeptical of man, of his motives, of justice, of life itself.

At Israel's death there was another novelist on the staff of New York's
Jewish Daily Forward, a promising younger writer who had produced a
single well-received novel and who wrote then and later under the pen
names Isaac Varshavsky, I. Segal, and Isaac Bashevis. As the junior by
eleven years of his famous brother Israel Joshua, Isaac had chosen to write
under pseudonyms rather than appear to be trading on the reputation of
I.J. Singer. A quarter of a century later, Isaac too began publishing memoirs and recollections, at far greater length than his brother. Because he
followed a road common to the overwhelming majority of modern Yiddish
writers, Israel Joshua may very well be the less interesting of the two
brothers. It is Isaac Bashevis, standing in lonely eminence outside the
great tradition, who is the more intriguing, the more puzzling, and the
more anguished.

To read the memoirs of the two brothers is to discover two contrasting
worlds, so different was the perception of each. Isaac's memoirs are fixed
lovingly on his father; to Isaac home was a place of emotional warmth,
wondrous tradition, soul-filling piety. Anchored in the timeless cosmos
of eternal Judaism, it was marvelously disdainful of "the world," indifferent to time and place, gloriously immersed in the sea of the Talmud,
in the wisdom of commentaries. It is this legacy of faith and Isaac's deeply
felt regard for it that permeates all his memories—that and the pain of
doubt. Israel Joshua left his pious world with scarcely a backward glance,
a feat that Isaac Bashevis found impossible. The opening pages of Isaac's
A Little Boy in Search of God (1976) sound these twin motifs that dominate
his memoir as well as his life and work: faith and doubt, *gloybn un tsveyfl*.
Gloybn un tsveyfl is, in fact, the name of the several series of reminiscences that ran twice weekly in the *Jewish Daily Forward* from 1975 to
1979, the second such series of recollections from which *A Little Boy in
Search of God* is excerpted. *Gloybn un tsveyfl* is hardly intended as a
narrative of events. It is more nearly a kind of Wordsworthian *Prelude,*
the story of the growth of a writer's mind and consciousness, the story

of a writer caught in the contradictions of past and present, faith and reason, piety and the Enlightenment. It is not really the story of Itchele, the little boy of Leoncin and Number 10 Krochmalna Street searching for God, but of Isaac Bashevis Singer, the writer of seventy, tracing once again in yet another autobiographical reprise the origins of his views, trying to convince himself of the consistency of their growth, retelling once again his quarrel with God, and once again hoping to exorcise the dybbuk of doubt, to justify at last the ways of Isaac to God. His early questions really should be more childish than they are; his youthful wisdom, less wise. But the essential truth, the tortured truth, emerges as he seeks again the vindication of Isaac. With what affection, admiration, and pride he describes his home and his family's status:

> I was born and reared in a home where religion, Jewishness, was virtually in the air that we breathed. I stem from generations of rabbis, Hasidim, and Cabalists. I can frankly say that in our house Jewishness wasn't some diluted formal religion but one that contained all the flavors, all the vitamins, the entire mysticism of faith. . . . [p. 1]
>
> In our house the coming of the Messiah was taken almost literally. . . . My father had published a book in which there was a family tree tracing our descent from Shabatai Cohen, from Rabbi Moshe Isselis, from Rashi, until King David. My [younger] brother Moshe and I would enter the palace where King David sat with crown on head on a golden throne and call him "Grandpa!" . . . [p. 3]

With what admiration Bashevis (1965) describes his father's unworldliness, which "even at that time . . . was rare" (p. 51), or his father's total rejection of doubt, total refusal to doubt: "Father warned Mother that if she didn't stop abusing [his Hasidic master] before the children they would proceed from doubting the Rabbi to doubting God" (p. 56). (Years later, Gimpel the Fool would discover that first you doubt Elke, then you doubt God.)

How Isaac's imagination glowed with vivid re-creations of Biblical scenes, with the mysteries his father discovered in the Cabala. How he rejoiced in the Purim carnivals on Krochmalna Street, in the intense Jewishness of that world. "I actually *felt* that there was a holy soul inside me, a particle of the Godhead" (p. 70). In this timeless Jewish universe, it was the surrounding world that was in exile. "In our home, the 'world' itself was *tref*"—unclean and forbidden. And then the aged, reminiscing writer adds, in words that understate the great regret, the lasting ache,

"Many years were to pass before I began to understand how much sense there is in this attitude" (p. 68).

The family's move to Warsaw in 1908, which began to open doors for Israel Joshua, had little effect on Isaac Bashevis, for whom it meant a move from one pious enclave to another. What was it, then, that undermined Isaac's faith? In his first memoir, *In My Father's Court* (1965), he had placed the blame on his brother. "My brother and his worldly books had sown the seeds of heresy in my mind" (p. 243). Other encounters in war-torn Warsaw helped foster doubt: experiences at a disinfecting station in 1916, and visits to his brother, who was hiding from the army in the studio of the sculptor Ostrzego, brought him into contact with the non-Jewish outside world. "Between Ostrzego's studio and the disinfecting station, the heder, Father's courtroom, and the study house lost their attraction for me . . ." (p. 259). The family's stay at his grandfather's in Bilgoraj, "a century behind" the times, restored some of his peace. "In this world of old Jewishness I found a spiritual treasure trove. I had a chance to see our past as it really was. Time seemed to flow backwards. I lived Jewish history" (p. 290).

In a later memoir, however, Isaac (1976) reports that the great blows which battered his faith were neither his brother's books nor the great world. His doubts had really begun earlier with his observation of the cruelties that both nature and man inflicted without reproof or punishment from the Almighty. His doubts were supported by his brother's views. "Nature demonstrated no religion. . . . It apparently didn't concern nature that the slaughterers in Yanash's Market daily killed hundreds or thousands of fowl. Nor did it bother nature that the Russians made pogroms on the Jews or that the Turks and Bulgarians massacred each other and carried little children on the tips of their bayonets" (p. 12). And "boys caught flies, tore off their wings, and tortured them in every manner only man could conceive while God the Almighty sat on his throne of Glory in seventh heaven and the angels sang His praises" (p. 20). He often felt "an unbearable pity for those who were suffering and who had suffered in all generations. . . . I lived in a world of cruelty. . . . I was a child, but I had the same view of the world that I have today—one huge slaughterhouse, one enormous hell" (p. 49). He could "find no answer in the Scriptures" (p. 55). Israel Joshua's memoir reports not a flicker of pain when doubts began to appear. For Isaac Bashevis, however, the experience was terrifying. "I am becoming a heretic!" (p. 57). Israel, who had given up trying to "fathom the truth of the world," urged Isaac to "eat, drink, sleep, and if it's possible, try to create a better order" (p. 71). Neither eating nor drinking nor improving the world held any attraction for Isaac then, nor do they now.

Isaac could neither secede from piety like his brother nor reject all doubt like his father. He continued to be tortured by God's dereliction from duty and by the question of "why people and animals must suffer so. This to me was the question of questions" (p. 77). Again and again the challenge, sometimes the very phrase reverberates in his memoirs. "The question of questions was the suffering of creatures, man's cruelty to man and animals. . . . Those were my feelings then, and those are my feelings still" (p. 88). The "problem of problems is still to me the suffering of people and animals" (p. 89). Isaac's conclusions deepened his doubts. "If God were indeed full of mercy and benevolence, He wouldn't have allowed starvation, plagues, and pogroms" (p. 91). The outcome of such heretical thoughts might well have been a denial of God such as his brother had embraced. But such denial was beyond Isaac's power. The only viable alternative was war. " 'God is evil,' I said, astounded at my own words. 'A good God wouldn't arrange it that wolves should devour lambs and cats should catch innocent mice' " (p. 102). Still, though God was evil, Isaac could not shed belief.

Some years later, witnessing a scene of anti-Semitic hooliganism in a railroad car,*

> I knew that what I was seeing now was the essence of human history. Today the Poles tormented the Jews; yesterday the Russians and the Germans had tormented the Poles. Every history book was a tale of murder, torture, and injustice; every newspaper was drenched in blood and shame. . . . At that moment I knew that there was only one true protest against the horror of life and that was to hurl back to God his gift. . . .
>
> Until that night I had often fantasized about redeeming the human species, but it became obvious to me then that the human species didn't deserve redemption. To do so would actually be a crime. Man was a beast that killed, ravaged, and tortured not only other species but its own as well. The other's pain was his joy, the other's humiliation his glory. [pp. 135–136]

When Israel Joshua was nineteen, he had concluded his business with God. Isaac Bashevis at nineteen was attempting to reestablish a relationship with God and man on a new basis that, in fact, was at once rejection and acceptance.

---

* *Editor's note*: I.J. Singer may have borrowed from Bashevis's recollection of this incident in writing the climax of his *The Brothers Ashkenazi* (1969). There one twin brother, soon after having saved the life of his unworthy sib, ironically is murdered on a train by some mindless hooligans.

I said to myself: I believe in God, I fear Him, yet I cannot love Him. . . . Nor can I deny God as the materialists do. All I can do is to the best of my limits treat people and animals in a way I consider proper. I had, one might say, created my own basis for an ethic—not a social ethic nor a religious one, but an ethic of protest. . . . The moral person protests not only when he is personally wronged but also when he witnesses or thinks about the suffering of others. If God wants or feels compelled to torment His creatures, that is His affair. The true protester expresses his protest by avoiding doing evil to the best of his ability. [pp. 127–131]

Indeed, he had related his philosophy of protest to Jewishness:

The Jew personified the protest against the injustices of nature and even those of the Creator. Nature wanted death, but the Jew opted for life; nature wanted licentiousness, but the Jew asked for restraint; nature wanted war, but the Jew, particularly the Diaspora Jew (the highly developed Jew) sought peace. . . . Even if he had to wage war against God, the Jew would not desist. . . . [pp. 179–180]

"With this view of life and in this mood," he wrote, "I went to Warsaw [in 1923] to become the proofreader of the *Literary Pages*" (p. 131). The resolution in this ethic of protest seems to have resolved nothing. The ethic of protest was only a name and a frame for continuing inner conflict, for a state of constant warfare with God and man—and self. It neither cured him of his desperate need to believe nor did it provide a solid foundation for renewed belief. It left him with "moments when I almost deny God, but I also have moments of exultation. . . ." And "in spite of the fact that I pray to God, I also sin against God" (Burgin, 1978, p. 46). Did the ethic of protest really give him the strength to endure the ravages of life? For all his bravado about standing up to God and life on behalf of righteousness, Singer admitted the terrifying proviso: "Well, but this kind of strength lay only within the Jew who observed the Torah, not in the modern Jew who served nature like the gentile, was subservient to it, and placed all his hopes upon it . . ." (pp. 179–180). Where in this confrontation of contending forces does Isaac Singer stand? He has said, "An artist is a person who is rooted in his milieu; he does not deny his parents and grandparents. . . . [My] identity I got at home. I know exactly who my father was—the rabbi in Warsaw. My grandfather was the rabbi in Bilgoraj, and so on and so on" (Rosenblatt and Koppel, 1979, pp. 23–24). But is this really Isaac's identity, embraced without qualification or conflict, or is it merely genealogy? Is he really a Jew who observes the Torah as did his pious forebears? His pious ancestors did not write novels, and modern Yiddish novelists are at best only intellectually enamored of their pious ancestors. Did Father Singer read even the Yiddish newspapers that printed both his sons' work? "Father said that the newspapers were full of blasphemy and heresy" (p. 59) and to the end of his days pretended that his sons were in the newspaper business, not writers for the Yiddish press.

War with God and war with the moderns who rejected Him created a predicament that left Isaac the Yiddish writer in almost total isolation, an exile from two worlds, forever caught between them, like a typical Singer character. In a passage revealing his own clear recognition of his state of exile, he observed:

> I often spoke with rage against God, but I never ceased to believe
> in His existence. I wrote about spirits, demons, cabalists, dybbuks.
> Many Yiddish writers and readers had cut loose from their Jewish
> roots and from the juices upon which they had been nourished.
> They yearned once and for all to tear away from the ghetto and its
> culture—some as Zionists, others as radicals. Both factions preached
> worldliness. But I remained spiritually rooted deep in the Middle
> Ages (or so I was told). I evoked in my work memories and emotions
> that the worldly reader sought to forget and factually had forgotten.
> To the pious Jews, on the other hand, I was a heretic and a blas-
> phemer. I saw to my astonishment that I belonged neither to my
> own people nor to any other peoples. Instead of fighting in my
> writings for the political leaders of a decadent Europe and helping
> to build a new world, I waged a private war with the Almighty.
> [1976, pp. 113–117]

A stranger, he belonged neither to the secular world of modern Yiddish culture nor to the world of Jewish religion. He had rejected the one and been rejected by the other. But it was the one that rejected him that stood at the heart of his yearning. Neither the new socialism nor the new nationalism could really resolve his dilemma. Indeed, he not only indicted God for permitting the cruelties he saw; he despised man for committing them.

Isaac closes the memoir of his early years on a note of bitter despair. In a dream he realized that

> that which we called life was death. . . . That which we called life
> was a scab, an itching, a poisonous toadstool that grew on old planets.
> The earth suffered from an eczema of its skin. . . . The symptoms
> of this eczema were quite familiar to the cosmic medicine—a little
> dust on the surface became ill and transformed into consciousness,

which in God's dictionary was a synonym for death, protest, goals, suffering, doubting, asking countless questions and growing entangled in endless contradictions. . . . [1976, pp. 206–209]

The bitter despair is rarely to be seen on the surface of the numerous novels and short stories that Isaac Singer has produced. Indeed, the greatest of his fictions—certainly the most ingratiating—may very well be the complex public persona he has created, a character of sometimes impish wit and charm, who skates lightly over surfaces and soars gracefully on the wings of clever phrases, an expert at verbal thrust and parry, the Nobel laureate whose ill-fitting dresscoat slyly mocks the practiced pomp, who modestly accepts his prize (with unspoken irony) on behalf of Yiddish literature. What ever happened to Itchele the rabbi's son of Leoncin and Number 10 Krochmalna Street, the terribly troubled, lonely, unbearably shy, dreadfully sinful, audaciously, guiltily doubting little boy, torn by Promethean rage and defiance and bodily hungers, who so desperately wanted to love the ways of his pious ancestors but could not make peace with their God? Behind the public disguise he is still the driving force of Isaac Singer's fiction, replaying in every work the central struggle, enunciating the central theme, and really resolving nothing, so that it all must be told again and again.

In contrast to Isaac's childhood, Israel's early experiences had left him with no faith in God, no faith in man, no faith in the justice of a class-divided society. His fiction became a mirror for man's capacity for delusion—of others, of self—and for grossness, moral degeneration, and defeat. Ironically, this secularist's gloom is pierced only by the possibility of faith in a morality embodied in and symbolized by traditional Jewish morality. This dubious note of the permanence only of the obligation to be moral in a universe of continuous change is his first and final vision of life. (How curiously similar to Isaac's ethic of protest!) It is this note that permeates and concludes his greatest work, *The Brothers Ashkenazi*. It is the center of his moral vision. His advice to young Isaac after he had given up trying to "fathom the truth of the world," the advice to "eat, drink, sleep, and if it's possible, try to create a better order," was counsel which he did not himself heed for long. There is no hedonism to be detected in his work (more nearly its opposite), and his hope for a better order becomes increasingly tentative, limited, and narrowly fixed. The skepticism—sometimes mocking, sometimes bitter, sometimes sad—pervades such larger fictions as *Steel and Iron* (his first novel), *The Sinner* (reissued as *Yoshe Kalb*), *The Brothers Ashkenazi*, *East of Eden*, and *The Family Carnovsky*, which ends on a note of only temporary suspension of his disbelief.

If the posture of the objective observer sadly recording folly, vice, and injustice in a world with an indifferent Nature and no God is the stance that suits Israel best, it is by no means one that Isaac can adopt. The tensions in Israel's fiction are those that arise in the struggle between man and man. The tensions that arise in Isaac's are those between man and himself. What to Israel is outside—the derelictions of men—is to Isaac the intensely personal, intensely painful dereliction of a man, himself, only a single example of the multitudinous sins of which he is capable.

However great was the cost of such a vision to Isaac the man, the gain to Isaac the artist was incalculable. From the very first he had his theme and his universe, his characters and his plots. Like Michelangelo's, his struggle was to liberate his works from the imprisoning marble. Each work springs from the inner tension, which it momentarily relaxes but which is never resolved. At the center of each fiction stands a simple moral-religious thesis: only a rigid conservatism of faith, only a probity as firm as that of his grandfather, the Rabbi of Bilgoraj, who single-handedly had held the world at bay during his lifetime, could serve to withstand the total moral anarchy that attends the slightest deviation from the path of the Torah. Only a rigid social and political conservatism makes sense in a world that is *tref*, unclean and forbidden, where change is impotent to change and therefore changes nothing, where man's nature and temptations are constant.

The unresolved psychic struggle leaves a state of unremitting tension, a heightened sense of his own audacity and guilt, of the enormity of the evil when bodily hungers are unleashed by loss or even diminution of faith, an acute sense of the awesome danger of doubt and a terrible awareness of the capacity—human and personal—for evil. The two sins of sex and slaughter, so common in his fiction, become opposite sides of the same coin. Add the inevitable third and there emerges the vicious trinity of sin—doubt, sex, and slaughter. These occupy the center of his fictions; they are forces to be chained by faith lest they run rampant to a crescendo of evil.

If many a story seems unresolved, if endings often seem inconclusive, it is because no resolution is possible for those who, like Isaac Singer, are tainted, who, though they hunger, can neither believe nor disbelieve, who are driven to doubt by the cruelty of God and man yet who cannot bear the guilt and the uncontrollable sin of doubt. The same story is repeated in endless disguises, but always "it's the same story you told us last time." "The little rogue," says Gimpel the Fool, "he was right."

The relations of the two brothers Singer to one another after their early years are recorded only in Isaac's later friendly reminiscences and in public tributes to his brother in recent years. Talk among contemporaries around the building of the *Jewish Daily Forward* on New York's East Broadway, where both were employed, confirms the amicable relationship. No matter. The collisions and caresses of later life are of far less importance to the creative life and vision, to the basic apprehension of the world and to responsive attitudes to it, than are the comets and asteroids whose impacts during the early years are beyond eradication.

REFERENCES

Burgin, R. (1978), Isaac Bashevis Singer's universe. *New York Times Magazine*, December 3.
Rosenblatt, P., & Koppel, G. (1979), *Isaac Bashevis Singer on Literature and Life*. Tucson: University of Arizona Press.
Singer, I.B. (1965), *In My Father's Court*. New York: Farrar, Straus, & Giroux.
———— (1976), *A Little Boy in Search of God*. Garden City, N.Y.: Doubleday.
Singer, I.J. (1936), *The Brothers Ashkenazi*. New York: Knopf; New York: Atheneum, 1980.
———— (1946), *Of a World That Is No More*. New York: Vanguard Press, 1970.

My first book, when it was published came out simultaneously with a book of his, both of them produced by the same publisher. They plastered a proud advertisement in all the Sunday newspapers which read: GLORIOUS PRESS FOR THE BROTHERS DURRELL.

Larry, when I showed this to him, read it carefully and then looked at me solemnly. "Congratulations," he said. "We are now a circus act; clad in sequined tights, three hundred feet above the ring, you will fling yourself into space, while I, hanging by my knees, will attempt to focus my bleary eyes sufficiently quickly to catch you by the ankles as you sweep past."—*Gerald Durrell, 1961*

That metaphor, like Clea's slap at Darley-as-Critic, is fit warning to those who would begin a study of Lawrence George and Gerald Malcolm Durrell, for it forces them to consider whether the Durrells can be linked or whether they are so far apart that comparison is artificial, a construct of this book of brothers. Clearly the project is, as Lawrence Durrell told me, "thorny," for the reason he gave: both brothers are alive. And for another, they work, in the main, in different rings, one as a novelist, poet, playwright, and essayist who, from *The Black Book* on, has condemned the "English way of death" with its "tea-cosy on reality," the other as a zoologist, reforming visions of animal conservation, and an extraordinarily popular popularizer of animals and family whose books, like Pirates or Pinafore, provide a rite of passage to just those Englishmen who join

12

Sideways Out of the House: Lawrence and Gerald Durrell

JANE LAGOUDIS PINCHIN

383

Iolanthe's lords in "bow, bow, you lower-middle-classes."

Studying siblings as writers is of course examining the biography of family, the webs we all weave. It becomes a very different tale if its subjects are alive. Thorny, indeed. In addition to most of the fifty odd books the Durrells have written and numerous works about them, this paper has been informed by three interviews. With family friend Alan Thomas, the well-known bookseller who edited *Spirit of Place*, at his London home. And with the Durrells themselves: a seven-hour conversation with Lawrence Durrell at his house in Sommières, in the south of France, and two and a half hours with Gerald Durrell at Les Augres Manor in Jersey. The disadvantages to interviewing are real. One comes away with a sure sense that it is foolish to presume one can understand the motivation or significance of lives still being lived. And I liked the Durrells, losing distance as I did. But the greatest disadvantage in dealing with living writers with living relatives is clearly the most obvious—some of what one hears in interview is, and should be, at one and the same time essential and private.

With these difficulties in mind and with the clear sense that one of the brothers views himself as a naturalist who hates writing—"if one makes love four hundred and two times and likes it only twice . . ."—I present to you, the Brothers Durrell.

They have of course a collective persona. A stewardess told Lawrence Durrell he was her favorite author and presented him with a copy of *My Family and Other Animals*, in which he wrote: "Signed in the absence of the author by a better author." They are sparring partners who know how to pull a beard or leg. Mostly, but not exclusively, because of Gerald's writings, a wide audience follows this public feud with great pleasure. Anglo-Saxons have always found it easier to accept affection between men when it exhibits itself through indirection. The punch that is the embrace. Even when the men are brothers. Which is one reason why the collective image of Lawrence and Gerald Durrell has such appeal. Theirs is a robust comedy—of duels with cobras in Hyde Park—of permissible love. Thus we enjoy Lawrence Durrell's *Spirit of Place* as it becomes Gerald Durrell's *Fillets of Plaice* and understand the juxtaposition of a dedication—"This book is for Larry who has always encouraged me to write and has rejoiced more than anybody else in what success I have had"—with what follows:

"The child is mad, snails in his pockets!"—*Lawrence Durrell, c. 1931*

"The man is mad, crawling about snake-infested jungles!"—*Lawrence Durrell, c. 1952*

"The man is mad, wanting to have a zoo!"—*Lawrence Durrell, c. 1958*

"The man is mad."—*Lawrence Durrell, c. 1972*

Lawrence (1981b) tells tales out of school of a brother who sold his books and of like retaliation. Gerald deflates the pompous balloon of his brother's Art.

These are, of course, public, if self-created, faces, part of the image of the zany Durrell family: Mother, age seventy-five, "clad in a leopard skin bikini rid[ing] a camel through Trafalgar Square" (G. Durrell, 1961). "One travelling Circus and Staff" (G. Durrell, 1956, p. 301). Like "the Animal's M.P.," or "the two fisted Irish mick in a mackintosh" (with which, Lawrence Durrell suggests, a press bored with sedentary artists has labeled him), these faces are useful, and they lie. They tell us most about what we, as an audience, rejoice in and what we fear. The Durrells elude us.

The purpose of this chapter is of course to find them, and to that end it will first examine biography—with particular attention to the early and to the shared years—and then, in its second and third parts, Lawrence Durrell as writer and Gerald Durrell as writer; focusing, in all three sections, on where the brothers touch and on how each views family and, through family, this world; knowing, in all three sections, that life exceeds our geometries.

It will become clear that the Durrells are not, for all their clowning, Punch and Karaghiosis, an illusory pair. Nor are they simply two brothers who write. They are siblings who write about the same place and the same people, and they write about each other. What is more, they use each other as fictive figures, characters who work to illuminate their authors' vision. And one, I will venture to guess, is responsible in no small measure for his brother's prose style.

Yet for all these bonds, no one who reads them can have missed the sense that the audiences they address and the tone, the moods they create, are so dramatically different that one wonders about the possibility of common origins: for Gerald Durrell domesticates everything, bringing all living creatures into the family, the circus, the zoo. While his brother makes the familial exotic, frightening, one with the strange world in which the alienated self, the artist, moves alone.

One wants to know why. Which leads to a fatal but human flaw—to the belief that we can turn our own vision to those characters and places about which both Durrells wrote and thereby learn their real history. That we can tell the truth and write biography.

Two Lives

> So once in idleness was my beginning.
> Little known of better then or worse
> But in the lens of this great patience
> Sex was small,
> Death was small,
> Were qualities held in deathless essence,
> Yet subjects of the wheel, burned clear
> And immortal to my seventh year.
>
> To all who turn and start descending
> The long sad river of their growth:
> The tidebound, tepid, causeless
> Continuum of terrors in the spirit,
> I give you here unending
> In idleness an innocent beginning
>
> Until your pain become a literature.
>   [L. Durrell, 1980a, p. 159]

Lawrence and Gerald Durrell were both born in India, in 1912 and 1925, the eldest and youngest sons of a family that had long been Anglo-Indian. There were, as their readers know, four children: Lawrence, then Leslie, Margaret, and Gerald, eight years younger than his sister. The classic British colonial family—a tribe, Lawrence Durrell called them, which conferred the appropriate rights and responsibilities on its son and heir when its father died. That father, Lawrence Samuel Durrell, a civil engineer of considerable talent who built the Tata Iron and Steel Works—"he for whom steel and running water / Were roads" (L. Durrell, 1980a, p. 160)—was remembered by his first-born as a decent if distant figure who could send his son a collection of Dickens when not himself drawn to literature. Gerald, only two when he died, noting that his father was reputed to be something of a martinet, carries of him one vivid image: that of crawling into the dying man's bed to be read a story. Their mother, of an Irish ancestry upon which the Durrells pin all their idiosyncrasies, is a character drawn for us in the *My Family* books and in Lawrence's *Bitter Lemons*. The portraits in those works are very close. Louisa Durrell is described as the archetypically benevolent maternal figure, feeding friends and entire villages—a portrait not far from the one Alan Thomas (1973b) draws of a warm-hearted woman given to loving tolerance.

In conversation the sons' visions of their mother are positive but not similar. Lawrence, speaking of Louisa Florence Dixie in her youth, talks of someone with a strong sense of self who had become a nurse, making their father wait three or four years before marrying him. Gerald, who by all accounts was very attached to his mother, when asked about her describes a more passive if possessive figure—"Larry and I have different views. He feels he was neglected. I was the lucky little bastard that got all the attention. I don't think it matters. She was the most marvellous non-entity: a great mattress for her children." Clearly she was an important figure in all her offsprings' lives and as adults they did not refrain from expressing affection toward her nor indeed from living with her. As Alan Thomas put it—most families run away from mother, theirs was a family in which everyone was fighting to have her.

> Pity these lame and halting parodies
> Of greater, better poems; . . .
> . . . I have fashioned them
> . . . .
> . . . from the memories of hours forlorn
> When I lived goodbyes, and crushed the stem
> Of conscious sadness, pillaging the sap
> Of tired youth.
> Strange yearning that I've had
> To climb the trough of some forgotten jest
> Or cry, and lay a tired head on your lap.
>
> [L. Durrell, 1980a, p. 25]

"A Dedication: To My Mother," written in 1931 by a very young poet, perhaps speaks to the unhappiness Lawrence Durrell felt when, from the age of twelve on, shortly before Gerald was born, he, with his brother Leslie, was "sent home" to England to be educated—at their father's insistence and against their mother's objections (Fraser, 1973, p. 20). Lawrence and Leslie went to different schools. With family still in India and letters a month away, the boys were under the care of a postmaster's wife who was, Lawrence suggested, "correct in a dull British way," but lacked the "solicitude of a mother." One is reminded of Felix Charlock's lines, at the opening of *Tunc*, "My parents I hardly remember. They hid themselves in foreign continents behind lovely coloured stamps" (L. Durrell, 1968, p. 12).

Lawrence Durrell speaks of St. Edmund's School, Canterbury, as "a shepherd's pie" of an experience. The staff uninteresting but not without kindness (again a remembered gift of words, French words for the young boy). It was "no snakepit," but it was certainly a difficult time. "Small

boys were the problem"; "Africans would have treated one better." With
the confidence of the first-born, "the son on whom the sun never set,"
and the ability to box, Lawrence survived. Leslie, his older brother suggests, had a harder time. Given to suppurating earaches, headaches, and
the head colds Gerald describes at the beginning of *My Family*, he was
miserable and more vulnerable to bullying.

In the late twenties, after her husband's death, Louisa Durrell settled
in England, finally in Bournemouth, with her younger children. Lawrence
and the painter Nancy Myer, with whom he was to be married, lived for
a while in Bloomsbury and then in a cottage in Sussex with friends, friends
who later moved on to Corfu, the island that was soon to figure so significantly in all the Durrells' lives. Nancy and Lawrence moved back into
his mother's Bournemouth household.

Alan Thomas, who first knew the Durrells in those days when he was
penniless and they prosperous, describes their generosity and the countless meals he had at Mrs. Durrell's table with Lotte, a Swiss woman, in
assistance. "All six members of the family were remarkable in themselves,
but in lively reaction to each other the whole was greater than the sum
of the parts. Amid the gales of Rabelaisian laughter, the wit, Larry's songs
accompanied by piano or guitar, the furious arguments and animated
conversations going on far into the night, I felt that life had taken on a
new dimension" (L. Durrell, 1969, p. 24). In *Spirit of Place* Thomas goes
on to describe an early encounter between Lawrence and Gerald: "I
remember Gerry, furious with Larry who, wanting to wash, had pulled
the plug out of a basin of marine life. Spluttering with ungovernable rage,
almost incoherent, searching for the most damaging insult in his vocabulary: 'You, you (pause), you AUTHOR, YOU' " (1969, p. 24). We feel
we are in *My Family and Other Animals*. And we believe every word.
As we do when Thomas, in conversation, tells about meeting the headmaster of a Bournemouth school and proudly identifying with the Durrells
and the pupil Gerald. "The most ignorant boy in the school," said the
headmaster in disgust.[1] Gerald himself remembers the days in Bournemouth as "charcoal drawings" beside the oils that were to follow.

Lawrence and Nancy decided to take their friends' advice and follow
them to Corfu. Mrs. Durrell and her family came to the island a little
while after. Corfu from 1935 until the war. With poems and essays as well
as four books—*Prospero's Cell, My Family and Other Animals, Birds,
Beasts and Relatives, Fauna and Family*[2]—and, in addition, segments of

---

[1] Gerald, in 1982, recalls the story with glee—and that he, the school's most distinguished
failure was asked back later to deliver an address.
[2] The English title is *In the Garden of the Gods*.

others, including Henry Miller's *Colossus of Maroussi*[3]—the reader must feel he knows Corfu in the days of the Durrells, in fact he is apt to join a large public for whom Corfu in the days of the Durrells is still, almost fifty years later, Corfu.

For both brothers were affected by the island's landscape and let its colors invade their prose. Both believed in its *deus loci*. Lawrence Durrell (1945) writes:

> Somewhere between Calabria and Corfu the blue really begins. All the way across Italy you find yourself moving through a landscape severely domesticated—each valley laid out after the architect's pattern, brilliantly lighted, human. But once you strike out from the flat and desolate Calabrian mainland towards the sea, you are aware of a change in the heart of things: aware of the horizon beginning to stain at the rim of the world: aware of *islands* coming out of the darkness to meet you. [p. 11]

From Gerald Durrell (1969):

> Corfu lies off the Albanian and Greek coast-lines like a long, rust-eroded scimitar. The hilt of the scimitar is the mountain region of the island, for the most part barren and stony with towering rock cliffs haunted by blue-rock thrushes and peregrine falcons. . . . The blade . . . is made up of rolling greeny-silver eiderdowns of giant olives, some reputedly over five hundred years old and each one unique in its hunched, arthritic shape, its trunk pitted with a hundred holes like pumice stone. [p. 37]

Both brothers also wrote about the people who inhabited the island in their day: Lawrence and Gerald themselves, their siblings, Mother, the learned naturalist–poet–family friend, Theodore Stephanides, and Spiro, Spiro "Americanos"—the taxi driver who adopted the Durrells, whom Lawrence (1945) saw as "a great drop of olive oil" (p. 21) and Gerald (1956) as "a great brown ugly angel" (p. 33), whose dying Henry Miller described in *The Colossus*. Their readers have met these figures over and over again. Later in this chapter we will examine how both Durrells use real names in known places to create the characters and settings of fictions.

Here we confront the necessarily difficult questions, what was Corfu really like, how does the fictive relate to the real? To answer, one goes to private orderings—to conversations and letters—and to one fat obvious

---

[3] See "The Birthday Party" in *Fillets of Plaice* and "Oil for the Saint: Return to Corfu" in *Spirit of Place*.

fact: there were two separate households on Corfu. One Lawrence and Nancy's, in a fisherman's house in the small northern village of Kouloura, talked about in letters home: "Well the north is flowering under the rain. . . . The iris and the flag stare at one like stone carved and coloured delicately everywhere. And the asphodel are going through their Victorian aspidistra stage. Moderate fishing. Ten miles south the family brawls and caterwauls and screams in the cavernous new Ypso villa" (L. Durrell, 1969, p. 44). And the other quartered nearer the town, that included Louisa Durrell, and Leslie, Margaret, and Gerald.

In his telling, Gerald Durrell created one home, moving Larry back into, and rubbing Nancy out of, the family portrait. Having said this I should add that, when asked, Lawrence Durrell said he and Nancy and their friends spent much time with the family. A letter he wrote in 1936 gives one some of the sense of familial adventure one finds in Gerald's books, although it does not mirror their mood.

> Margaret picked up a couple of jongleurs in Kerkyra and brought them to the family villa in the car. They sat on the porch and played turgid Greek jazz with a guitar, a mandolin, and their strong voices in unison. *Tha geiresis*—I think it means I will come back. One was a sharp featured boy with black eyes and a corrugated forehead, and one a queer humpy man in a cloth cap, with a strong, absolutely flawless voice. He was blind. I was reminded of them putting out birds' eyes to make them sing. Very queer melodies under the olives, with the old plectrum smacking away at the mandolin, and their right toes tapping in time. Afterwards we took them back into town, and went by car, royally, with music along the roads by the sea. [1969, p. 45]

For all the Durrells, this seems to have been a particularly good time. For Lawrence it was a productive one as well, for in Corfu he wrote the *Black Book* (1938), the novel in which he first heard his own voice, a voice that T.S. Eliot said gave him hope for the future of English prose. After a return visit to the island with his third wife in 1964, Lawrence recounts looking at old pictures: "Who was this good-looking and rather cocksure young man who stared out at me, fishing trident in hand? What had he been so damned sure about anyway? It is hard to say. The world he lived in, like our own, had existed under the threat of sudden doom. Everybody had known it" (1969, p. 295).

War came and with it the separations that those of us who have not lived through collective tragedies find difficult to imagine. Mrs. Durrell and her household moved back to England. Lawrence Durrell on to

Athens and Kalamata where, quite dramatically—in a caique filled with others fleeing Greece—he, Nancy, and their infant daughter made the crossing to Crete and then Egypt. To Cairo, where Theodore Stephanides, now a medical officer, searched for and found them, and to Alexandria—"Here at the last cold Pharos between Greece / And all I love" (L. Durrell, 1980a, p. 154)—where Durrell worked as Foreign Press Officer and Press Attaché. His marriage did not survive the war.

A year after it dissolved Durrell met the woman who was to become his second wife, the Alexandrian Eve Cohen—part Nefertiti and part gazelle is how Alan Thomas described her—with whom, happy, he traveled to Rhodes, where again he had an official job, wrote, and collected the material for an island book.

The brothers Durrell no longer shared the same landscape. Louisa Durrell and her children had been quite well off when they had first settled in Bournemouth. But funds were not well handled. The houses got smaller and smaller, and somewhat seedier. Lawrence, returning after the war, and coming from the world of the foreign service, was, Alan Thomas suggests, shocked and concerned.

Although it is clear that Gerald Durrell has seriously contemplated what life might have been like if, as he put it, his father had lived and he'd been sent to hideous schools and been more formally trained as a scientist, as a young man—though he may have been thought ill-trained—he had little difficulty finding his way in the world. In 1945 he spent a year as a student keeper in Whipsnade Zoo and two years later organized his first animal collecting expedition to West Africa. He knew that he had two serious interests: animals and travel. In June 1947, Lawrence wrote to Henry Miller from 52 St. Alban's Avenue, Bournemouth. "By the way Gerald—you remember my youngest brother—has turned out a zoologist as he wanted and is leaving for Nigeria in September. Margaret (who is married to an airman) sends her love. At present, I am sharing mother's house with her until I know for certain what my plans are" (1969, pp. 240–241). Those plans included a year in Argentina—a place he hated and Gerald, traveling there a bit later, enjoyed: "Whereas Larry is a European, I don't mind where I go. Larry was miserable when he was in Argentina and longed for Europe. But I loved Argentina. When you're interested in animals, people are generally kind wherever you are because they think you must be feeble-minded" (Weatherby, 1961).

In the early fifties, Lawrence Durrell was with the British Embassy in Belgrade—another place he minded very much indeed, a place where his politics moved to the right,[4] where one suspects it had always really

---

[4] "As for Communism—my dear Theodore, a short visit here is enough to make one decide that Capitalism is worth fighting for" (1969, p. 100).

been. In Yugoslavia, faced with the choice of a new posting to Russia or
Turkey, Durrell chose to leave the Foreign Service and turn to a com-
patible landscape, to Cyprus, and writing. "Heaven knows how we'll keep
alive," he told Henry Miller (L. Durrell, 1963), "but I'm so excited I can
hardly wait to begin starving" (p. 291). But before leaving Belgrade his
wife Eve suffered a breakdown and was sent to England.

> Truly though we never speak
> The past has marked us each
> In different lives contending for each other:
> We bear like ancient marble well-heads
> Marks of the ropes they lowered in us.
> [L. Durrell, 1980a, p. 230]

With his infant daughter, Sappho-Jane, Lawrence went on to Cyprus.

Gerald Durrell, during the early fifties, met and married Jacqueline
Rasen, a young woman from Manchester, and began a career writing
about his travels, at, she suggests, her instigation: "Larry Durrell was
quite a successful author and had, from all accounts, always encouraged
Gerry to write. If one Durrell could write and make money at it, why
should another not try? So began Operation Nag. Poor Durrell suffered"
(J. Durrell, 1967, p. 30). The venture, like James Fenimore Cooper's,
has an improbable ring. Still, the book Gerald wrote, *The Overloaded
Ark*, was an immediate popular success. In her own book, *Beasts in My
Bed*, Jacquie Durrell (1967) says of Gerald's first work: "I began to have
a sneaking feeling that it might make us quite a bit of money." *Beasts in
My Bed* clearly suffers from the attempt to be the satellite of a best-seller
and to adopt a wifely narrative voice that would suit the comic expectations
of her audience. But it does chronicle Gerald's string of successes, the
business manager's functions Jacquie took on, the travels—first to Argentina and Paraguay and then to film at Lawrence's village home on
Cyprus—and the accompanying, quite clearly terrifying, need to keep
forever one book ahead.

Lawrence, who had by all accounts encouraged his brother to write,
clearly had not himself made money at it. And on Cyprus, although he
had the help of his mother, who had come to care for the child, he could
not give up wage-earning for full-time writing: indeed his job as Chief
Information Officer put him on the world stage during the mid-fifties'
ENOSIS crisis. On Cyprus Lawrence Durrell met the French Alexandrian, Claude-Marie Vincendon, a translator and fledgling novelist, and
he wrote and finished the first novel in *The Alexandria Quartet: Justine*.

It was not until 1957, after he and Claude-Marie had moved on to the south of France, that Lawrence Durrell, in the words of a *Life* magazine subtitle, "burst from poverty and obscurity to wealth and fame" (Dennis, 1961), for in that year both *Justine* and his book about Cyprus, *Bitter Lemons*, were published within months of one another. This was what Faber and Faber, his publishers, called "Durrell's annus mirabilis." Critical success had of course come earlier (Durrell said in conversation that the reporter from the *Manchester Guardian* didn't mean much to him after Miller or Eliot). Still, wealth and fame are to be reckoned with—and they came earlier to Gerald than to his brother. Thomas (1973b) remembers those days:

> Durrell had been writing for over twenty-five years before his books reached the general reading public; whereas his younger brother Gerald became widely popular overnight. . . . When *Reflections on a Marine Venus* received some good reviews, an old lady telephoned my bookshop: "I want to order a book by a Mr. Durrell, not THE Mr. Durrell, it's not about animals at all." [p. 78]

It is a measure of their affection and of Lawrence Durrell's generosity that he greeted his brother's early windfall with serious, if wistful, pleasure. In January of 1954 he wrote to Henry Miller:

> My youngest brother Gerry has scored a tremendous success with his first book and is making a deal of money. He collects wild animals for zoos and writes up his adventures afterwards. The one pays for the other; how marvellous to have one's career fixed at 25 or so and to be able to pay one's way. The perpetual nibbling of money worry is the worst of curses when one has children or can't bear squalor; and the lack makes it so hard to see and enjoy one's friends properly. [1963, p. 300]

To Richard Aldington he wrote in March, 1957:

> My brother Gerry? He is delightful, Irish gift of the gab on paper—but *loathes* writing and puts all his money back into expeditions. At the moment the little fool is down with bad malaria in the Cameroons and due home in June-July. I'm trying to persuade him to do a popular book on [Jean Henri] Fabre's life—to come down here and do it. Do you know these blasted books about animals sell thousands of copies. My agent says that it is the only sure-fire steady *eternal* market. I wish I liked animals enough—or even felt like Whitman about them. [1981a, p. 15]

Gerald's "gift of gab on paper" had produced, in 1956, *My Family and*

Other Animals, his best and best known work. The next few years were
extraordinarily successful ones for both brothers. For Gerald there was
of course the ongoing travel,[5] expeditions and filming for the BBC, but,
more important, it was during this period that he established the Jersey
Zoological Park, on advances from his publishers ("he's always been more
willing to risk his money than I have," said his brother), and, in 1963,
the Jersey Wildlife Preservation Trust devoted to practical and theoretical
work to save endangered species.

Lawrence Durrell finished *The Alexandria Quartet*, working incredibly
quickly, with a purpose and intensity for which he credits his wife Claude,
who clearly managed the world surrounding his writing and was his
reader: "You only need an audience of one." Their lives in the south of
France do not seem to have been changed greatly by money. Except that
they bought the big nineteenth-century house in Sommière Durrell now
lives in, and neither of them needed to find undesired jobs.

Louisa Durrell, who had moved to Jersey to live with her son Gerald,
died in 1964.

After a short illness, the seriousness of which no one seems to have
suspected, Claude Durrell died on January 1, 1967. A letter, written from
Paleokastritsa, Corfu, in June of that year speaking about Claude—and
about Athenaios the peasant, who, in *Prospero's Cell*, stays up late to
discover Homer—speaks to the death of so many things, including the
idyll of prewar Corfu that both brothers, celebrating innocence, had
drawn.

> There's hardly a soul about except for Durrells and there are rather
> too many of those about—Margaret is also here spreading sweetness
> and light. Theo as well. I've been round about a good deal looking
> up old friends—it's been melancholy in a way. Claude was so very
> much loved here that it's been watering-cans all the way. This last
> three years so many friends, etc., have died that I feel ringed about
> with graves. Another sad epilogue—that peaceful house at Kouloura
> with its gay and industrious family—I noticed that it was all shut-
> tered and barred, through my heavy glasses. Today I learned that
> Athenaios, that sweet man, in despair at the paralysis gaining on
> him committed suicide. He drank the olive spray insecticide—terribly
> painful death. Little Kerkyra has abandoned the house and gone to
> Jannina to live with her daughter. Spiro, the boy, my godson, has
> gone to sea again on the China run. I went up yesterday and sat
> about on the rock below the house. Niko, the sailor, was away. *Pas
> un chat.* How strangely things turn out. I expect you feel rather as

[5] Trips to the Cameroons, Argentina, and Sierra Leone.

I do, vague and scattered—as if one were convalescing from a major operation. Damn everything. [L. Durrell, 1969, p. 155]

That was in 1967, sixteen years ago. Years which have in many ways been productive for both Durrells. For Gerald there were more expeditions—Mexico, Australia, and five years later Mauritius, then Assam and a return to Mexico—and a stream of books, some now fictive, some that circle *My Family*, one—*Birds, Beast and Relatives*—evincing extraordinary skill. For Lawrence, *The Revolt of Aphrodite*, including *Tunc* and *Numquam*, and the planned quincunx of which *Monsieur* and *Livia* are out and, it would seem, *Constance in Love* soon to come.

But one wrestles with success on the threshing floor. Gerald, a public personality recognizable to many a man on the London street and all in Jersey, taking on the Trust's fund-raising, extended the begging bowl to, one suspects, many who robbed him of privacy and vital energy.

And earning one's living by writing demands a certain number of books a year. Three, says Lawrence Durrell. Who claims he no longer has "a wife to protect me" against writing the bad ones—*The Greek Islands* and *Sicilian Carousels*. The dangers that come with paying one's household bills in books are the dangers that can accompany self-imitation, of which both Lawrence Durrell and his brother have been accused.

One suspects it takes great will and courage to continue on as a writer. Not the rather melodramatic courage spoken of in the early Henry Miller–Lawrence Durrell correspondence, where the artist is a young god in motley conquering the—female—world, but rather the mature courage of a craftsman who believes in his work against the nattering of reviewers who have made Lawrence Durrell a moving target, perhaps for the reason Alan Thomas gives—he's stayed away from England and hasn't been "in any log-rolling clique"—perhaps because, as Durrell himself believes, England in hard times does not take kindly to exiles. Or perhaps because he is an artist of scale, of large canvases. "There is something in the English temper that loves a shortage, be it of words . . ."—so Durrell (1980a) quotes the *Times Literary Supplement* in his "Ode to a Lukewarm Eyebrow" (p. 262). And in the modern temper. One thinks of the Aldington-Durrell correspondence (L. Durrell, 1981a), in which Lawrence was so helpful to another writer, and would wish Lawrence Durrell Lawrence Durrells.

Gerald Durrell's life has changed dramatically since 1979. He has been divorced and is now remarried, to Lee McGeorge, an American animal behavioralist trained at Duke University, with whom he is presently collaborating on a book, which may indeed change the direction of his prose.

Lawrence Durrell

I said in the introduction to this piece that one is struck by a difference in tone in the works of Lawrence and Gerald Durrell so great as to throw doubt upon the possibility of common origins. One domesticates all people and wild animals; the other makes the familial wild. That is true but perhaps no more interesting than the split one finds within the writing of Lawrence Durrell himself.

A part of Durrell is of course extraordinarily playful, as this letter makes clear:

> My beastly brother has started a Zoo in Bournemouth and travels everywhere with a giant ape called Chumley. Dreadful scenes in the dining car of the Bournemouth Belle; but I must admit it is a good way to call on one's publishers when asking for money. Our techniques are widely different. I find that Fabers get awfully scared when I put imaginary titles to books. For a long time I convinced them that *Justine* was to be called Sex and The Secret Service or Not Now Your Husband's Looking. This worried them into a defensive position; they were so relieved when they got the MS they offered quite a decent contract. Gerry, who is cruder (with Hart-Davis one must be tougher I suppose), always threatens to write a life of Jesus.
>
> I expect they'll come down here and make my life a cicada ridden mystery before long; my sister enjoyed ten days of courses libres. I'm expecting my ballet dancer daughter to appear too for a short while. Money! I must press on. [1981a, p. 30]

A recent reviewer (Jenkins, 1981) of the Aldington correspondence says of Durrell's letters: "On the family side, it is true there is an impression of enormous warmth. But this is translated, on the literary side, into a persona of *Boy's Own* enthusiasm, only one which goes in for fiction rather than, say, flying biplanes or trekking to the Poles." There is something here—some sense of a created persona. But it is an argument that extends itself into an old complaint, one that sees Durrell as the writer who cares about being a writer but not about what he writes, who gives us the idea of a great novel but not that novel, for whom, in Wood's words (1975), "the only question is whether the overtheatrical or unreal comes off or not—the criterion being not verisimilitude or probability or even artistic necessity, but something akin to acrobatic excellence, an ability to stay on the high wire" (p. 17). The sense of the sleight-of-hand-man to which Durrell so easily lends himself.

What is interesting about this complaint as it focuses on family is that it points us toward, not the lie it suggests—bourgeois comfort playing with blackness—but rather a division at the very center of Lawrence Durrell's perception. The Durrells are a vital, large family, and Lawrence is their love poet; and, at one and the same time, he is a writer who speaks to desertion and treachery within family, to the sense that one seeks out one's sibling not to discover self but to know that most radically different Other. There is of course much posing. When Lawrence Durrell gets tired he does not stand quietly, he struts. But both sides of Durrell's vision of family come out of his experience and color his work. One does well to very briefly trace these two strains—in Durrell's poems, in the island books, and in the novels.

The celebratory is strong in Lawrence Durrell. We find it in rather gentle musings, as in one of his earliest poems, "The Gift":

> Now that I have given all that I could bring
> Slit the wide, silken tassel of the purse
> . . . .
> Will you remember it and, mother-wise
> Thank me in these chill after-days
> When I am empty-handed . . . with your eyes?
> [1980a, p. 17]

Or in the better poem, "To Ping-Kû, Asleep": "The turning of a small blind mind / Like a plant everywhere ascending. / . . . / Invent a language where the terms / Are smiles" (1980a, p. 104).

It often comes forth in humor, as in the youthful Christmas poem, "Ballade of Slow Decay," that creates the image of a *My Family* family:

> When Winifred my manuscript destroys,
> And dearest little Bertie mis-employs
> His time by crying when he sees my nose—
> It makes me want to stamp and make a noise:
> I wish that George would pay me what he owes.
> [1980a, p. 32]

This sense of songs of praise, like the words dedicated to his mother—"quaint offerings / Each one some little magic that belongs to you" (1980a, p. 25) is balanced by another strain in the poems about family: the feeling that death or distance or difference leaves one finally standing alone. In "Wheat-Field: For Leslie"—an early poem which is, as Durrell himself said, strongly imitative of D.H. Lawrence—he writes, "I have been so in dreams: rooted / And standing with the warm male sperm in me, /

Hideously wary of death" (1980a, p. 35). And in the 1938 "Poem to
Gerald" one finds, amid false literary posturing, real quaverings: against
the power of death and, sadly, the female power of birth. The sense of
three brothers and their necessary bonding is strong, for they must escape,
wander, to ward off the wrath of fate in this fatherless world. The contest
with life is a man's affair.

> The father is in death.
> Let him now enter into the sun's attic,
> Enter the floating chambers of the sea.
> Who will bear witness how foreign,
> How musical with the silence
> And alphabets we three be?
>
> . . . .
> O conjure, my brothers, the pelican
> That its monstrous egg is not laid here
> Lest dogs snap the poisoned yolk.
>
> The father is strangled in his vine.
> We will go sideways out of the house
> Leaving only by the oven to nestle
> A small rabbit on her perch-grass:
> She is too soft a thing, too abhorred
> A morsel for the twelve angers,
> The pestle and mortar of the Lord.
> [1980a, p. 64]

"Poem to Gerald" was written in Greece, midst other, better work—"On
Ithaca Standing" (1937), for example: "Tread softly, for here you stand /
On miracle ground, boy" (1980a, p. 111). Or the wonderful, Hopkins-like
"Carol on Corfu" (1937), celebrating the sounds of English and its fine,
hard monosyllables which the Greek language Durrell was hearing daily,
for all its honey, does not have.

> I, per se I, sing on.
> Let flesh falter, or let bone break
> Break, yet the salt of a poem holds on,
> Even in empty weather
> When beak and feather have done.
> [1980a, p. 56]

Corfu was, of course, also responsible for the first of the island books,
Prospero's Cell (1945).

"And here we are," says the Count . . . "each of us collecting and arranging our common knowledge according to the form dictated to him by his temperament. In all cases it will not be the whole picture, though it will be the whole picture for you. You, Doctor [Theodore], will proceed under some title like *The Natural History, Geology, Botany and Comparative Ethnology of the Island of Corfu*. You will be published by a learned society in Vienna. . . . As for you, Zarian, your articles . . . will present a ferocious and lopsided account of an enchanted island which has seduced every historical figure of note from Nero to Napoleon. . . ."

"And I?" I say. "What sort of picture will I present to Prospero's Island?"

"It is difficult to say," says the Count. "A portrait inexact in detail, containing bright splinters of landscape, written out roughly, as if to get rid of something which was troubling the optic nerves. You are the kind of person who would go away and be frightened to return in case you were disappointed; but you would send others and question them eagerly about it. You are to be forgiven really, because you have had the best of your youth in the island." [p. 107]

Perspective—and the difference that comes when one changes the lens—has always been crucial to Lawrence Durrell, as it has to most writers of his generation; one need hardly mention *The Alexandria Quartet*. But it is interesting to see the Count D. play with the notion here, as it relates to Corfu, for we will contend with two Corfus by the Brothers Durrell.

Lawrence's island is seen through prisms, dated journal entries, that often focus on comic anecdotes about, or musings of, a small group of literati whom the island makes friends. Most prominent among the group is Theodore Stephanides, the "Ionian fawn" (p. 116) "in whom there lives a vague Edwardian desire to square applied science with comparative religion" (p. 99). Theodore, poet and zoologist but, in temperament, understated, professorial, the antithesis of the Durrells. Lawrence credits him with much of the data in *Prospero's Cell*, but, more important, he uses him to heighten its gentle, bemused tone. The prisms involve the island's history told through anecdote and myth; its landscape and images—"the little early grapes, delicately freckled green, and of a pouting teat-shape. The sun has penetrated their shallow skins and has confused the sweetness with its own warmth; it is like eating something alive" (p. 101); and its peasant life and lore: the poetry of professional mourners, the shadow-play of Karaghiosis (" 'the triumph over causality' is considerably older than Breton—and indeed an integral part of all peasant art" [p. 53]).

Lawrence Durrell works hard to create the illusion that his book it-self—with its actual names, places, and anecdotes—is unordered: life not art, and the device of the dated journal entry is his primary tool, with its supposedly unpolished prose, its unexplained, unannounced cast of char-acters who move in and out of a frame that can shift in time and space without transition.[6] But, having thoroughly grounded us in the real, Dur-rell moves us, unsuspecting, to the world of dreams. I think Fraser (1973) is exactly right when he says

> The war is looming over all these characters, and in a sense each is playing his part in a *commedia dell'arte* improvisation, delighting in the absurdities of his mask. Nothing disastrous, and indeed noth-ing painful in the sense of satirical or corrective comedy, is going to happen within the confines of the book; the comedy is to be wholly sympathetic. The lyrical elements, like the glimpses of N. (Nancy) with her fair beauty, her nereid quality, her doe-like ears, more water-nymph than human being, hardly with a speaking part, enhance the sense of the green or golden world, of Shakespearian romantic magic. [pp. 75–76]

The Durrell family does not play a major role in *Prospero's Cell*, but like "N." Leslie is here, as part of the romantic magic, as "L." helping to uncover an underwater villa, or in conversation with a man in a boat, who was on weekend leave from prison ("I am a murderer" [1945, p. 92])—a scene Gerald gives himself in *My Family*—or viewed at a distance: "My brother's boat *Dugong* lies just off Agni, heading for the house. I can see his characteristic pose, legs stretched out, head on one side and eyes closed against the smoke of his cigarette. He has stowed his guns in their leather cases under the half-decking where the faithful Spiro sits scanning the horizon for something to shoot at" (p. 120). And this book ends as all the Durrell Corfu books do—with that final metaphor for well-being, a small feast on the beach at which Spiro tends the fire. "We picnic for supper on these warm nights by the Myrtiotissa monastery. Spiro lights a fire of pine-branches and twigs, and the three wicker hampers

---

[6] "A Landmark Gone" (1949), an essay written while Durrell was working on *Prospero's Cell* ("I have been trying for a year to rebuild the white house by the water's edge in a book"), is itself an earlier, less successful draft of a number of the passages in *Prospero's Cell* including its opening: "You are aware not so much of a landscape coming to meet you invisibly over those blue miles of water, as of a climate." Interestingly, in this short piece, people who float into the book unannounced are here defined, become "Dorothy and Veronica, two ballet-dancers." "A Landmark Gone" was written less than a year after Durrell fled Greece. It was not published in *Middle East Anthology* until a year after the 1945 publication of *Prospero's Cell*. One hundred twenty-five copies were privately reprinted.

of the Count are brimmed with food and drink. In the immense volume of the sea's breathing our voices are restored to their true proportion—insignificant, small and shrill with a happiness this landscape allows us but does not notice" (p. 128).

Gerald and their mother do not appear in *Prospero's Cell*, but they do make their ways into *Bitter Lemons* (1957a), set on Cyprus. Written a year after Gerald's *My Family*—"my brother's wicked pen portrait of the genius at the age of twenty-one" (L. Durrell, 1981a, p. 120)—it was a book which clearly gave Lawrence much pleasure.

Bitter Lemons is a pained work with none of the innocent joy of *Prospero's Cell*, although it seems at first to use family as a minor motif: a brief comedy, in the style of *My Family*, set against a terrible moment in time, for the family it portrays is of one fabric with Gerald's fictive vision.

> My mother has arrived for a holiday, full of energy and malapropisms, and totally convinced that yet another of the family follies is in full swing. But the beauty of the house contents her, and she is able to establish something like a regular domestic routine with the help of Xenu, the huge porpoise of a maid. . . .
>
> Meanwhile the work on the house went on unflaggingly under my mother's rather variable direction. She had a passion for folklore and ghost stories and I was rather glad she had never managed to learn Greek as all would be lost if she and Michaelis once got together. But she had taken to over-feeding the workmen in her large compassionate way . . . so that lunch hour had begun to resemble a rather original sort of garden party. [L. Durrell, 1957a, pp. 109, 111]

Gerald himself seems to take a more uproarious part, even before he appears on the scene. He becomes the ruse in a taverna debate about the English with a belligerent villager.

> "My brother. He died at Thermopylae, fighting beside the Greeks."
> This was a complete lie, of course, for my brother, to the best of my knowledge, was squatting in some African swamp collecting animals for the European zoos. I put on an air of dejection. [p. 40]

The evening ends in drinks celebrating the *palikars* of all nations. "My brother at Thermopylae" becomes a much repeated echo throughout the first half of the book, even when Gerald resurrects himself and, in the flesh, dances with a grace and agility that surpasses that of the Cypriot village youth. Gerald brings film and the villagers "nourish absurd dreams of Hollywood" and of course he collects "every foul creeping thing the Creator invented to make our lives uncomfortable here below. No one who has not smelt an owl at close quarters, or seen a lizard being sick, will have any idea what I mean!" (p. 151). We seem to be in Corfu and *My Family*, but island war, guerrilla war, that has at its inception "the air of good-natured farce," interrupts and ends comedy.

> "Still in the operatic phase": the phase has much to commend it.
> "But what happens," asked my brother idly, "when in the middle of the opera a real shot rings out and an actor falls dead?"
> "It will never reach that pitch," I said.
> "I wish I could be sure," he said.
> So did I but I could not say so. [p. 179]

Gerald, precisely as comic symbol of brotherly love and a philhellenism that can resurrect itself, works in the end to illuminate the tragedies of Cyprus. For here, in the middle of the book, actors do fall dead, for real and forever.

The world of *The Alexandria Quartet* is, for all its horrors, at its close not so sad as that of *Bitter Lemons*, for here wounds have been healed, and we feel "happily ever after" might accompany the "once upon a time" Darley can finally write. But one of the *Quartet*'s most telling and indeed tragic moments is the death of Narouz. Durrell has always been, is still, interested in siblings in his fiction, in incest, in doubles, in the Jocas and Julians, paired opposites with alliterative names. But although siblings are central to *The Revolt of Aphrodite* and to *Monsieur* and *Livia*, there is nowhere so interesting a portrait as that of the Hosnanis.

Actually there are three brothers, for Mountolive in his love for Leila joins Nessim and Narouz. In one of her letters to him—her art for an audience of one—this perfect mother, lover, writes: It was a shock "to suddenly see Nessim's naked body floating in the mirror, the slender white back so like yours and the loins. I sat down and, to my own surprise, burst into tears, because I wondered suddenly whether my attachment for you wasn't lodged here somehow among the feeble incestuous desires of the inner heart" (L. Durrell, 1958, pp. 53–54). Mountolive and Nessim, for all the chasm of nationality and politics, are a matched pair: elegant, cultured men of the world. They have had Leila's love. Narouz is their opposite. Harelipped, bearlike, with a "gentle savagery," he is a man of the land and the hunt, who receives only the afterthoughts of his mother's affection.

However tempting the alliteration of Larry and Leslie, I do not mean to suggest biographical parallels. I don't know enough. And I suspect Durrell doesn't take photographs. What one does clearly see here is a writer who understands sibling jealousies and affections and the family politics of position. He understands what it means to be the first son expecting to be followed, wounded by the separate self your brother becomes. Durrell is finally able to enter both skins—indeed to have the dullard become the poetic mystic touching a truth as coiled as the whip he carries—to have us move beyond judgment. But the triumph is not in Durrell's delineation (and our understanding) of conflict, or even of the flirtation with fratricide.

It is in Narouz: so thoroughly the embodiment of unrequited love. His is explicitly a love for Clea but, behind that, a son's call for his mother. Durrell pictures him murdered in a vast landscape, utterly alone. " 'Then he must really die?' he asked Nessim sadly, 'without his mother?' " (1958, p. 309). The kindly lie, Balthazar's ventriloquism (of whose voice finally?)—"He whispered in Arabic: 'Rest, my darling. Easily, my loved one' "—underlines the loss, and as Narouz, in dying, roars "Clea," we hear its echoes. "So nude a word, her name, as simple as 'God' or 'Mother' . . ." (p. 312).

In one of his most recent books, *A Smile in the Mind's Eye*, Lawrence Durrell (1980b) describes a visitor's approach to his house in Sommières:

> It is, I suppose, the most beautiful [village] in the Languedoc, with its girdle of medieval walls and ravelins and its tumpy Roman bridge across the green Virdoule. . . . My abandoned garden with its tall trees and hidden pool also met with his approval. . . . For a while we sat in quiet affability, watching the maid get through her routine—she only spares me an hour a day, which is just enough to maintain the balance of things in the bat-haunted old Provençal house I inhabit, more often than not alone. [p. 4]

"My image of home," said Lawrence Durrell, sitting in the kitchen of that large sparse house he inhabits "more often than not alone," "is a hotel, a hotel with bar." Here too Lawrence Durrell described himself as "a failed mystic who has disguised himself as Hemingway." And again one thinks of the lines from *Tunc*: "My parents I hardly remember. They hid themselves in foreign continents behind lovely coloured stamps. Most holidays I spent silently in hotels (when the aunts went to Baden). I brought introspection to a fine art." Or one thinks of a fine poem Lawrence Durrell wrote in 1946 about Jean Henri Fabre, a turn-of-the-century naturalist, a popularizer of science, who lived in the south of France, to whose works Lawrence introduced a young Gerald.

The ants that passed
Over the back of his hand,
The cries of welcome, the tribes, the tribes!

Happier men would have studied
Children, more baffling than pupae,
Their conversation when alone, their voices,

The dream at the tea-table or at geography:
The sense of intimacy when moving in lines
Like caterpillars entering a cathedral.

He refused to examine the world except
Through the stoutest glasses;
A finger of ground covered with pioneers.

A continent on a bay-leaf moving.
If real women were like moths he didn't notice.
There was not a looking-glass in the whole house.

Ah! but one day he might dress
In this black discarded business suit,
Fly heavily out on to the lawn at Arles.

What friendships lay among the flowers!
If he could be a commuter among the bees,
This pollen-hunter of the exact observation!
[1980a, p. 157]

Gerald Durrell

Lawrence Durrell may be intrigued by a figure like Fabre, and he may
move from people to place for reasons Fabre would understand, but he
is not a naturalist, and Gerald Durrell seems justified in suggesting the
brothers experience little conflict about their work because they are "poles
apart." But they are both writers, and, I would suggest, it is precisely
because Gerald is not himself a literary figure that his brother has had
a strong influence on his prose. Gerald Durrell reads widely in zoology
but, I would guess, there is only one twentieth-century creative writer
whose works have shaped his own. And he knows them well. When he
discussed his brother's writing he was given to much exact observation
and to frequent quoting. We talked about the Fabre Gerald once wanted

to write a BBC film about—a figure planting a flower in his top hat and putting it in the central square—and I asked him if he knew his brother's poem; he gave me: "Fly heavily out on to the lawn at Arles." And he knew the prose.

Later I will examine the important ways in which Lawrence Durrell the writer has been mentor to, elder brother to, Gerald Durrell writer, as well as the ways in which Gerald has brought science into his fictive world. But first, remembering Count D. in *Prospero's Cell*, another "Account of the Durrell Family of Corfu."

We can of course look at Gerald Durrell as family biographer recording data on a friendly tribe, for they are all there in the *My Family* books. The central figures: Mother—"whose maxim in life was always defend your young regardless of how much in the wrong they were" (1969, p. 25); Mother, capable of saying "You will do as you're told" (p. 33), but needing to only once in all those books, and then only to protect her wayward daughter. And Larry, "designed by Providence to go through life like a small, blond firework, exploding ideas in other people's minds, and then curling up with cat-like unctuousness and refusing to take any blame for the consequences" (1956, p. 15). Leslie, who seems never, in anyone's telling, to have moved without a gun in hand, "short, stocky, with an air of quiet belligerence" (1956, p. 20), and Gerald's Mrs. Malaprop, Margo. Theodore Stephanides and Spiro are at the center too and, surrounding them, an endless series of cameo portraits: Lugaretzia the hypochondriacal maid, lecherous Captain Creech (who first appears in *Birds, Beasts* and has about him something of the *Quartet*'s Scobie), Doctor Androuchelli, Larry's stream of eating artists, and Gerald's tutors, including Kralefsky, the teller of autobiographical tales: "It was a wonderful story, and might well be true. Even if it wasn't true, it was the sort of thing that *should* happen, I felt; and I sympathized with Kralefsky if, finding that life had so far denied him a bull-terrier to strangle, he had supplied it himself" (1956, p 239).

Gerald's extraordinarily popular story may well be true. But truth is, after all, not an important concern. Gerald Durrell is after fiction. Moreover, he is after a particular kind of fiction: "The sort of thing that *should* happen." *My Family* is at its core a utopian tale. Actual names and known places are the real illusion, for they allow us to willingly enter an island idyll.

The perspective from which the stories are written is an interesting one. They are told in the first person by a man looking back to his boyhood days, but there is no line between manhood and boyhood, no sense that the child's is a partial or distorted vision, nor that there is a fictive moment when experience makes the child adult. Indeed, in Gerald Durrell's books the bemused boy is wiser than the adults in whose company we find him, and always has been. And, unlike a Huckleberry Finn, young Gerry knows it. Nor does Durrell equate wisdom with goodness. Adult foibles are examined with amusement and forgiveness, without satire. One thinks of what Fraser said about *Prospero's Cell*—*commedia dell'arte* characters in a wholly sympathetic comedy. Lawrence also created an idyll. But *Prospero's Cell* has its "Epilogue in Alexandria." We hear the Wallace Stevens line, "No winds, like dogs, watched over them at night." All its characters know that time and place are indifferent to their comedy and may, unintentionally, cause it to end.

In *My Family*, a small boy brings all the strays, all the world, safely home. He doesn't have to light out for the territory, because excitement occurs around him and it clearly can, and does, occur over and over again. Alan Thomas suggested *My Family* has great appeal because it allows those of us who have compromised with life, become middle-aged straphangers, to withdraw into Arcadia. He is in part right.

But Gerald Durrell's vision is really a boy's dream: the dream of a world in which no one says no. Which presupposes the right parents, and here is the trick: Gerald Durrell makes Lawrence Durrell a figure fit for Greek shadow-play: the grouch with the heart of gold; the roaring, raging, ineffectual father whose wrath is to be avoided by benign deception. Call it displaced oedipal impulses if you will. The boy wins. And the stern father provides no more of an obstacle to him than—is indeed in power subordinate to—everyone's favorite mom.

Hard cop, soft cop, but really there is no policing at all. Nor is there need, for all adults—including those with expertise or ego, like Theo or Larry—treat the boy with easy equality; learning is never forced, always spun out of his interests, sometimes with great ingenuity on the part of his tutors; and nothing is denied him. For the adolescent who has gone to bed by ten, had one messy pet and no serious adult conversation, unwillingly studied trigonometry, and seldom gotten the better of his dad, Durrell creates heaven.

It is a heaven that teaches tolerance. Lawrence Durrell, uncomfortable with middlebrow attention, would wish as his audience members of the Tribe, fellow artists whom he admires. Gerald Durrell understands the fascination and fears of middle-class people. Part of the success of his books comes from both brothers' fame: one reads about these real people the way one looks at Vanessa Bell's photograph album, staring at those who've lived and talked better than most. But his audience knows Gerald's Bloomsbury was born in Bournemouth. Never fear. Declaring himself one of their number and subject to their misapprehensions, Gerald nevertheless takes those things middle-class English people shun—art, homosexuality, mental illness, the foreigner—and brings them into the family. No one is denied access to Mother's table.

One can argue that he creates stereotypes, but, although autobiography lends them the appearance of full-blown characters, the figures in *My Family* are, like Punch or Karaghiosis, not meant to be rounded. Surprise comes from situation not character; in fact comedy relies on our anticipation of varied but predictable greens in a new pot. So that Sven, the homosexual artist who plays the accordion, is no less fully human than Leslie polishing his guns; both are two-dimensional and drawn with affection.

There's a substantial cast in *My Family*, but for all the siblings, at its center Gerald Durrell gives us only one fully drawn figure: an only child with no contemporaries, with many Nigger Jims but no Tom Sawyers, which at first seems surprising for a book that has strong adolescent appeal. Here too one sees the child's dream, and this aspect of Gerald's utopian novels is not class bound: for he pictures a world in which one need never compete for parental affection, for mother-love.

Another might have suggested loneliness, or even the melancholy that wraps one in "a most humorous sadness," but for all that Durrell begins with Shakespeare's lines, his tone is steadily affirming. "So once in idleness was my beginning. / . . . in the lens of this great patience / Sex was small, / Death was small, / Were qualities held in deathless essence."

Young Gerry is portrayed as a boy who does not want for companions, he has the family and its friends, he has the local peasants, and his own entourage: Roger and the Other Animals.

It is important to examine how the animals—Ulysses, the Magenpies, Achilles, Quasimodo, Cicely, Alecko—are given to Durrell's readers. For, one would suspect, Durrell the naturalist cared about those sketches. Gerald Durrell described himself as an amalgam: a "failed poet" and a "failed scientist" whose strength is that he can combine the two, a kind of "striped toothpaste." And, for all that Gerald suggests he one day realized he was too "slovenly" to be a good scientist, it is clear that he's felt more ambiguity and, at least early on, resentment about his informal education than the *My Family* books show.

He may be, as he says, neither fish, flesh, nor fowl (his third talent, like his brother's, is for the visual arts), but his accomplishments as a self-trained naturalist have been extraordinary. This slowly becomes apparent when one travels to Jersey. The zoo that he founded is, at first glance, simply pleasant: the store given to toys that would have suited the Coney

Island of my youth; the architecture, landscaping, signs, pleasing but visually unimaginative. But one doesn't have to read *The Stationary Ark* (1976) to begin to realize that Durrell and the others who created the park created it for animals, for their future preservation and current well-being. Here are living experiments in animal communication and the reproduction of endangered species and, one would guess, among the best kept animals in the world. The books may rely on a knowledge of middle-class values, fund-raising clearly does, but the zoo itself faithfully avoids the human yardstick and is a magnificent achievement by any measure.

The crusade against viewing animals as "Uncle Fred and Aunt Freda in a fur coat" (1976, p. 38) is clearly important to Durrell; one wishes his own prose worked harder to avoid the anthropomorphic turn. This is difficult for someone who loves metaphor and who portrays the animals in the *My Family* books as a boy's friends. Still one would wish for more of the animal's-eye view given us in, say, a few passages of Hemingway's "The Short Happy Life of Francis Macomber," or even the sense of humans taking on the perceptions and coloring of wild animals that Margaret Atwood suggests at the close of *Surfacing*. People are never obviously *more important* than animals in Durrell's books—Roger is as companionable and foolish as Sven—but all move gently toward the domestic, toward the home toad Deidre shares "with her husband Terence Oliver Albert Dick" (1978, p. 126).

It would be an overstated generalization to suggest that in Gerald Durrell's telling we all stay at home in mother's kitchen, whereas, in the works of Lawrence Durrell, protagonists are required to wander, to do what the three sons do in "Poem to Gerald": "We will go sideways out of the house / Leaving only by the oven to nestle / A small rabbit on her perch-grass." Still, if we are careful not to see them as Tennyson's Telemachus and Ulysses, we come close to the truth. Their perceptions of home have made them very different writers.

"My brother is a classic back to the womber," said Gerald Durrell, to my surprise. "He once told me what he'd like to do is design a room with the minimum in it to sustain life. I like opulence." There *is* something of the minimalist in Lawrence Durrell. He seems to live in his home in Sommières a little bit as if he were camping out, as if he could pack all his books in a van and be off. "Extreme sensuality and intellectual asceticism. . . . It is a national peculiarity of the Alexandrians to seek a reconciliation between the two deepest psychological traits of which they are conscious" (L. Durrell, 1957b, p. 87). Lawrence Durrell, like his Alexandrians, has these two strains within him—but the strain that moves toward opulence is the more dominant in his prose, and it is from this that his brother, as writer, has learned.

The Booster, published in Paris in the late thirties, a monthly put together by the likes of Henry Miller, Alfred Perlès, Anais Nin, and Lawrence Durrell, included in one of its numbers a prose-poem by an eleven-year-old boy. It is about a patient on an operating table, and is thick with animal metaphors, with faces like cuttlefish and blue lace handkerchiefs in butterflylike hands: "The scalpel whispered as if it were cutting silk, showing the intestines coiled up heatly [sic] like watchsprings. The doctor's hands moved with the speed of a striking snake, cutting, fastening, probing. . . . Then the sewing-up, the needle burying itself in the soft depth and appearing on the other side of the abyss, drawing the skin together like a magnet. The stretcher groaned at the sudden weight" (G. Durrell, 1937).

Lawrence Durrell is supposed to have at first thought his brother's tutor had written the piece, to which Patrick Evans is said to have replied: "Do you suppose . . . that if I could write as well as that I would waste my time on being a tutor?" (Thomas, 1973a, p. 207). It *is* extraordinary prose for one so young, showing a clear predisposition to write and, in the scalpel on silk, as Gerald Durrell himself pointed out, a borrowed metaphor.

It is hard to tell, when people have lived together and write autobiographical prose, what is borrowing. More important, neither Lawrence Durrell nor Gerald Durrell would care; they have both created original fictions. Nor are they as frightened of self-imitation as their critics. Neither would mind hearing echoes of his own images in his brother's prose.

The structure of *Prospero's Cell* and the texture of Lawrence's language have seriously influenced Gerald's work. Before examining these, we would do well to look at more direct, and less essential, teaching and borrowing.

It seems likely that, more than a decade after *My Family* was published, when Gerald sat down to write its sequel, *Birds, Beasts, and Relatives*, he reread not only his own earlier Corfu book but his brother's, as well as the works *Prospero's Cell* mentions in its text and bibliography. All five of the quotations that begin the separate parts of *Birds, Beasts*—from *The Tempest*, Homer, Professor Anstead's 1863 *The Ionian Islands*, Edward Lear, and Napoleon—come from works Lawrence Durrell sends us to in *Prospero's Cell*.

As for anecdote, here, for the second time, we meet the murderer in a boat, the young peasant with dynamite, and the eerie tale of night fishing. In Lawrence's telling Lawrence is with Anastasios, in Gerald's

Gerald is with one "Taki Thanatos" (Mr. Death), but in both the peasant first spears the rare scorpion fish and then catches an octopus which he kills dramatically by plunging his teeth into the animal.

None of this very much matters except as it shows us how both of the Durrells work. They are writers for whom a good image has a vitality of its own, that easily leads to repetition. Thus in Lawrence's *The Black Book* (1938) one finds images that also live in his *Prospero's Cell* (1945): "Lost the grapes, black, yellow, and dusky. Even the ones like pale nipples, delicately freckled and melodious"; and "The fishermen complain that they cannot see the fish any more to spear them. Well, the rufous sea scorpion and the octopus are safe from their carbide and tridents" (p. 19).

In the same way two images from *Prospero's Cell* seem to take on a later life. Describing olive-gathering, Lawrence writes that "the long lines of coloured women come, bearing their baskets full of the sloe-shaped fruit, now covered in bloom" (1945, p. 94). He sees a procession which includes "rows of priests in their stove pipe hats, each wearing a robe of unique colour and design—brocade of roses, maize, corn, grass-green, kingcup-yellow. It is like a flower bed moving" (p. 31). Gerald seems to have been caught by the image and, in *Birds, Beasts* (1969), he sees olive-picking in which "the peasants gathered under the trees looked like a moving flower bed . . ." (p. 132). Writing a decade later, in *Fauna and Family* (1978), Gerald allows the same image, which has become his own, to surface, and this time, I would bet, has unconsciously linked it to priests as Lawrence first did: "The gangplank was lowered, the band struck up blaringly, the army came to attention, and the crowd of church dignitaries moved forward like a suddenly uprooted flower bed" (p. 112).

Lawrence and Gerald Durrell are writers whose prose is richly imagistic and given to metaphor, as is their speech. It is here, of course, that young Gerald learned from a mentor who did not move, with the dignitaries of his day, all dressed in gray and brown. That quality and the sympathetic comedy of *Prospero's Cell*—with its characters who unfold their individual anecdotal tales, with its use of biography and fact as the perfect mask for fiction—are Lawrence's gifts to Gerald, who took them and, making them his own, returned with another gift, the "wicked pen portrait of the genius at the age of twenty-one" (L. Durrell, 1981a, p. 120).

There are costs of course to the makers of metaphor, for when they get tired or sloppy, they overwrite. At the end of *Livia* one finds a line about Blanford that could do, as Lawrence well knew, for both brothers: "It was a bad sign he thought, frowning, to see metaphors everywhere" (L. Durrell, 1979, p. 262). One particularly wishes that Gerald would work with other literary tools. Still, when he is good, this naturalist who disclaims writing is very good indeed, and one thinks of his brother's praise: "Don't you think the little devil writes well? His style's like fresh, crisp lettuce" (Weatherby, 1961).

> Summer gaped upon the island like the mouth of a great oven. Even in the shade of the olive groves it was not cool and the incessant, penetrating cries of the cicadas seemed to swell and become more insistent with each hot, blue noon. The water in the ponds and ditches shrank and the mud at the edges became jigsawed, cracked and curled by the sun. The sea lay as breathless and still as a bale of silk, the shallow waters too warm to be refreshing. You had to row the boat out into deep water, you and your reflection the only moving things, and dive over the side to get cool. It was like diving into the sky. [G. Durrell, 1969, p. 186]

Words for the Count D.

A personal note. When I was eighteen and traveling alone I visited my father's brother, whom I'd never met before, in Johannesburg, South Africa. The men had been separated for forty-five years and were deeply divided in ideology, but their resemblances—in temperament and mannerisms—were uncanny. Meeting the Durrells I was reminded of that August twenty years ago. Members of a family inherit mannerisms and manners, and both Durrells greeted a stranger with the same gestures, the same drinks, and a magnanimity for which they are known.

It is hard to trust the perceptions one makes after only two visits, however long, but I came away with the strong sense that the Durrells are linked in temperament, in humor, in metaphoric speech, and I felt that these brothers know and care about one another; that Lawrence has high hopes for Gerald's next twenty years; that Gerald can still experience pleasure when he recalls Lawrence's recent praise of a story that moves in a new direction, over which he'd taken some time.[7]

One sees, of course, differences as well. I met Lawrence Durrell where he lives alone. Gerald Durrell was surrounded by people, an extraordinarily genial group, in a comfortable, not opulent, living room in Les Augres Manor set in the zoo, from which even on a cold and windy day in January, he can emerge only as a public person.

They are both, without any doubt, large figures with something of the strengths of first or only children. Perhaps they are like the band of

---

[7] "The Entrance," in *The Picnic and Suchlike Pandemonium* (1979).

brothers Lawrence wrote about in an early, now lost, story called "The Large Field." Alan Thomas (1973b) describes it as about brothers with "an intense mutual attraction," "all writers and each the leading authority on his subject. Reviewers of their vast publications invariably used the phrase '. . . he covers a large field' " (p. 175). Certainly the Brothers Durrell are like the figures Lawrence applauds in the poem "Mythology."

> All of my favorite characters have been
> Out of all pattern and proportion:
> . . . .
> . . . . No judgment
> Disturbs people like these in their frames.
> [1980a, p. 115]

REFERENCES

Dennis, N. (1961), The rise of the king of novelists. *Life*. International edition, January 16.

Durrell, G. (1937), In the theatre. *The Booster*, 2(8):8.

———— (1956), *My Family and Other Animals*. Harmondsworth: Penguin Books, 1981.

———— (1961), Lawrence Durrell. *Evening Standard*, October 5, p. 8.

———— (1969), *Birds, Beasts and Relatives*. Glasgow: William Collins, 1981.

———— (1971), *Fillets of Plaice*. Glasgow: William Collins, 1980.

———— (1976), *The Stationary Ark*. Glasgow: William Collins, 1977.

———— (1978), *Fauna and Family: An Account of the Durrell Family of Corfu*. New York: Simon & Schuster.

———— (1979), *The Picnic and Suchlike Pandemonium*. Glasgow: William Collins.

Durrell, J. (1967), *Beasts in My Bed*. London: William Collins.

Durrell, L. (1938), *The Black Book*. London: Faber & Faber, 1977.

———— (1945), *Prospero's Cell*. London: Faber & Faber, 1978.

———— (1949), *A Landmark Gone*. Privately printed. Los Angeles: Reuben Pearson.

———— (1957a), *Bitter Lemons*. London: Faber & Faber, 1978.

———— (1957b), *Justine*. London: Faber & Faber.

———— (1958), *Mountolive*. London: Faber & Faber.

———— (1963), *Lawrence Durrell and Henry Miller: A Private Correspondence*, ed. G. Wickes. London: Faber & Faber.

———— (1968), *Tunc*. London: Faber & Faber.

———— (1969), *Spirit of Place: Letters and Essays on Travel*, ed. A.G. Thomas. London: Faber & Faber.

———— (1979), *Livia*. London: Faber & Faber, 1981.

———— (1980a), *Collected Poems: 1931–1974*, ed. J.A. Brigham. London: Faber & Faber.

———— (1980b), *A Smile in the Mind's Eye*. London: Wildwood House.

———— (1981a), *Literary Lifelines: The Richard Aldington–Lawrence Durrell*

Correspondence, ed. I.S. MacNiven & H.T. Moore. London: Faber & Faber.

—— (1981b), Foreword, *Fine Books and Book Collections: Books and Manuscripts Acquired from Alan G. Thomas*, ed. C. de Hamel & R.A. Linenthal. Leamington Spa: James Hall, p. vii.

Fraser, G.S. (1973), *Lawrence Durrell: A Study*. London: Faber & Faber.

Jenkins, A. (1981), Anti-home thoughts from abroad. *The Times Literary Supplement*, November 27, p. 1397.

Thomas, A.G. (1973a), Bibliography. In: *Lawrence Durrell: A Study* by G.S. Fraser. London: Faber & Faber.

—— (1973b), Recollections of a Durrell collector. In: *Lawrence Durrell: A Study* by G.S. Fraser. London: Faber & Faber.

Weatherby, W.J. (1961), The Durrell brothers. *The Guardian*, May 6, p. 4.

Wood, M. (1975), Play it again, Sam: *Monsieur* by Lawrence Durrell. *New York Review of Books*, March 6, p. 17.

NAME INDEX

Note: Listed here are technical writers, i.e., literary critics and behavioral scientists. Creative writers, their friends and relatives, are listed in the Subject Index.

418

SUBJECT INDEX

addiction, drug, 31
alcoholism, 31, 219
androgyny, theme of, in novels, 209
anxiety, separation, 212
appendectomy, in childhood, 203-204
betrayal, preoccupation with, 202-203
children, in fiction, 204
conflict, preoedipal, 211
cruelty, personal, 200, 205
delusions, paranoid, 29-31, 200-202, 213, 221-223
dental problems, 29
depression, 29, 31, 200, 206, 219
drugs, addiction to, 31
failure, fear of, 206
fantasy, sexual, 207-208
fathers, in fiction, 211
fibrositis, 29
fixation, on mother, 202-203
hallucinations, 29, 200
hemorrhoidectomy, 29
homosexuality, 200, 209-210
    in fiction, 33, 210-211, 213
hypochondria, 31
identity, sexual, 207-208
insomnia, 23, 29, 31, 200, 219
jealousy, 195
memory, failing, 29
mother, feelings toward, 211, 213
narcissism, 203, 208
orality, 219
paralysis, hysterical, 204
paranoia, 29-31, 200-202, 206, 207, 213
psychotic episode, 218-219
religion, importance of, 200, 205, 206-207, 220
rheumatism, 29
Rossetti, identification with, 32
satire, use of, 223
self-hatred, 206
sex, confusion about, 207-208
sibling
    absence of, in fiction, 211
    rivalry with, 3, 8, 16, 194, 195, 199-200, 203
suicide, attempt at, 30, 206
Tito, paranoid ideas of, 208
victim as hero, theme of, 202-204
women, in novels, 210
see also Individual works
Waugh, Evelyn Gardner, first wife, 208
Waugh, Peter, Alec's son, 195
Weaver, Harriet Shaw, 24
    Joyce, J., financial support of, 97, 106
Wharton, Edith, 327

White Hotel, The, 6
White Lies (White Liars), 278-279, 296
Wickerman, The, 279
Wicker Man, The, 279
Wilkinson, J.J. Garth, 303
Wilde, Constance, Oscar's wife, 134
Wilde, Isola, sister of Oscar and Willie, 117
Wilde, Lady, 35
    letter to Oscar about Willie, 127, 128-129
    in London, 120, 121
    as model for Lady Bracknell, 116
    physical stature, 116
Wilde, Oscar, 115-136, 147
    Beerbohm, M., influence on, 143
    childhood, 117-118
    homosexuality, 33-34, 115, 133
    obesity, 25, 117
    in Reading Gaol, 134
    review of Knight's *Dante Gabriel Rossetti*, 269
    Rossetti, attitude to, 22
    sibling
        rivalry, 3, 7, 125
        support, financial, to Willie, 35, 125-126
    see also Individual works
Wilde, Willie, 115-136
    alcoholism, 25, 32, 115, 123, 134
    childhood, 117-118
    critic, drama, 120
    depression, 25, 32, 124
    impotence, sexual, 35
    journalist, 120-121
    masochism, 125
    narcissism, 125
    obesity, 25, 117
    poetry of, 118-119
    sibling
        anger, toward Oscar, 127-128
        dependence, financial, on Oscar, 35, 125-126
        rivalry, 3, 7, 125
Wilde, Sir William
    children, illegitimate, 116
    death, 117
    father, of Oscar and Willie, 115-116
    promiscuity, sexual, 116
Winner Take All, 8
Withered Murder, 278
Woman of No Importance, A, 125
Woman's World, The, O. Wilde as editor of, 121
Woolf, Leonard, 332, 345, 357